These Principles are intended to serve as a guide by which radiologic technologists may evaluate their professional conduct as it relates to patients, colleagues, other members of the medical care team, health-care consumers, and employers and to assist radiologic technologists in maintaining a high level of ethical conduct.

Principle 6

Radiologic Technologists shall apply only methods of technology founded upon a scientific basis and not employ those methods that violate this principle.

Principle 7

Radiologic Technologists shall not diagnose, but in recognition of their responsibility to the patient, they shall provide the physician with all information they have relative to radiologic diagnosis or patient management.

Principle 8

Radiologic Technologists shall be responsible for reporting unethical conduct and illegal professional activities to the appropriate authorities.

Principle 9

Radiologic Technologists should continually strive to improve their knowledge and skills by participating in educational and professional activities and sharing the benefits of their attainments with their colleagues.

Principle 10

Radiologic Technologists should protect the public from misinformation and misrepresentation.

Basic Medical Techniques
and Patient Care
for Radiologic Technologists

Basic Medical Techniques and Patient Care for Radiologic Technologists

THIRD EDITION

Lillian S. Torres, R.N., B.S., M.Ed., M.S.N., N.P.
Division Chairperson for Allied Health, Chaffey College, Rancho Cucamonga, California

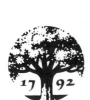

J. B. LIPPINCOTT COMPANY
Philadelphia

Cambridge • New York • St. Louis • San Francisco
London • Singapore • Sydney • Tokyo

Acquisitions Editor: Charles McCormick, Jr.
Indexer: Irene Glynn
Production: Till & Till, Inc.
Compositor: David E. Seham Associates, Inc.
Printer/Binder: The Murray Printing Company

Library of Congress Cataloging-in-Publication Data
Torres, Lillian S.
    Basic medical techniques and patient care for radiologic
technologists / Lillian S. Torres. — 3rd ed.
        p.   cm.
    Bibliography: p.
    Includes index.
    ISBN 0–397–50935–9
    1. Radiology, Medical.   2. Nursing.   3. Radiology technologists.
I. Title.
    [DNLM: 1. Technology, Radiologic.   WN 160 T693b]
RC78.T67 1989
616.07′57—dc19
DNLM/DLC
for Library of Congress   88-12880
                                                                CIP

The author and publisher have exerted every effort to ensure that
drug selection and dosage set forth in this text are in accord with
current recommendations and practice at the time of
publication. However, in view of ongoing research, changes in
government regulations, and the constant flow of information
relating to drug therapy and drug reactions, the reader is urged to
check the package insert for each drug for any change in indications
and dosage and for added warnings and precautions. This is
particularly important if the recommended agent is a new or
infrequently employed drug.

To Joseph

Preface

It has been 10 years since the first publication of *Basic Medical Techniques and Patient Care for the Radiologic Technologist*. The success of this textbook is complimentary to all members of the radiologic technology profession because they have recognized the growing need for safe and competent patient care in radiology and have worked to make this the rule. The expanded scope and technological preparation for radiologic technology emphasize the need of the RT for a more complete understanding of every aspect of the patient's medical care and desired treatment outcomes.

The RT must be knowledgeable in the areas of assessment, therapeutic communication, and teaching because these areas of patient care are now considered to be basic skills for all health-care professionals. Infection control has also become an increasingly significant part of basic health care as the diseases with which all health workers must deal become more virulent and difficult to detect.

The term *radiologic procedures* is not always accurate at this time, so I have chosen to use new terminology in this text. All radiographic procedures and other imaging techniques will be referred to as *diagnostic imaging procedures,* a term more in keeping with the new technology.

The format of the third edition of *Basic Medical Techniques and Patient Care for Radiologic Technologists* is unchanged. Patient assessment, therapeutic communication, and teaching are discussed in some depth. There are a greater number of medical procedures discussed, and more time is spent explaining the scientfic rationale for each procedure. Infection control has been emphasized and is in keeping with the latest Centers for Disease Control guidelines for health-care workers.

A chapter has been added to the new edition of this book, which includes patient care needs during special procedures, magnetic resonance imaging, sonography, and external radiation therapy. At the request of a number of persons in radiology professions, I have included some basic information concerning cardiac monitoring. RTs working in the special procedures area are in constant contact with cardiac monitors and should have some understanding of their significance.

The needs of the patient receiving external radiation therapy are included because I have had the privilege of caring for a number of persons who have received external radiation as treatment for cancer in recent years. They have related their problems during these treatments, and I felt that their suggestions for improvement of care in this area could not be ignored.

Nothing that was discussed in the previous editions of this text has been omitted, but has simply been augmented as the professional needs of the RT have grown. It is my trust that every aspect of patient care needed to enhance the RT's professional service is presented here.

Lillian S. Torres

Acknowledgments

Writing a textbook such as this is not an individual effort, and this one is no exception. There are a number of persons who willingly gave of their time and professional expertise to whom I shall always be grateful.

The Chaffey Community College Radiologic Technology Class of 1989 used this book in an incomplete condition and helped to edit and revise it as the course progressed. The students' assistance, good humor, and suggestions were of great value.

The Radiologic Technology faculty at Chaffey were a resource on whom I am always dependent. TerriAnn Linn–Watson was a supportive technical advisor. Gordon Lockwood, Don Fincher, and Andrea Dutton were there to advise and help whenever asked.

Special thanks go to the following:

My photographer, Jay Cordary, who was always ready to take one more picture, even on Saturday mornings.

Daniel M. Dorsey, M.D., whose assistance with the medical aspects of radiology and review of Chapter 12 were extremely helpful.

B. Don Ahn, M.D., who assisted and advised me on the technical aspects of cardiac monitoring and ECG.

Richard Steidl, M.D., ACR, who again allowed us to use the Kaiser Foundation Hospital Radiology Department for observation and photographs.

Tada Sato, M.D., who advised me on the clinical use of anti-infective drugs in pediatrics.

Ernest Sellers, RT, Administrative Assistant of Radiology at Pomona Valley Hospital Medical Center, who introduced me to magnetic resonance imaging and allowed us to take photographs in the magnetic resonance department.

Sidney R. Shearing, RT, supervisor of the Cardiac Catheterization Laboratory at St. Vincent Hospital, Los Angeles, California, who instructed me in patient care during cardiac catheterization.

Judy Lakritz, RN, and Roberta Justice, RN, who were generous in sharing their professional expertise in cardiac catheterization and cardiac care.

Sylvia Pompura, M. ED., RN, and Marion Carter, M.S., R.N., who were there any time I needed help with photographs.

Laureen Harley, Sylvia Cortez, and Gail Baeskens, my student secretaries.

The operating room staff and all at Kaiser Foundation Hospital, Fontana, California, who allowed us to take photographs there at our convenience.

And last, to Bernice Heller, retired Developmental Editor of J. B. Lippincott Company, who helped me through the previous editions of this book. Her past direction was a help throughout this work. She is fondly remembered.

Contents

Basic Medical Techniques and Patient Care for Radiologic Technologists

Chapter One
The Radiologic Technologist and Professionalism

Goal of this chapter:

The radiologic technology student will understand the extent of his professional commitment and will be aware of the patient as an individual with emotional as well as physical needs that may be met by therapeutic communication.

Behavioral objectives:

When the student has completed this chapter, he will be able to do the following:
1. Differentiate between the ethical and legal aspects of radiologic technology
2. List and explain the ethical and legal obligations that the RT has toward his patients and his colleagues
3. List the basic physical and emotional needs of the patient
4. Make an accurate assessment of the patient's needs when assigned to him
5. Describe problem-solving techniques that may be used in planning patient care
6. List the patient's rights when entering a health-care institution for treatment
7. List the expectations that a patient might have of the RT assigned to his care
8. Define, list, and demonstrate techniques of therapeutic communication.

Glossary

Adhere to stay fixed or firm

Anxiety uneasiness of mind, often over anticipated illness or surgery

Assess to evaluate; to determine the significance of data

Basic needs those absolute essentials without which life cannot continue

Biases a mental learning of a particular view or prejudice

Commitment a pledge to self or others to do something

Common law decisions and opinions of local law courts, based on customs and habits of the area within a particular country or state

Continuum continuous whole whose parts cannot be separated

Diagnostic imaging modern name for radiography, which encompasses all specialties devoted to producing a picture of a body part

Effective communication produces a satisfying result through an exchange of information

Grieving process an emotional state one must go through when a loss is experienced, to maintain stable emotional health

Litigation lawsuit

Regressive behavior gradual movement to earlier patterns of thinking and acting; a returning to undesirable behavior

Self-actualization complete development of one's abilities or ambitions

Self-esteem respect for oneself

Statutory law established law enacted by a legislative body, which is legally punishable

Terminal illness a disease for which there is no known cure, which ends in death

Therapeutic healing

Unethical not conforming to the standards or conduct of a given profession or group

Profession a calling requiring specialized knowledge and intensive academic preparation

The student who has made the decision to enter the profession of radiologic technology must understand that with this decision comes a commitment to accept the code of ethics of the profession and all that it entails. Health professionals are faced daily with situations that may have ethical and legal implications for them. The student must also understand that this aspect of health care is oriented to the diagnosis and treatment of human disease. For this reason, the RT will be working in intimate contact with people on a daily basis.

Most health care is oriented toward effective communication. Persons choosing health-care professions must develop a way of communicating with patients that is therapeutic. This means that the health worker must leave his patient feeling that the situation has been improved, not worsened, by contact with the health worker.

In the practice of his profession the RT will be working with patients who have serious, often terminal illness. He must be able to relate to these people in an understanding and sensitive manner. Competence in this area of communication requires an understanding of the phases of the grieving process and an understanding of one's own feelings about death and dying.

The student contemplating a career in radiologic technology must examine the reasons why he has chosen this profession. He must ask himself the following questions:

Am I prepared to accept and practice the profession of radiologic technology and support the ethics of this profession?

Am I prepared to accept and practice the profession of radiologic technology and avoid violations of law?

Am I willing to learn to relate to my patients in a professional and therapeutic manner?

If your answers to these questions are positive, you are ready to proceed.

Professional ethics

RTs are members of a team of health-care professionals who work in consort to maximize patient wellness. As a member of this health-care team, the RT is governed by a Code of Ethics and Principles of Professional Conduct that incorporate all members of the profession. These principles have been formulated by the American Society of Radiologic Technologists and the American Registry of Radiologic Technologists and must be followed at all times.

As a member of this profession the RT obtains information about patients that is considered to be privileged. It is unethical for the RT to reveal to anyone not professionally involved in the care of a patient the patient's name, the examination performed, or the results of an examination. This prohibition extends to relatives and friends of the patient. Any questions about the nature of treatment or diagnosis should be referred to the radiologist in charge of the case.

It is also unethical for an RT to offer personal criticism or make judgments concerning the professional practice of physicians, nurses, or other health-team members to any patient or other person. If the RT observes any illegal or unethical practice by his co-workers, it is his duty to report such practice to the proper person (usually the supervisor of the department). If this is not effective, he should present the matter to his professional organization for consideration.

The RT must not be wasteful of materials and medications used for patient care or take them for personal use. Medications should be kept in a safe place from which they cannot be stolen.

The RT, as a member of a health profession, has the responsibility of keeping abreast of the changes and growth of knowledge in his profession. It is also his ethical responsibility to be a member of his local and professional organizations and to expand his professional education so that he can be a contributing member of his profession.

Legal aspect of radiologic technology

All patients who present themselves for care in a health-care institution are protected by The Patient's Bill of Rights. This bill delineates the rights that the patient has as a consumer of health care. All health workers are required to adhere to the provisions of this bill. The RT should be aware of areas of his practice in which he might possibly infringe on patient rights and be held legally liable.

There are many types of laws that affect people in daily life; however, statutory law and common law are most significant for the RT in his professional practice. Statutory laws are derived from legislative enactments. Common laws usually result from judicial decisions. Two major classifications of the law are criminal law and civil law.

An offense is regarded as criminal behavior if it is an offense against society or a member of society that has been prohibited by common or statutory law. If the accused party is found guilty, he is punished.

One breaks a civil law if he offends another per-

CODE OF ETHICS FOR THE PROFESSION OF RADIOLOGIC TECHNOLOGY

Principle 1

The Radiologic Technologist functions efficiently and effectively, demonstrating conduct and attitudes reflecting the profession.

1.1 Responds to patient needs.
1.2 Performs tasks competently.
1.3 Supports colleagues and associates in providing quality patient care.

Principle 2

The Radiologic Technologist acts to advance the principle objective of the profession to provide services to humanity with full respect for the dignity of mankind.

2.1 Participates in and actively supports the professional organizations for radiologic technology.
2.2 Acts as a reresentative for the profession and the tenets for which it stands.
2.3 Serves as an advocate of professional policy and procedure to colleagues and associates in the health-care delivery system.

Principle 3

The Radiologic Technologist provides service to patients without discrimination.

3.1 Exhibits no prejudice for sex, race, creed, religion.
3.2 Provides service without regard to social or economic status.
3.3 Delivers care unrestricted by concerns for personal attributes, or nature of the disease or illness.

Principle 4

The Radiologic Technologist practices technology founded on scientific basis.

4.1 Applies theoretical knowledge and concepts in the performance of tasks appropriate to the practice.
4.2 Utilizes equipment and accessories consistent with the purpose for which they have been designed.
4.3 Employs procedures and techniques appropriately, efficiently, and effectively.

Principle 5

The Radiologic Technologist exercises care, discretion, and judgment in the practice of the profession.

5.1 Assumes responsibility for professional decisions.
5.2 Assesses situations and acts in the best interest of the patient.

Principle 6

The Radiologic Technologist provides the physician with pertinent information related to diagnosis and treatment management of the patient.

6.1 Complies with the fact that diagnosis and interpretation are outside the scope of practice for the profession.
6.2 Acts as an agent to obtain medical information through observation and communication to aid the physician in diagnosis and treatment management.

Principle 7

The Radiologic Technologist is responsible for protecting the patient, self, and others from unnecessary radiation.

7.1 Performs service with competence and expertise.
7.2 Utilizes equipment and accessories to limit radiation to the affected area of the patient.
7.3 Employs techniques and procedures to minimize radiation exposure to self and other members of the health-care team.

Principle 8

The Radiologic Technologist practices ethical conduct befitting the profession.

8.1 Protects the patient's right to quality radiologic technology care.
8.2 Provides the public with information related to the profession and its functions.
8.3 Supports the profession by maintaining and upgrading professional standards.

Principle 9

The Radiologic Technologist respects confidences entrusted in the course of professional practice.

9.1 Protects the patient's right to privacy.
9.2 Keeps confidential, information relating to patients, colleagues, and associates.
9.3 Reveals confidential information only as required by law or to protect the welfare of the individual or the community.

Principle 10

The Radiologic Technologist recognizes that continuing education is vital to maintaining and advancing the profession.

10.1 Participates as a student in learning activities appropriate to specific areas of responsibility as well as to the Scope of Practice.
10.2 Shares knowledge with colleagues.
10.3 Investigates new and innovative aspects of professional practice.

Developed by The American Society of Radiologic Technologists.

PRINCIPLES OF PROFESSIONAL CONDUCT FOR RADIOLOGIC TECHNOLOGISTS

"Principle 1:

Radiologic Technologists shall conduct themselves in a manner compatible with the dignity and professional standards of their profession.

Principle 2:

Radiologic Technologists shall provide services with consideration of human dignity and the needs of the patient, unrestricted by consideration of age, sex, race, creed, social or economic status, handicap, personal attributes, or the nature of the health problem.

Principle 3:

Radiologic Technologists shall make every effort to protect all patients from unnecessary radiation.

Principle 4:

Radiologic Technologists should exercise and accept responsibility for independent discretion and judgment in the performance of their professional services.

Principle 5:

Radiologic Technologists shall judiciously protect the patient's right to privacy and shall maintain all patient information in the strictest confidence.

Principle 6:

Radiologic Technologists shall apply only methods of technology founded upon a scientific basis and not employ those methods that violate this principle.

Principle 7:

Radiologic Technologists shall not diagnose, but in recognition of their responsibility to the patient, they shall provide the physician with all information they have relative to radiologic diagnosis or patient management.

Principle 8:

Radiologic Technologists shall be responsible for reporting unethical conduct and illegal professional activities to the appropriate authorities.

Principle 9:

Radiologic Technologists should continually strive to improve their knowledge and skills by participating in educational and professional activities and sharing the benefits of their attainments with their colleagues.

Principle 10:

Radiologic Technologists should protect the public from misinformation and misrepresentation."

These Principles are intended to serve as a guide by which radiologic technologists may evaluate their professional conduct as it relates to patients, colleagues, other members of the medical care team, health-care consumers, and employers and to assist radiologic technologists in maintaining a high level of ethical conduct.*

* Reprinted with permission of the American Registry of Radiologic Technologists.

---

son's private legal rights. The person who is found guilty of this type of violation is usually expected to pay a sum of money or restore the damage done.

It is possible for the RT to be gound guilty of criminal law in his professional practice. Generally, however, in professional practice, the RT is more apt to be legally liable for malpractice in the commitment of a tort. A *tort* is a wrongful act that involves personal injury or damage resulting in civil action or lawsuit to obtain a sum of money for damages incurred. A tort may be committed intentionally or unintentionally.

An example of an intentional tort would be assault: threatening to perform a medical procedure that the patient has refused; or battery: actually performing a procedure that the patient has refused. An example of an unintentional tort might be forgetting to protect a patient from radiation while making a radiographic exposure.

Anyone may be found guilty of a tort who causes, by an intentional or unintentional negligent act, injury to another person by failure to act in a reasonable and prudent manner. An RT or any other health-care professional may be found guilty of medical malpractice by negligence in carrying out professional responsibilities, whether intentionally or unintentionally, and may be required to pay damages if found guilty.

THE PATIENT'S BILL OF RIGHTS

The American Hospital Association presents a Patient's Bill of Rights with the expectation that observance of these rights will contribute to more effective patient care and greater satisfaction for the patient, his physician, and the hospital organization. Further, the Association presents these rights in the expectation that they will be supported by the hospital on behalf of its patients, as an integral part of the healing process. It is recognized that a personal relationship between the physician and the patient is essential for the provision of proper medical care. The traditional physician—patient relationship takes on a new dimension when care is rendered within an organizational structure. Legal precedent has established that the institution itself also has a responsibility to the patient. It is in recognition of these factors that these rights are affirmed.

1. The patient has the right to considerate and respectful care.
2. The patient has the right to obtain from his physician complete current information concerning his diagnosis, treatment, and prognosis in terms the patient can be reasonably expected to understand. When it is not medically advisable to give such information to the patient, the information should be made available to an appropriate person in his behalf. He has the right to know by name the physician responsible for coordinating his care.
3. The patient has the right to receive from his physician information necessary to give informed consent prior to the start of any procedure and/ or treatment. Except in emergencies, such information for informed consent should include but not necessarily be limited to the specific procedure and/or treatment, the medically significant risks involved, and the probable duration of incapacitation. Where medically significant alternatives for care or treatment exist, or when the patient requests information concerning medical alternatives, the patient has the right to such information. The patient also has the right to know the name of the person responsible for the procedures and/or treatment.
4. The patient has the right to refuse treatment to the extent permitted by law, and to be informed of the medical consequences of his action.
5. The patient has the right to every consideration of his privacy concerning his own medical care program. Case discussion, consultation, examination, and treatment are confidential and should be conducted discreetly. Those not directly involved in his care must have the permission of the patient to be present.
6. The patient has the right to expect that all communications and records pertaining to his care should be treated as confidential.
7. The patient has the right to expect that within its capacity a hospital must make reasonable response to the request of a patient for services. The hospital must provide evaluation, service, and/ or referral as indicated by the urgency of the case. When medically permissible, a patient may be transferred to another facility only after he has received complete information and explanation concerning the needs for and alternatives to such a transfer. The institution to which the patient is to be transferred must first have accepted the patient for transfer.
8. The patient has the right to obtain information as to any relationship of his hospital to other health-care and educational institutions insofar as his care is concerned. The patient has the right to obtain information as to the existence of any professional relationships among individuals, by name, who are treating him.
9. The patient has the right to be advised if the hospital proposes to engage in or perform human experimentation affecting his care or treatment. The patient has the right to refuse to participate in such research projects.
10. The patient has the right to expect reasonable continuity of care. He has the right to know in advance what appointment times and physicians are available and where. The patient has the right to expect that the hospital will provide a mechanism whereby he is informed by his physician or a delegate of the physician of the patient's continuing health-care requirements following discharge.
11. The patient has the right to examine and receive an explanation of his bill regardless of source of payment.
12. The patient has the right to know what hospital rules and regulations apply to his conduct as a patient.

No catalogue of rights can guarantee for the patient the kind of treatment he has a right to expect. A hospital has many functions to perform, including the prevention and treatment of disease, the education of both health professionals and patients, and the conduct of clinical research. All these activities must be conducted with an overriding concern for the patient and, above all, the recognition of his dignity as a human being. Success in achieving this recognition assures success in the defense of the rights of the patient.*

* A Patient's Bill of Rights, American Hospital Association, Chicago, 1973. Reprinted with the permission of the American Hospital Association.

Informed consent

Many procedures performed in diagnostic imaging departments require special consent forms to be signed by the patient or, in the case of minor children or other special cases, by their parents or legal representative. The RT must familiarize himself with the procedures that require special consent and not confuse these with the blanket consent forms that are often signed when the patient enters the hospital because these are not valid if an informed consent is required.

Although these special consent forms are usually signed before the patient comes to the diagnostic imaging department, it is the RT's duty to recheck the patient's chart to be certain that this has been accomplished. He should also ascertain that the patient understands what is going to be done and the essential nature of the choices available to him. If the patient, his parents, or legal representative denies knowledge of the procedure, the RT must notify the radiologist of this, and the procedure should be postponed until the matter is satisfactorily resolved. If the case is an emergency and it is not possible to obtain consent from the patient, his parents, or a legal representative, the health-care professionals performing the procedure are able to proceed under what is called implied constructive consent.

Medical records

Consent forms are part of a record of medical care that is maintained for every patient. This record is called a *chart*. All patient visits, treatments, medications, and medical procedures are documented on this chart. When a patient is admitted to the hospital, a record is begun the moment he is admitted and is kept up-to-date until he is discharged.

The purpose of the chart is to transmit information about the patient from one health worker to another, to protect the patient from medical error, to provide information for medical research, and to protect the health worker in case of litigation. The chart includes all physicians' orders, around-the-clock nurses' records of patient care, laboratory and radiology reports, medical history, progress notes, and any other data pertinent to patient care. Any treatment, procedure, or medication received by the patient while he is in the diagnostic imaging department must be included on the patient's chart. It is usually the nurse or physician who does this documentation; however, the RT must be certain that the records are complete before the patient leaves the department. If there is something omitted, he must bring it to the attention of the physician.

Insurance

All RTs should carry their own malpractice insurance even if their employer carries insurance for them. An RT could possibly be named in a lawsuit in which the legal expenses for his defense are not completely covered by his employer. It is not wise to place oneself in this type of professional jeopardy when a professional malpractice policy may be purchased for a reasonable price.

Communication

Health is a perceptual state of being. All persons have a unique way of defining their own state of being healthy. Health is often seen as being on a continuum. At the positive end of the continuum, all body organs are in top working function with one's mental faculties working at their best. At the negative end, a person is close to death or in a state of despair. In the middle are persons in all states of mental and physical well-being ranging from good health to illness and death.

All persons have basic needs that govern their lives. When their basic needs are met, other needs emerge that are called higher needs. Abraham Maslow, a renowned psychologist, placed the needs of man in the following order:

1. *Physiologic needs.* The basic needs are for food, shelter, air, water, sleep, and sexual fulfillment. If these basic needs are not satisfied, a person is unable to pursue other needs.

2. *Safety and security.* After the individual has satisfied his most basic needs, he begins to seek a place where he can be free from harm and can be sure of being able to earn a living.

3. *Love and belongingness.* When primary needs are met, the person begins to seek someone with whom to share his life and a social group in which he feels accepted.

4. *Self-esteem and the esteem of others.* Everyone thrives on self-regard and the feeling of being favorably regarded by others beyond his immediate family or circle of significant others.

5. *Self-actualization.* When all of the foregoing needs have been met, the individual begins to grow spiritually. He begins to desire to accomplish deeds that will make him feel that he has attained the ultimate growth in his life.

Persons whose state of mental and physical health are at the most positive end of the health—illness continuum have their basic needs met and are pursuing self-actualization. When illness, whether it be physical or emotional, overtakes an individual, he loses his state of well-being. He no longer perceives himself as one whose basic needs for food, water, air, love, belonging, and self-esteem are being met. Illness may mean the loss of one's ability to maintain social and economic status. One's place in his social group is threatened. As illness progresses, the realization of unmet basic needs increases, and feelings of great anxiety overwhelm the ill person.

This is often the patient's state when the RT meets him. Persons who are in need of diagnostic imaging procedures may have been feeling ill for a long time and are presenting themselves for diagnosis and treatment after a long period of feeling unwell. Others may have been well until minutes before they come to the department and have just met with a serious accident that is threatening their state of well-being. When one's level of wellness has been compromised and the satisfaction of his basic needs is threatened, whatever the cause, regressive behavior may result. A person in such a state has difficulty communicating effectively. He may resort to aggressive demands or may withdraw in silence and not be able to make his needs known at all. Whatever the case, it will be the RT's first obligation to assess his patient's needs and be able to communicate with him in a therapeutic manner. He must remember that his patient is feeling threatened and is not functioning at his best. He must do everything possible to reassure and comfort the patient while providing care.

Communication defined

Communication is a constantly changing process made up of both spoken and unspoken messages that go from the sender to the receiver. It has been theorized that there are six components of communication. The first is the *message,* that which the communicator hopes to convey. The second is the *source,* or instigator, of the communication. The *channel,* or vehicle, that carries the message is the third component. This might be a written page, a spoken command, a television message, a film, radio, and so on. The fourth component is the *receiver* of the message. The *context,* the fifth part of the communication, is the set of circumstances that surrounds a particular communication and may completely change the meaning of the message. The sixth part of communication is *feedback.* The sender of the message receives a response to the message, which he then interprets. This response will usually indicate to the sender whether his message has been understood or misinterpreted. Feedback serves several very important purposes. It prevents misunderstandings, acknowledges receipt of the message, and clarifies, or, if necessary, continues the communication.

RT-patient communication

All members of the health-care team must learn to communicate clearly, effectively, and therapeutically with their patients. Any problem of communication, whether major or minor, has an impact on the patient's health care. If a patient leaves your department feeling confused or misunderstood, he may choose not to receive further health care. On the other hand, if he leaves the department feeling that he has been treated with dignity and respect, he will probably continue the needed treatment. Most feelings about health care result from communication between the health worker and the patient.

Health care is centered around communication. As an RT you will be faced with receiving, interpreting, carrying out, and giving directions. You will also be called on to offer consolation and to reassure your patients. For these reasons, being able to communicate effectively is as important to the RT as knowing the correct use of the complex equipment in the radiology department.

In order to become a successful communicator, one must develop skills in listening, observing, speaking, and writing. The student might feel that since he can hear, see, talk, and write, he is already skilled in the art of communication. Unfortunately, this may not be so. All of us are limited in our abilities to perceive others because of our learned attitudes. In order to communicate in a therapeutic manner, the RT must first understand himself. He must become aware of his own limitations and understand any feelings and attitudes that might lead to bias or discrimination in interactions with others. Biases are brought about by attitudes. Attitudes are a set of beliefs that a person holds toward issues or persons that cause the person to respond in a predetermined manner and may eventually affect his general behavior.

Human beings are born free of attitudes, beliefs, and biases. But, from the first day of life, these begin to develop from exposure to a particular set of people called *significant others.* These significant others may be mother, father, or other relatives in the home, or they may be persons who assume the role of parents. The person is constantly exposed to these others. Their environment, their religious beliefs, their food preferences, and their preferences in people become the person's own. As a person grows older, he seeks friends and mates who are in accord with the attitudes and beliefs that have been learned, in order to maintain the balance, or harmony, that is an essential part of existence.

This need for harmony eventually affects every aspect of a person's manner of perceiving and reacting to the world. No two people see the world in the same way. For this reason, a person reacts not to a particular event, but to a personal perception of that event, a perception that is the result of learned attitudes. The RT must understand this and not expect patients to feel as he does in any situation. For instance, the patient who is experiencing pain will react to pain in a manner learned from past life experience.

The RT student will be better able to understand and communicate with others in a therapeutic manner if he examines his own background and considers the source of his own attitudes, beliefs, prejudices, and values. Then, with a new understanding of himself, he can try to put aside his own biases and look at each patient as an individual, with needs and perceptions different from his own.

Nonverbal communication

There is more to communication than the spoken word. The unspoken or nonverbal aspects of communication can be defined as all stimuli other than the spoken word involved in communication. In order to understand nonverbal communication, the RT must depend on what he *sees* the patient doing as he speaks, what he *hears* in speech other than the spoken words, what he *feels* (if he is touching the patient during the communication), and what he *smells* as he comes closer to the patient. These nonspoken messages can often indicate how the patient feels more quickly than any words do. Nonverbal communication functions in the following ways:

It may repeat or stress the spoken message. In this case the face or body movements are in agreement with what is said. For instance, a patient who states that he is in pain and who is protecting the painful body part and wincing or grimacing as he speaks is stressing his message.

It may contradict the spoken word. As the patient speaks of his severe pain he may smile and seem to enjoy his experience. This nonverbal behavior is obviously not in agreement with what is being spoken.

It may accent the spoken word. As the patient says "no," he slams his fist on the table to make the message more clear or to give it stress.

It may regulate the spoken word. If, as a person is speaking, the receiver is nodding his head and giving

the speaker an interested look, it is an indication to continue. Conversely, if the receiver is looking away and seems uncomfortable or uninterested, the speaker has a cue to stop speaking.

It may totally substitute in some instances for verbal communication, as in the case of a frown or a nod. A person may get his message across without saying a word.

The perceptive health worker can learn a great deal about a patient by other types of nonverbal communication. The manner in which a person moves his body and his face can say a great deal. The person with a frown and a set jaw is determined or angry about something. The patient who does not look the RT in the eye may feel insecure or mistrustful of him. The way in which your patient carries his body may tell you how he feels about himself. The person who walks or sits proudly erect probably has a positive feeling about himself. The person who has a poor self-concept or who is depressed may walk slowly and with his head down and his shoulders slumped. While sitting, he will draw his body in and look away from the room.

Social and economic status may also be suggested in nonverbal cues. There may be obvious signs such as those indicated by the clothing worn or by posture. Less obvious status cues might be the patient's manner of speech or the manner in which he enters a room or addresses those in his environment.

Cultural variations

The RT must be aware of cultural differences in verbal and nonverbal communication so that he will not offend or be offended, misunderstand or be misunderstood. For instance, in some cultures it is considered courteous to place one's body very close to the body of another person during communication. In the United States people are very protective of the space close to their bodies and might be offended if one with whom they are not on very friendly terms invades this "personal space."

Nonverbal symbols such as a nod, meaning "yes," or the shake of the head, meaning "no," do not mean the same thing in all cultures. Symbols also have different meanings to different age groups. People of one age group may not understand the symbols of another. A safe rule when communicating with a patient is to use speech instead of symbols if there is any possibility of being misunderstood. Another frequent cause of cultural misunderstanding is the use of humor. Although humor is often an effective communication tool, it must be used with care when there are cultural or age differences. Humor can be an effective means of releasing tension or conveying a difficult message, but it should not be used in life-threatening situations, when there is a possibility of legal action, or when there may be a cultural misunderstanding. The RT must remember too, that a patient's age may affect a common understanding of humor. In other words, if there is any doubt concerning its appropriateness, do not use humor.

Other factors that affect communication

The rate at which one speaks, along with the volume, fluency, and vocal patterns, is categorized under the term *para-language*. Para-language has to do with the sound of the speech, rather than the content. The correct pauses and inflections are extremely important if the communication is to be understood. If one speaks without proper inflection, a question will not sound like a question, or the words may run together and be difficult to sort out. Poor knowledge of correct grammatical usage may also make it difficult to understand what is being said.

The RT's first obligation is to know the material that he wants to communicate thoroughly so that he can transmit the message correctly. He must assess the patient-receiver's age; sex; educational, social, and economic levels; cultural background; and physical ability or disability before beginning so that he may adapt his communication to the patient. If the patient has difficulty hearing, the RT will want to speak in a normal tone of voice but speak more closely to the patient's ear. A patient unable to stand comfortably should be placed in a position in which he is comfortable enough to listen to the message without the distraction of pain. If the patient is accompanied by another person or group of persons, the RT must be certain that the patient hears the message.

Feedback

In order to be certain that the message you are transmitting has been correctly received, feedback must be obtained. This might be done by having your patient repeat to you the directions that you have given, or by simply observing him to be certain that he is doing as he was instructed. If the message was misunderstood, the patient will not respond in the manner that was anticipated. If he does not, it will be the RT's responsibility to restate the message in such a manner that the patient will understand and will demonstrate understanding by giving the correct feedback.

Developing a harmonious working relationship

The most important responsibility of the RT as a communicator is to develop a harmonious working relationship with the patient. Although interactions with a patient will often be brief, the patient should be made to feel that he is a partner in the examination process, for indeed the patient is the most important member of the health team. He should be made to feel that he is sharing in the process. The RT creates this therapeutic relationship through communication that conveys the message that he is a concerned and caring person. If the patient is made to feel that he is an unimportant object being passed through the radiology department in order to get the job done, he will leave with a feeling of discontent. This atmosphere of discontent is created primarily through communication and is called a *nontherapeutic relationship*. There are a series of communication techniques that the RT student should cultivate that will help him to become a therapeutic member of the health team. They include (1) establishing communication guidelines, (2) reducing distance, (3) listening, (4) using therapeutic silence, (5) responding to the feeling and the meaning of the patient's statements, (6) restating the main idea, (7) reflecting the main idea, (8) making observations, (9) exploring.

ESTABLISHING COMMUNICATION GUIDELINES

Since many of the RT's relationships with patients are brief, in order to make the best use of the time allowed, guidelines for the interaction should be set by the RT. Establishing guidelines will include an introduction of yourself to the patient and an explanation of the examination or treatment to be performed. What will be expected of the patient and what he can expect of the radiology staff should be included in this interaction.

REDUCING DISTANCE

In order for the communication to be therapeutic, the physical distance between the RT and the patient should be reduced. This closer distance also makes the patient feel included and involved. Physical barriers or a noisy environment should be avoided. The RT should face the patient and make direct eye contact as he speaks and the patient responds.

Crossing arms or legs during a communication creates a physical barrier that nonverbally conveys a lack of receptiveness from the health worker. Performing other tasks while attempting to communicate also indicates that there is something more important than what the patient is trying to convey.

LISTENING

Listening in a therapeutic manner is vital. When your patient is speaking, you must be able to "shut out" your own feelings and assume a totally nonjudgmental attitude. While your patient is speaking you should not be anticipating your own responses, comparing, or interpreting. Your goal is to gather accurate information. If you are planning your response instead of listening, you cannot do so.

USING THERAPEUTIC SILENCE

Related to listening is the therapeutic use of silence. Short periods of silence give the patient a chance to arrange his thoughts and consider what he wants to say. These periods will also give the RT an opportunity to assess the patient's nonverbal communication as well as his own.

RESPONDING TO THE UNDERLYING MESSAGE

When a patient expresses a feeling of frustration, anger, joy, or relief there is no better way of letting him know that you understand him than by responding in a manner that lets him know that you comprehend what he has said and understand how he feels about the situation. An example of this type of response follows:

PATIENT: *"I'm really discouraged. I'm not sure that being so sick following these treatments is worth it."*
RT: *"You feel disheartened because you're sick after the treatments and you aren't certain that they're making you better."*

RESTATING THE MAIN IDEA

Restating or repeating the main idea expressed by your patient is a useful communication technique. It serves to validate the RT's interpretation of the message received and also informs the patient that he is being heard. Consider the following dialogue:

PATIENT: *"I am having a lot of pain in my left hip, and I might need help to get up on the examining table."*
RT: *"You think you'll need help getting up on the table because your left hip is hurting?"*
PATIENT: *"Yes. Could you please help me?"*

REFLECTING THE MAIN IDEA

Reflecting or directing back to the patient the main idea that he has stated is another useful technique. It keeps the patient the focus of the communication and allows him to explore his own feelings about the

matter he is discussing. The RT in this instance helps the patient to make his own decision. For example, consider the following dialogue:

PATIENT: *"Do you think that I should continue this therapy? It's so expensive, and I'm not sure it's doing me any good."*
RT: *"Do you think that you should stop the therapy?"*

SEEKING AND PROVIDING CLARIFICATION

Seeking clarification is another therapeutic technique that the RT might use. It indicates to the patient that the RT is listening to what is being said but is not sure that he has received the message clearly. In such a situation the RT will simply say, "I'm not sure that I understood you. Will you please repeat that?" or, "I'm not sure that I follow what you've said." The RT may also clarify directions that he has given a patient.

RT: *"In order to prepare for this examination, you will have to take all of this medicine at bedtime tonight."*
PATIENT: *"How much of this should I take at bedtime?"*
RT: *"Before you go to bed tonight, take all of the medicine in the bottle at one time."*

MAKING OBSERVATIONS

Making observations or verbalizing what you perceive to be your patient's feelings is another useful communication technique. You might say, for example, "You seem to be very tense, Mr. Smith. Are you concerned about this examination?"

EXPLORING

The patient may offer information about himself that you wish him to pursue more extensively. To do this, you may use the technique of exploring. An example of this might be as follows:

PATIENT: *"Every time you give me this medicine it makes me feel funny."*
RT: *"Tell me what it's like when you have this medicine."*

These are a few of the techniques that may be used to communicate with your patient in a therapeutic manner. The guiding principle of therapeutic communication is to keep the communication focused on the patient by asking open-ended questions, questions that allow the patient to expand his answers to your questions. Avoid "what" and "why" types of questions, or questions that require only a yes-or-no answer. It is important to keep the conversation focused on the patient and not on yourself.

Keep your verbal responses minimal, and always redirect the communication to the patient. For example:

PATIENT: *"Do you have a family, young lady?"*
RT: *"Yes, I have a husband and two children. And you?"*

Blocks to therapeutic communication

There are several factors that actually block or destroy the possibility of creating a therapeutic atmosphere in communication. Distracting your patient by speaking rapidly, using complex medical terminology that you assume he understands, and providing a distracting environment such as a noisy waiting room or a crowded hallway for directing him are serious barriers to communication. The RT should deliver messages to the patient in a quiet area of the department in a simple and direct manner. He should make sure that the patient understands English. If the patient does not understand English, an interpreter should be made available.

Obtaining incomplete answers or failing to explore the patient's description of a problem are also detrimental to communication. It is essential that the RT listen to what the patient tells him. If he is not certain of the message received, he must explore by further questioning until he is certain that he understands. Failure to do this may result in harm to the patient.

Some other blocks to therapeutic communication that may leave the patient alienated are making judgmental statements and offering false reassurance. Judgmental statements place the patient in the position of feeling that he must gain the approval of the health worker in order to be cared for. These statements can be simple, such as, "That's good," or "That's bad." Or they can take the form of stereotyped comments such as, "We have to take the bad with the good, you know." Another nontherapeutic communication is falsely reassuring the client who expresses fear or concern by making a comment such as, "Now don't you worry. Everything will be just fine."

Defending, another block to communication, is an attempt by the health worker to protect himself, another person, or the institution. This type of communication rejects the patient's opinion and prevents him from continuing to communicate. For instance:

PATIENT: *"I'm not sure Dr. Jay knows what to do with me."*
RT: *"Dr. Jay is an experienced physician, and he has taken care of many people with problems just like yours."*

This type of nontherapeutic answer ends the communication with the client feeling rejected and unworthy. How much better it would have been had the RT simply restated the patient's comments and allowed him to complete his expression of concern.

Changing the subject when the patient is speaking is a nonverbal means of informing him that what he is saying is unimportant.

Also to be avoided are giving advice, offering subjective interpretations of a patient's statements, disagreeing, probing, and demanding explanations, all of which interfere with communication.

The grieving process

Loss of a loved one, social status, a loved material possession or changes in one's body as a result of the aging process, disease, or physical injury that leaves one disabled in some way alters a person's self-concept. If these changes are extreme and permanent, a process of grieving occurs. In the course of his work, the RT will often care for patients who are grieving the loss of a body part or body function. He may also care for persons with illnesses that will lead to death.

Before the RT can interact in a therapeutic manner with a patient who is grieving, he must examine his own feelings about death and loss of something or someone of major importance to his well-being. Consider past reaction to a loss and how you were able to cope with the situation. It is not unusual for a health worker to be filled with emotion when he cares for a person who has suffered a tremendous loss. It may be therapeutic to discuss these feelings with a colleague or a counselor. All persons grieve in an individual manner based on learned attitudes and values that are the result of cultural and environmental factors.

Behavioral theories of the grieving process are complex and diverse. In this text I shall use the general theory of Dr. Elisabeth Kubler-Ross to summarize the phases of the grieving process in a concise manner. The student must remember that the picture of the grieving person given here is general and will differ somewhat with each individual. It will improve your ability to care for the grieving patient if you assess him prior to beginning care to determine which phase of the grieving process he may be going through.

Phase I: denial

When a human being has an illness that will ultimately lead to death, he usually senses that he is dying before he is informed of this fact by his physician. It is in the physician's realm to inform the patient of approaching death, and no other member of the health team should assume this responsibility. Often a sensitive physician will wait for the patient to bring up the matter. When verification of a terminal illness or permanent disfigurement is made to the patient by his physician, the initial response is usually one of shock and denial. This first response is used by the patient as a defense until he can become accustomed to the idea. The idea of one's own death is difficult to face. Death happens to other people, "not me." If the RT is questioned about the possibility of death or permanent disability, he should respond with reflective answers and give support without being unrealistic. For example:

PATIENT: *"Do you think my disease is incurable?"*
RT: *"You feel that you have an incurable disease?"*

Phase II: anger

If the illness preceding death is lengthy, or as the recognition of disfigurement and handicap is verified, the patient moves into the second phase of the grieving process. In this phase, the client becomes angry. He may hurl criticism and abuse at family members or at health workers. He feels that he has been done a serious injustice, and hopeless rage is his only defense. If the RT is insulted or verbally abused, he should not take the abuse personally. He should be matter-of-fact and understanding in his responses. Releasing anger is therapeutic to these patients and should be permitted.

Phase III: bargaining

The third phase in the grieving process is a period of bargaining. The patient becomes a "good patient." He tries to follow all medical advice and become submissive. He may feel guilty for his outbursts of anger. He has hopes that if he is "good" he will be spared. Perhaps, he thinks, there will be a miraculous cure or, at least, less pain and suffering.

Phase IV: depression

The fourth phase in the grieving process is a period of depression. The patient accepts the reality of his impending death, permanent disability, or disfigurement. He begins to mourn for his past life and all that he has lost or is losing. He is often silent and retiring at this time. Quiet support is the best response of the health worker during this period.

Phase V: acceptance

The fifth phase in the grieving process is a period of acceptance. If the patient is dying, he will lose interest in the outside world and become interested only in his immediate surroundings and the support of persons near him. He deals with his pain and illness and begins to disengage from life. The health workers should be quietly supportive during this time. Communication should be reflective, and the client should be allowed to discuss whatever he desires.

If the client is facing a permanent handicap or disfigurement and not death, this is the time when he makes his first attempts at rehabilitation. He faces the reality that he must make the most of his life. This does not mean that the handicap is forgotten or totally accepted. The handicapped person may have a longer grieving period than the person who suffers the loss of a loved one because he is constantly reminded that he is no longer the person that he once was. The RT must remember this and approach him with consideration and understanding. Allow the rehabilitating patient to direct his own care as much as possible. He will inform you of the assistance that he needs. Stand by to assist; do not take the lead. Be matter-of-fact as you care for the handicapped patient and comply with requests for assistance.

Problem solving

When the RT is assigned to a particular patient, he must decide how to perform the assigned task quickly, efficiently, and as comfortably as possible for the patient. Before beginning a diagnostic imaging procedure, he must go through a problem-solving process. This may be done in writing initially and may later become a simple thought process.

The first step in the problem-solving process is data gathering. Data that affects how the procedure will be performed will include the following:

Subjective data: Subjective data includes anything that the patient might say that is pertinent to the procedure. For instance, the patient might say, "The last time I had an x-ray, they gave me some medicine in my vein that made me itch all over" or "When I move it hurts my back." Either of these statements may be significant for some diagnostic imaging procedure. Anything the patient, or a person who accompanies the patient, to the department says that can in some way affect what is to be done there must be considered as important subjective data.

Objective data: Anything that the RT sees, hears, smells, feels, reads on a hospital chart, or is reported to him about the patient by another health worker who has cared for the patient is objective data. After the data has been gathered, it should be analyzed (*e.g.*, the patient is unable to stand, he has difficulty breathing, he is disoriented). Irrelevant data should be disregarded and relevant data listed in priority order.

Potential problems should also be listed. A goal should then be set, and a plan for achieving the goal should be formulated. Patient involvement in setting the goal and planning to achieve the goal is recommended because the patient will be more willing to cooperate to achieve the goal if he feels that he is partially responsible for a successful examination or treatment.

The use of systematic problem solving allows the RT to accomplish his work assignment in a minimum amount of time with the least amount of effort for him and the greatest amount of comfort and safety for the patient. After each procedure is complete, it should be evaluated. The RT should ask himself the following questions: How did the plan work? What problems arose that I did not anticipate? What must I do differently next time? If this type of evaluation is done after caring for each patient, you will rapidly grow in professionalism and skill.

Summary

Radiologic technology has become a complex and highly specialized profession. The person who selects this profession must be aware of the ethical and legal constraints that will govern his practice as a member of that profession and be willing to accept these constraints. The RT must learn the Principles of Professional Conduct for Radiologic Technologists and adhere to those principles. The RT must also be aware of the rights of the hospitalized patient and treat each patient as a human being with dignity and worth.

The patient who comes for a diagnostic imaging procedure is often fearful and anxious because his basic needs are threatened. Grieving and handicapped patients present particular problems that must be recognized and dealt with. By means of therapeutic communication techniques, the RT can decrease the patient's anxiety. Effective communication is often the key to a successful examination or treatment; therefore, it is essential for the RT to become a successful communicator.

The RT will need to plan the patient's care before he begins to work. A systematic problem-solving process that includes assessment, data analysis, setting a goal, establishing a plan to achieve the goal, and evaluating the work done is required for efficiency and safety in completing assignments.

Chapter 1, pre-post test

_____ 1. Professional ethics may be defined as
  a. Rules and regulations made up by the department in which you work
  b. Standards for any professional person
  c. The same as not violating the law
  d. A set of standards made up by a particular profession to be abided by members thereof

_____ 2. An RT comes to work daily without bathing and in a soiled uniform. This is an example of
  a. Illegal behavior
  b. Unethical behavior

_____ 3. Which of the following is an example of privileged (confidential) information?
  a. Your friend buys a new car and asks you not to tell anyone about it yet.
  b. A colleague discusses his stock market holdings with you.
  c. You assist with a diagnostic study and a large adherent mass is discovered in the colon.
  d. A fellow student is told that he has the highest grades in the class.

_____ 4. Following completion of a radiologic technology program you are employed at the local community hospital in the diagnostic imaging department. You are approached by a colleague who asks you to become a member of the local chapter of your professional organization. You know that you will be expected to pay yearly dues. Which would be your best response to your colleague?
  a. You explain that you have just begun your first job and money is in short supply at this time.
  b. You laugh and say, "No thanks, I've had all of the organization I can take for a while."
  c. You join in 1 or 2 years when your financial status improves.
  d. You join at once because you feel that it is an obligation to be a member of your professional organization.

_____ 5. You are the RT assigned to the special procedures area to assist with an arteriogram this morning. Mr. Contrast, the patient, arrives by gurney, in the room where the examination is to take place. He asks you what this examination is for and what the doctor has planned. You check his chart and find that the consent for the procedure has been signed. The next thing you must do is

a. Explain the procedure to Mr. Contrast
b. Remind the patient that he has signed the consent form; therefore, he must understand what is going to happen
c. Explain the problem to the physician who is about to treat Mr. Contrast and ask him to review the procedure with the patient
d. Tell the patient not to worry because he is in capable hands

_____ 6. All persons have basic needs that must be met. Match the situations listed below with the basic physiologic need that is not being satisfied:
a. A patient waiting alone on a gurney in a corridor. Everyone rushes by and does not offer explanation or communicate with him.
b. No food was allowed prior to this examination since dinner the previous evening. The examination is late; it is now 11:00 AM.
c. A middle-aged gentleman who is having a lower GI series has an involuntary evacuation of barium on the examination table.
d. A young mother is studying music in her leisure time.
e. A child is taken from his parents into the diagnostic imaging department for examination. The parents will wait outside.
1. Physiologic need
2. Safety and security need
3. Love and belonging need
4. Self-esteem need
5. Self-actualization need

_____ 7. Jack Sprat has been coming to the diagnostic imaging department in which you work for several months for a series of radiation treatments for metastatic carcinoma. He has returned this morning for another treatment. He enters the treatment room in which you are working. You greet him and he does not respond. Your best response to this would be
a. "It seems that you aren't feeling very well today, Mr. Sprat."
b. Do not say anything; just get to work.
c. "Don't worry, Mr. Sprat. We'll have you feeling better in no time."
d. "Why do you think you're feeling so bad today, Mr. Sprat?"

_____ 8. Mr. Sprat says, "I wonder why I keep coming here for these treatments; they don't seem to help." Your best response would be
a. "You have to give them a chance, Mr. Sprat."
b. "You're feeling discouraged because these treatments don't seem to be making much difference."
c. Silence
d. "Maybe I can call your doctor to discuss this with you."

_____ 9. Mr. Sprat tells you that he has decided that he wants to go home without receiving treatment today. Your best approach to this would be
a. To tell him that he should have the treatment no matter how he feels about it
b. To quickly give him the treatment before he leaves
c. To allow him to make his own choice

d. To leave the room and refuse to discuss the decision with the patient

_____ 10. A 19-year-old male paraplegic patient has come to the diagnostic imaging department for treatment. He looks sullen, and when you address him, he responds with a sarcasm. You accept this because you realize that this patient is still going through the grieving process over his newly acquired handicap. You know that he is in the stage of
a. Denial
b. Depression
c. Bargaining
d. Anger

_____ 11. Before you begin to care for any patient, you go through the problem-solving process. The data that you collect from what the patient tells you is called
a. Subjective data
b. Objective data
c. Situational data
d. Basic data

_____ 12. After you have collected the data that you need to plan the care of your patient, you
a. Set a goal and plan the work on your own
b. Set a goal and plan your work with the patient's collaboration
c. Assess your options and go for it
d. Set a goal and plan your work with your colleague

_____ 13. The last step in the problem-solving process is
a. Implementation
b. Organization
c. Evaluation
d. Orientation

_____ 14. A patient might go through the grieving process for which of the following reasons:
1. Losing an executive position
2. Having a fractured clavicle
3. Being unable to maintain his own home and moving to a residence for the elderly
4. Receiving a job promotion
5. Losing a spouse
6. Having a home destroyed by fire
a. 1, 2, 3, and 4
b. 1, 3, 5, and 6
c. 1, 4, 5, and 6
d. 3, 4, 5, and 6
e. 2, 3, 4, and 5

15. List the five phases of the grieving process.

_____ 16. Information about a patient's condition or prognosis
a. May be freely discussed with close relatives
b. Must always remain confidential
c. Should always be open to discussion since "a well-known fact is no secret"
d. Should be discussed only on a co-worker–interdepartmental basis

17. List five steps in the problem-solving process.

18. List six rights of patients who are seeking health care.

19. List six professional obligations of the RT.

Laboratory reinforcement

1. In the school laboratory, pick a fellow student and have a 5-minute discussion with him about his background and immediate concerns. When the 5-minute discussion is complete, write a report of the subjective and objective data that you collected from your colleague during the discussion. Evaluate the information with the student chosen for the discussion for completeness and accuracy of content.

2. The RT student will select a patient and interact with him following the techniques of therapeutic communication. A written report using the format described below will be handed to the instructor for evaluation based on the criteria listed in the chapter.

   A. *Introduction.* Explain the setting, using the patient's initials only, and give his approximate age. Record the patient's sex and include a brief explanation of his background (*i.e.,* his culture and social history).

   B. *Dialogue.* Divide a sheet or two of 9 × 12 inch paper in half. On one side of the paper write the RT's verbal comments with an explanation of the technique of communication used. If a nontherapeutic comment was made, include it. Write an explanation of why the comment was or was not therapeutic. On the other half of the paper write the patient's responses or comments.

   C. *Analysis.* Briefly discuss what you felt during the communication. Describe the nonverbal communication. Describe the nonverbal communication that you observed in your patient and yourself. Explain what changes you would make during the next assignment to improve your communication skills.

Chapter Two
Infection Control

Goal of this chapter:

The radiologic technology student will learn techniques for controlling infection during patient care and will accept responsibility for infection control in his professional practice.

Behavioral objectives:

When the student has completed this chapter, he will be able to do the following:
1. Define the terminology used in this chapter
2. List and describe four types of microorganisms
3. List and define three elements needed to produce an infection
4. List and explain four means of transmitting microorganisms
5. Describe 12 methods that the RT can use routinely to control infection in his daily practice of radiologic technology
6. In the school laboratory, demonstrate the correct method of hand-washing for medical asepsis
7. Define the seven category-specific methods of isolation
8. In the school laboratory, demonstrate the correct method of entering and leaving an isolation room by means of strict isolation technique

Glossary

Amoeboid action movement of a one-celled animal; changes shape to obtain nourishment and access to small openings

Chronic a disease or condition lasting a long time, showing little change

Contaminate to make unclean, to introduce microorganisms into an area where they did not previously live

Convalescence period of recovery at end of disease process

Cyst wall abnormal sac formed by microorganisms when dormant or inactive, which may also serve as a reproductive structure

Cytotoxic drugs chemical substances used to destroy or prevent multiplication of particular cells; used in cancer therapy

Flora plant life adapted for living in a specific environment; may be microscopic in size

Globulin a group of simple proteins found in body tissue, soluble only in saline solution

Immunosuppressive drugs drugs that interfere with normal immune response

Intravenous within a vein

Parasite organism that lives upon or within another organism called the host; does not contribute to survival of host

Pathogenic capable of producing a disease

Pseudopod temporary protruding of processes in protozoa for the purpose of obtaining nourishment and aiding in locomotion

Remission period when symptoms of disease are not apparent

Transducers any of various devices that transmit energy from one system to another

Infection control in health-care institutions is essential to the safety of patients, their families, and health-care workers. All health workers are taught the concepts and procedures for infection control before they begin to work in their various specialty areas, and all are responsible for complying with infection-control precautions. To overlook this aspect of health care is a violation of professional ethics, because the violator is disregarding the safety of his patient, his coworker, and himself.

Patients who seek care in a hospital or any other type of health-care facility are also responsible for complying with infection-control measures while in that institution. Their visitors must also comply. This has become a standard regulation because infractions in technique by one person affect the safety of all others in that institution.

People come to the diagnostic imaging department from many different environments, and the possibility that they will bring disease with them is perhaps even greater here than elsewhere in the hospital. Though some patients arrive in apparent good health, all must be regarded as potential carriers of disease. Every piece of equipment must be thoroughly cleaned after each use, and the RT must use every means available to protect his patient, his coworkers, and himself from infection.

Nosocomial Infections

In spite of increasing use of infection-control measures in health-care institutions, the incidence of infections acquired by patients while in these institutions has increased. When a patient acquires such an infection, it is labeled a *nosocomial infection.* The continued increase in this type of infection is due to a rise in the severity of illnesses and injuries for which people are hospitalized, the increased number of elderly persons who make up the hospital population, the increased use of potent immunosuppressive and cytotoxic drugs, and radiation.

Another contributing factor is that the antimicrobial drugs used to treat infections change the normal bacterial flora of the body. This encourages the growth of *hospital bacteria* that have learned to resist antimicrobial drugs.

The most frequent site of nosocomial infection is the urinary tract and is associated with the use of indwelling catheters. Wound infections following surgical procedures are the second most frequent cause of nosocomial infections, and respiratory tract infections are the third most frequent cause. The use of intravenous catheters, respiratory therapy equipment, and transducers requires meticulous infection-control technique because they are frequently implicated as the cause of nosocomial infections.

Microorganisms

In order to fully understand the process of infection control, the RT must have an idea of the nature of microorganisms. A brief description of the major types of microorganisms follows.

There are basically four major groups of microorganisms: bacteria, fungi, viruses, and protozoas. Within these groups there are many different species that may produce infections in man and many that are useful or not harmful. Some microorganisms that are natural flora in one area of the body produce infection if they are accidentally relocated into other than their natural habitat. For example, *Escherichia coli,* which normally inhabits the human intestinal tract, will not cause disease there; however, should it gain entrance to the urinary bladder, it can cause urinary tract infection.

Many microorganisms make the world in which we live a better place. They are used in food and drug processing, destroy waste, and contribute positively to our environmental comfort.

Bacteria

Bacteria are minute, one-called organisms without a typical nucleus. They contain both deoxyribonucleic acid (DNA) and ribonucleic acid (RNA). DNA carries the inherited characteristics of a cell, and RNA constructs cell protein in response to the direction of DNA.

Bacteria are classified according to their shape, which may be either spherical (cocci), oblong (bacilli), or spiral (spirilla). They may be classified according to their divisional grouping as diplococci (groups of two), streptococci (chains), or staphylococci (grapelike bunches) (Fig. 2-1). Bacteria may also be classified by their reaction to various staining processes in the laboratory. They may be gram-positive, which means that the bacteria take the stain; gram-negative, which means that they do not take the stain; or acid-fast, which means that the bacteria are resistant to decolorization by acid-alcohol.

Some types of bacteria form spores. A spore is a protective coat that surrounds the nucleic material of a bacteria. Spores are formed to protect the bacteria when it is in an unfavorable atmosphere for growth and reproduction. When the environment is again suitable for life and function, the spore germinates, and the bacteria resumes its normal life. Spores are

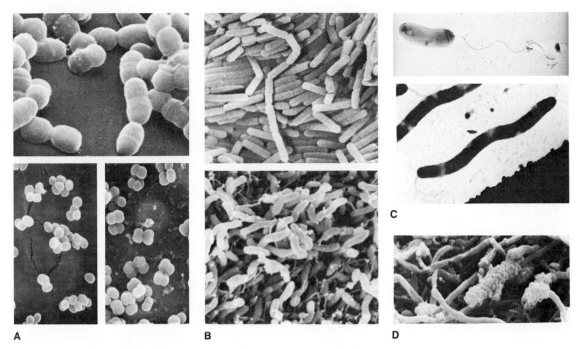

A   B   D

Figure 2-1.   *Forms of bacteria.* **(A)** *Cocci.* **Top: Streptococcus mutans,** *demonstrating pairs and short chains (×9400).* **Bottom left:** *Single cells and small clusters of* **Staphylococcus epidermidis** *(×3000).* **Bottom right:** *Pairs, tetrads, and regular clusters of* **Micrococcus luteus** *(×3000).* **(B)** *Bacilli.* **Top:** *Single cells and short chains of* **Bacillus cereus** *(×1700).* **Bottom:** *Flagellated bacilli (unnamed) associated with peridontitis (×3700).* **(C) Top:** *A cell of* **Vibrio cholerae;** *note curved cell and single flagellum (×8470).* **Bottom:** *The spirillum* **Aquaspirillum bengal;** *note polar tufts of flagella (×2870).* **(D)** *Variety of organisms in dental plaque after 3 days without brushing (×1360). (Volk WA, Benjamin DC, Kadner RJ et al: Essentials of Medical Microbiology, 3rd ed. Philadelphia, JB Lippincott, 1986)*

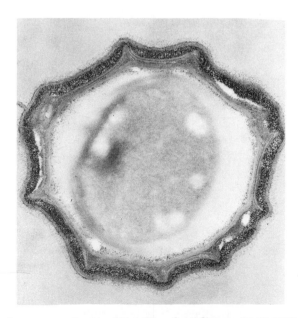

Figure 2-2.   *Spore of* **Bacillus fastidiosus** *(×53,590). (Volk WA, Benjamin DC, Kadner RJ et al: Essentials of Medical Microbiology, 3rd ed. Philadelphia, JB Lippincott, 1986)*

more difficult to destroy than are the vegetating bacteria; therefore, many methods of destroying pathogenic bacteria do not affect their spores (Fig. 2-2).

Bacteria are often opportunists. That is, they are able to adapt to any situation and carry on their lives. They may also learn to resist or thrive in the presence of antimicrobial drugs and disinfectants.

Some common diseases produced by bacteria are diptheria, tuberculosis, streptococcal infections of the throat, boils, abscesses, wound infections, and Salmonella.

Fungi

Fungi exist in two forms, yeasts and molds. Yeasts are one-celled animals, whereas molds have many cells. Some fungi have the characteristics of both yeasts and molds. Fungi reproduce by budding or spore formation (Figs. 2-3 and 2-4). Fifty percent of all fungi may cause disease in humans, but they require moisture and darkness in order to do so. Many pathogenic fungi infect the skin and scalp of humans

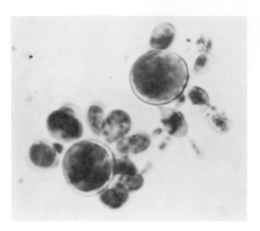

Figure 2-3.   Yeast cells of **Paracoccidioides brasiliensis** *with multiple buds. (Volk WA, Benjamin DC, Kadner RJ et al: Essentials of Medical Microbiology, 3rd ed. Philadelphia, JB Lippincott, 1986)*

and are difficult to cure because they produce spores that remain under the outer skin and reproduce when environmental conditions are favorable. Fungal infections affect body systems and are difficult to treat because most antimicrobial drugs are not effective against fungi.

Common diseases caused by fungi are those caused by *Candida albicans:* thrush, "black hairy tongue" infections, and vulvovaginitis. Frequently contracted systemic fungal infections are histoplasmosis and coccidioidomycosis (also known as *valley fever*).

Viruses

Viruses are minute microorganisms that cannot be visualized under an ordinary microscope. Their genetic material is composed of either DNA or RNA,

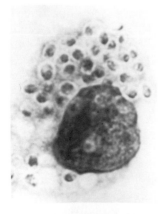

Figure 2-4.   Yeast cells of **H. capsulatum** *in a macrophage are shown in this example from a Giemsa-stained tissue smear (human case). (Volk WA, Benjamin DC, Kadner RJ et al: Essentials of Medical Microbiology, 3rd ed. Philadelphia, JB Lippincott, 1986)*

but never both. This genetic material is protected by a capsid or outer coat until they invade a host cell. They must invade a host cell in order to survive and reproduce (Fig. 2-5).

The capsid acts as a vehicle of transport to different host cells. When the virus selects a host, it attaches itself to the cell at receptor sites on the cell's surface and then penetrates the cell. Once inside, the capsid disintegrates and releases its nucleic acid into the host cell. The virus then replicates, and the newly produced nucleic acid and proteins assemble into new viruses and leave the host cell. As they leave, they sometimes destroy the host cell by rapid release of the new viruses. At other times, the new viruses are slowly excreted and leave the host cell intact.

Viruses may infect plants, animals, or humans. Some viral diseases that affect humans are influenza; measles; mumps; hepatitis A, B; non-A non-B hepatitis; herpes zoster; herpes simplex; acquired immunodeficiency syndrome (AIDS); and the common cold.

Protozoa

Protozoa are more complex one-celled microorganisms than those described in the preceding paragraphs. They are often parasitic and are able to move from place to place by pseudopod formation, by the action of flagella, or by cilia.

Pseudopod movement is an amoeboid action in which a part of the cell is pressed forward and the rest of the cell rapidly follows. Flagella are whiplike projections on the protozoa, which move the cell by their swift movements. Cilia are smaller and more delicate hairlike projections on the exterior of the cell wall, which move swiftly and in a synchronous manner to move the microorganism (Fig. 2-6). Many protozoa are able to form themselves into cysts, which are protected by a cyst wall in adverse conditions to prolong their existence.

Many of the diseases in humans caused by the protozoa affect the gastrointestinal tract, the genitourinary tract, and the circulatory system. Some of the common protozoal diseases are amebiasis, giardiasis, trichomoniasis, malaria, and toxoplasmosis.

The body's defense against disease

The human body has both specific and nonspecific methods of warding off contamination and infection. The RT should be aware of these defenses, because this knowledge will play a role in his professional and personal life.

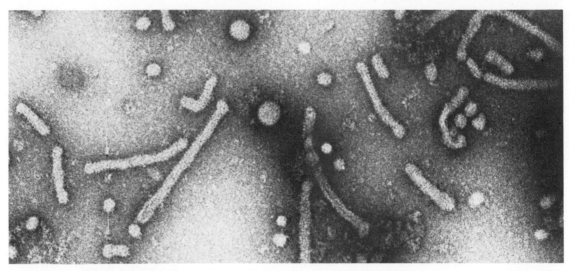

Figure 2-5. Fraction of the blood serum from a severe case of human hepatitis; the patient's immune system failed to counteract the infection. The larger spherical particles, or Dane particles, are 42 nm in diameter and are thought to be the complete hepatitis B virus. The smaller, more numerous spherical particles may be the cores (HB$_c$Ag) of the larger ones. Also evident are filaments of capsid protein (HB$_s$Ag). (Volk WA, Benjamin DC, Kadner RJ et al: Essentials of Medical Microbiology, 3rd ed. Philadelphia, JB Lippincott, 1986)

The nonspecific defense system is not selective when dealing with foreign material, usually a protein, or microbes that attempt to invade the body. The skin, the hair, ciliated mucous membranes in the upper respiratory tract, and the acidic condition of the mucoid linings of body organs all react to any foreign substance or microbe to prevent infection from beginning. The composition and flowing action of urine prevents urinary tract infections. Lysosome in human tears protects the eyes against infection. In the bloodstream, white blood cells called macrophages and neutrophils try to destroy foreign antigens. In the tissues, wandering tissue macrophages rush to an area of contamination and indiscriminantly destroy the invading molecules.

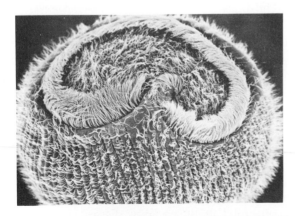

Figure 2-6. Scanning electron micrograph of the ciliate **Stentor coeruleus** *(× 336). (Volk WA, Benjamin DC, Kadner RJ et al: Essentials of Medical Microbiology, 3rd ed. Philadelphia, JB Lippincott, 1986)*

The human body also has a highly complex immune system that reacts to specific invaders that are able to bypass the nonspecific body defenses by forming an antigen (a foreign protein). When an antigen is present in the body, a specific antibody is formed to act against it. An antibody is a protein globulin produced by specific cells in the immune system when stimulated by an antigen. Antibodies form to react against an invading antigen to produce an immunity to further infection by that particular antigen. We are born with immunity to some diseases, and we may also acquire an immunity by actually having the disease and producing antibodies that prevent another infection or by being vaccinated with dead or weakened strains of the infecting microorganism (attenuated vaccine) or their products. These methods of achieving immunity all refer to what is called *active immunity.*

Passive immunity may be acquired by injection of antibodies of a particular infection into an individual, or they may be passed from mother to fetus *in utero* to protect the infant until his own immune system is mature enough to function. Passive immunity is a short-term immunity, because as the injected or transmitted antibodies are broken down, they are not replaced.

Occasionally antibodies function as antigens and produce diseases called *autoimmune diseases.* This occurs when substances identical to one's own tissues stimulate antibody production and these substances react with the host's tissues in an adverse manner. In other words, one's own antibodies destroy healthy tissue.

Multiplication of viruses is impeded in the body by an agent released by cells in response to viral invasion called interferon. It, along with the other immune responses, is instrumental in inhibiting multiplication of viruses.

Interferon is one of a group of agents discovered in the last century to be produced by the body, which increases, directs, and restores the body's immune system following attack by foreign agents. As a group these newly discovered substances are called *biologic response modifiers*. They also react against tumor cells present in the body to restrict their growth. Biologic response modifiers are now being produced in laboratories and tested clinically as cancer treatment.

The process of infection

Infection invades the body in a progressive manner. Although some diseases are considered to be infectious (contagious or communicable) during only one or two of their stages, it would be safer for the RT to deal with diseases as if they were highly infectious at all stages.

The first stage in the course of an infection is the *incubation* period. This is the period that begins when a pathogenic microorganism enters the body and ends when the actual symptoms of the disease begin. It is not possible to detect a particular disease during the incubation period, but some diseases are contagious during this period. The RT should use infection-control measures for all patients, since any one of them might be incubating a communicable disease.

The second phase of an infection is the *prodromal* phase. During this phase, early signs and symptoms of the disease are demonstrated.

The third phase of an infection is the *active* or *full* stage. During this time, all of the characteristic signs and symptoms of the disease are at their peak.

The fourth phase is *convalescence*. During this phase, symptoms begin to diminish and eventually disappear or, as is the case with some chronic infections, go into a phase of remission. Although many infectious diseases are not communicable during this phase, the RT should continue to assume that they are for his own, his coworkers', and his patient's safety.

Elements needed to produce infection

Infection cannot begin unless three elements are present: a source, a host, and a means of transmission.

A *source* is a person with or incubating a disease. This person might be a patient, a health worker, or a hospital visitor. It might also be a person who has large colonies of bacteria on his body. The RT should not work when he is ill or when he knows that he could be incubating a contagious disease, because he could easily infect others.

A *host* is any susceptible person. Persons who are particularly susceptible to infection are those who are fatigued or poorly nourished. Those at greater risk are people with chronic illnesses such as diabetes mellitus, cancer, and uremia. Also at high risk are patients who are undergoing radiation therapy, the elderly, postoperative patients, patients who are in shock or are comatose, and patients with traumatic injuries.

Means of transmission can be by direct and indirect contact, by droplet, by vehicle, by vector, or by airborne route. Contact is direct when a person or an animal with a disease, his blood, or body fluids are touched. This contact can be by hands, by kissing, or by sexual intercourse.

Indirect contact is defined as the transfer of pathogenic microbes by touching objects (called *fomites*) that have been contaminated by an infected person. These objects include dressings, instruments, clothing, dishes, or anything containing live infectious microorganisms.

Droplet contact involves contact with infectious secretions that come from the conjunctiva, nose, or mouth of a host or disease carrier as he coughs, sneezes, or talks. Droplets can travel from approximately 3 to 5 feet and should not be equated with the airborne route of transmission, which will be described in a later discussion.

Vehicles may also transport infection. Vehicle route of transmission includes food, water, drugs, or blood contaminated with infectious microorganisms.

The airborne route of transmission indicates that residue from evaporated droplets of diseased microorganisms is suspended in air for long periods of time. This residue is infectious if it is inhaled by a susceptible host.

Vectors are insect or animal carriers of disease. They deposit the diseased microbes by stinging or biting the human host.

Techniques of infection control

Controlling infection or breaking the *cycle of infectivity* is the duty of all health workers. Medical aseptic practices should become routine for the RT. Many persons wrongly believe that there is little need to be concerned about spreading disease because there is an antimicrobial drug available to conquer every infection. This is not so. Diseases caused by viruses, fungi, bacteria, and protozoa are becoming increasingly pathogenic and difficult to cure.

People who are ill are particularly susceptible to infection. It is the RT's duty to practice strict medical asepsis at all times in his work. There is a difference between medical asepsis and surgical asepsis. *Medical asepsis* means that so far as possible, microorganisms have been eliminated through the use of soap, water, friction, and various chemical disinfectants. *Surgical asepsis* means that microorganisms and their spores have been completely destroyed by means of heat or by a chemical process. It is not practical or necessary to practice surgical asepsis at all times, but one must always adhere to the practice of strict medical asepsis.

Dress in the workplace

Jewelry, such as rings with stones, and cracked or chipped nail polish harbor microorganisms that are difficult to remove. These items should not be worn by the RT when involved in patient care. A plain wedding band and a wristwatch are the only pieces of jewelry that are acceptable for the health worker to wear in the patient-care setting.

The RT should always wear freshly laundered washable clothing when working with patients. Uniforms are recommended because they will not be worn for other purposes. Short sleeves are recommended because cuffs of uniforms are easily contaminated. If a laboratory coat is worn to protect clothing, it should be buttoned or zipped closed and removed when one is not in the work area.

Laboratory coats and uniforms must be washed daily with hot water and detergent. A chlorine bleach is recommended for clothes that have become heavily contaminated.

A protective gown should be worn when working with any patient who may soil your clothing or if blood or body fluids may contaminate clothing. Gowns for isolation patients will be discussed later in this chapter.

Hair

Hair follicles and filaments also harbor microorganisms. Hair is also a major source of staphylococcus contamination. For these reasons, hair must be worn short or in a style that keeps it up and away from your clothing and the patient. Hair should be shampooed frequently.

Hand-washing

Microbes are most commonly spread from one person to another by human hands. It follows that the best means of preventing the spread of microorganisms is hand-washing. Correct hand-washing procedure before and after handling supplies used for patient care and before and after each patient contact is required even if gloves have been worn for the procedure. All blood and body fluids (secretions and excretions) must be treated as if they contain disease-producing microorganisms and be disposed of correctly. Then hands must be washed. Any exposed breaks in your skin must be covered by a waterproof protective covering.

There is a specific hand-washing technique that is accepted as medically aseptic that should be followed by the RT when working with patients. This technique must not be confused with the surgical scrub procedure, which will be described later in this text. The medically aseptic hand-washing technique is as follows (Figs. 2-7 through 2-10):

1. Approach the sink. Do not allow your uniform to touch the sink because the sink is considered contaminated.

2. Turn on the tap. A sink with foot or knee control is most desirable but is not always available. If the faucet is turned on by hand, use a paper towel to touch the handles, then discard the towel.

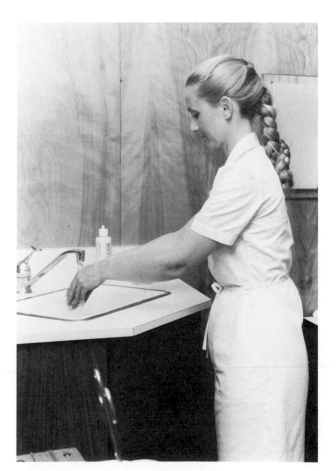

Figure 2-7

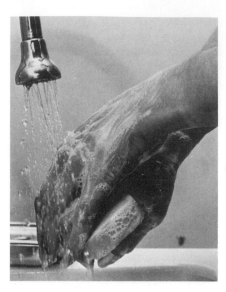

Figure 2-8.   Your hands and knuckles and the areas between your fingers are cleaned with a firm rubbing motion. Continue to hold the soap while doing this.

3. Regulate the water to a comfortably warm temperature.

4. Regulate the flow of water so that it does not splash from the sink.

5. During the entire procedure, keep your hands and forearms lower than your elbows. The water will drain by gravity from the area of least contamination to the area of greatest contamination.

6. Wet the hands and soap them well. Liquid soap is most convenient. When using bar soap, rinse

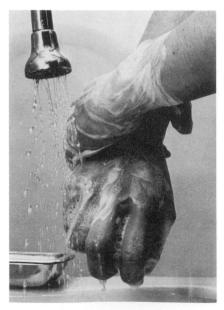

Figure 2-9.   Clean your wrists and forearms with a firm, circular motion, then drop the soap into the soap dish.

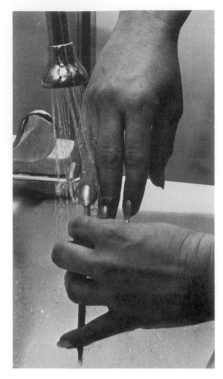

Figure 2-10.   Clean your fingernails under running water to flush away dirt and microorganisms.

the bar before using it and hold it during the entire procedure. The soap dish is considered contaminated; if the soap bar is replaced during the procedure and then reused, the hands will be recontaminated. Soap tissues are the most desirable method of applying soap for handwashing.

7. With a firm, circular rubbing motion, wash the palms, the backs of the hands, each finger, between the fingers, and finally the knuckles.

8. Rinse the hands well under running water.

9. Wet the wrists and forearms to the elbows. Apply soap and rub with the same circular motion.

10. Rinse, allowing the water to run down over the hands.

11. Clean the fingernails with a brush or an orange stick carefully once each day before beginning work, and again if the hands become heavily contaminated.

12. Rinse the fingers well under running water.

13. Repeat the washing procedure as described above.

14. Rinse the soap well and replace it in the dish. Do not touch the sink or the soap dish.

15. Turn off the water. If the handles are hand-op-

erated, use a paper towel to turn them off in order to avoid contamination of the hands.

16. Dry the arms and hands using as many towels as necessary to do the job well.

17. Use lotion frequently on the hands and forearms. It helps to keep the skin from cracking and therefore helps prevent infection.

The foregoing procedure should be performed at the beginning of each working day, when in contact with patient's blood or body fluids, when preparing for invasive procedures (injections, catheterization of the urinary bladder, etc.), before touching patients at greatest risk of infection, and after caring for patients with known communicable diseases. A 30-second hand-washing should precede and follow each patient contact. Time does not allow for a 2-minute hand-washing every few minutes.

Gloves

Disposable, single-use gloves are to be worn any time that the RT feels that he might touch a patient's blood

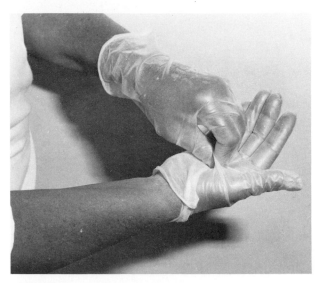

Figure 2-12

or body fluids in the course of a procedure. These gloves should be readily available in containers in each treatment room (Fig. 2-11). Since these gloves are to be used for medical aseptic purposes and not for surgically aseptic purposes, they may be donned simply by pulling them on after hand-washing. When they are no longer needed, the gloves should be removed by use of the following technique to prevent contamination of the RT's hands or clothing (Figs. 2-12 through 2-16).

1. With the gloved right hand, take hold of the upper, outside portion of the left glove and pull it off, turning it inside out as you do so (Fig. 2-12).

2. Hold the glove that you have just removed in the palm of the remaining gloved hand (Fig. 2-13).

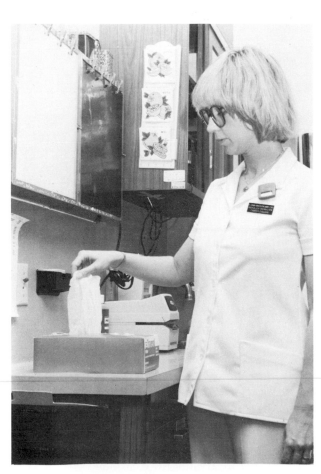

Figure 2-11

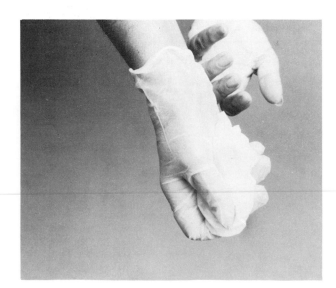

Figure 2-13

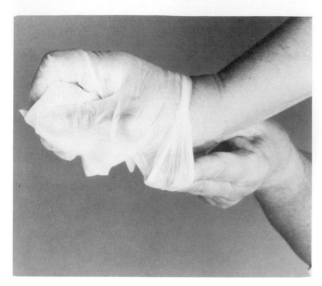

Figure 2-14

3. With the clean, bare index and middle fingers reach inside the top of the soiled glove and pull it off, turning it inside out and folding the first glove inside it as you do so. Be careful to only touch the inside of the glove (Figs. 2-14 and 2-15).

4. Drop the soiled gloves into a contaminated waste receptacle (Fig. 2-16).

5. Wash your hands.

Eye protection

There is evidence that the eyes may be a port of entry for pathogenic microorganisms. For this reason, if the RT is in a patient-care situation in which there may

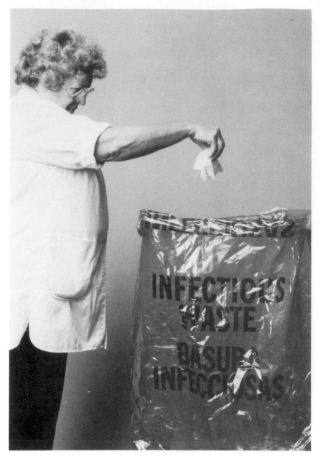

Figure 2-16

be a spattering of blood or body fluids, he must wear goggles or eye glasses to protect his eyes from becoming contaminated (Fig. 2-17). Hands must be kept away from eyes during the course of work so that infection is not introduced into them.

Cleaning and proper waste disposal

Not all disinfectants are equally effective. Before a disinfectant is chosen for the radiology department it should be thoroughly studied by an infection-control consultant. Microorganisms begin to grow in disinfectant solutions left standing day after day. This is also true in liquid-soap containers. If such items are used, they should be changed and cleaned every 24 hours. A more detailed description of disinfection and sterilization methods will be presented in Chapter 9. The following are guidelines for the disposal of waste or the cleaning of equipment after each patient use in the diagnostic imaging department:

1. Wear a fresh uniform each day. Do not place your uniform with other clothing in your per-

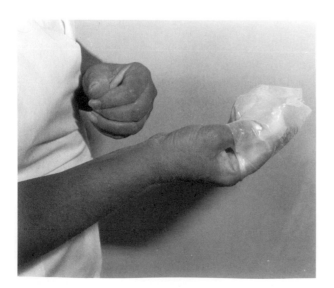

Figure 2-15

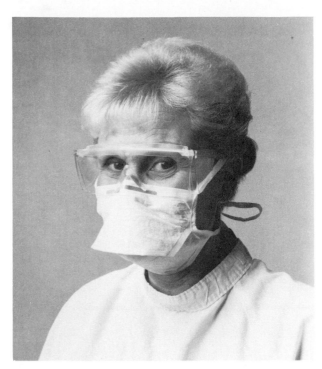

Figure 2-17

sonal closet. Shoes should be cleaned and stockings should be fresh each day.

2. Pillow coverings should be changed after each use by a patient. Linens used for drapes or blankets for patients should be handled in such a way that they do not raise dust. Dispose of linens after each use by a patient.

3. Flush away the contents of bedpans or urinals promptly unless they are being saved for a diagnostic specimen.

4. Rinse bedpans and urinals and send them to the proper place (usually a central supply area) for resterilization if they are not to be reused by the same patient.

5. Use equipment and supplies for one patient only. After the patient leaves the area, supplies must be destroyed or resterilized before being used again.

6. Keep water and supplies clean and fresh. In the radiology department it is best to use paper cups and dispose of them after a single use.

7. Floors are heavily contaminated. If an item that is to be used for patient care falls to the floor, discard it or send it to the proper department to be recleaned.

8. Avoid raising dust because it carries microorganisms. When cleaning, use a cloth thoroughly moistened with a disinfectant.

9. The radiographic table should be cleaned with a disposable disinfectant towelette or sprayed with disinfectant and wiped clean and dried from top to bottom after each patient use.

10. When cleaning an article such as a radiographic table, start with the least soiled area and progress to the most soiled area. This prevents the cleaner areas from becoming more heavily contaminated. Use a good disinfectant cleaning agent and disposable paper cloths.

11. Place dampened or wet items such as dressings and bandages into waterproof bags and close the bags tight before discarding them in order to prevent those handling these materials from coming in contact with bodily discharges.

12. Do not reuse rags or mops for cleaning until they have been properly disinfected and dried.

13. Pour liquids to be discarded directly into drains or toilets. Avoid splashing or spilling them on clothing.

14. If in doubt about the cleanliness or sterility of an item, do not use it.

15. When an article that is known to be contaminated with virulent microorganisms is to be sent to a central supply area for cleaning and resterilizing, it should be placed in a sealed, impermeable bag and marked "contaminated." If the outside of the bag becomes contaminated while the article is being placed in the bag, a second bag should be placed over it (Fig. 2-18).

16. Needles and syringes used in the diagnostic imaging department should always be treated as if they are contaminated with virulent microbes.

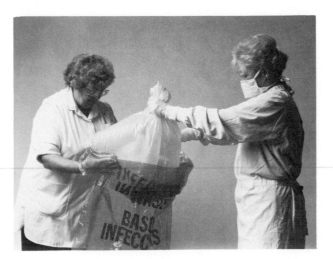

Figure 2-18

Needles should not be recapped or touched after use and should be placed immediately (needle first) in a puncture-proof container labeled for this purpose. No attempt should be made to bend or break used needles because they may stick or spray the health worker in the process (Fig. 2-19).

17. Specimens to be sent to the laboratory should be placed in solid containers with secure caps. If the specimen is from a patient with a known communicable disease, the outside of the container must be labeled as such. Avoid contaminating the outside of the container, and place the container in a clean bag. If a container should become contaminated, it must be cleaned with a disinfectant before placing it in the bag. Specimens must be sent to the laboratory after collection for examination (Fig. 2-20).

18. Medical charts that accompany patients to the diagnostic imaging department must be kept away from patient-care areas to prevent contamination.

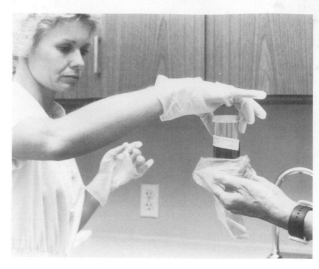

Figure 2-20

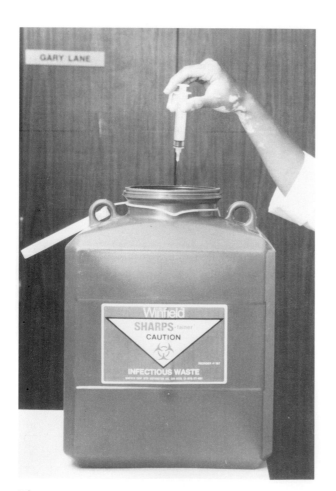

Figure 2-19

Disinfection

Disinfection is a term used to describe the removal, by mechanical and chemical processes, of pathogenic microorganisms, but frequently not their spores, from objects or body surfaces. Usually in reference to body surfaces, the term *antisepsis* or *antiseptic* is used rather than disinfect or disinfectant. Items are disinfected when they cannot withstand the process necessary to sterilize them or when it is not practical to sterilize. This is often the case with objects leaving an isolation unit. If an object leaving an examining room or isolation unit has been contaminated, it is cleaned first by vigorous scrubbing (mechanical means) and then disinfected by wiping it with, or soaking it in, a chemical selected by the institution for this purpose.

When a patient enters the diagnostic imaging department and the RT knows or suspects that the patient has a contagious disease, it is his responsibility to prevent the spread of infection. If the patient is coughing and sneezing, the RT must provide him with tissues and a place to dispose of them. He should instruct the patient to cough and sneeze into the tissues and then discard them safely. The patient should be removed from a crowded waiting room in order to prevent infecting other persons. The RT should put on a gown in order to protect his uniform and a mask, if necessary.

After the patient has been cared for and leaves the department, the RT must wash his hands thoroughly and then disinfect the radiographic table and anything in the room that the patient has touched. This can be accomplished with a disinfectant solution. The RT should then remove his gown and scrub his hands again.

Isolation technique

Although infection-control measures are to be used when caring for all patients, particular precautions are instituted when a patient is known, or is suspected of having, a disease that is contagious (communicable) and could be spread throughout the institution. These precautions are called *isolation precautions* or *protective asepsis.*

Isolation precautions separate the patient who has a contagious illness from other persons in the hospital. This separation may be accomplished in a hospital ward or in a private hospital room depending on how the pathogenic microorganisms are spread and the relibility of the patient with the disease in adhering to the precautions for prevention of the spread of his disease. If a disease can be transmitted only by direct contact, the patient may remain in a ward with other patients. If the disease is spread by airborne route, a private room is necessary. Two or more patients who have the same disease may share an isolation room.

There are two categories of isolation precautions currently recommended by the Centers for Disease Control, and each institution chooses the one that is preferable for its patient population. These categories are called *category-specific isolation* and *disease-specific isolation.*

The disease-specific isolation method defines certain practices to be followed for each communicable disease depending on the route by which the disease is transmitted. For instance, if a patient has varicella (chickenpox), strict isolation technique is used.

The category-specific isolation method groups diseases requiring similar isolation precautions together according to their commonality of route of transmission. For instance, hepatitis B and AIDS are both categorized with diseases requiring blood and body fluid precautions.

In this text, we will follow category-specific isolation technique. Several diseases requiring each category will be listed. The RT will be expected to familiarize himself with these classifications and the reasons for their use, because when a patient cannot come to the diagnostic imaging department from his hospital room, the RT may be expected to go into an isolation unit to make radiographic exposures. Therefore, he must be able to use the various isolation methods.

Whatever category of isolation technique is used, the RT must always adhere to four basic principles when dealing with patients who have a communicable disease. They are as follows:

1. Hands are washed using the procedure prescribed earlier in this chapter.

2. All items used for patient care are sterilized, disinfected, or disposed of to prevent spread of infection.

3. Items removed from isolation rooms are bagged and labeled as contaminated before being sent for disinfection.

4. All hypodermic needles must be placed in labeled, puncture-resistant receptacles used only for this purpose. Needles must not be bent or recapped after use.

The categories of isolation are drainage-secretion precautions; enteric precautions; AFB isolation (acid-fast bacillus; respiratory, contact, blood and body fluid precautions; and strict isolation.

Drainage-secretion precautions

Drainage-secretion precautions are used to prevent infections that are transmitted by direct or indirect contact with purulent material, drainage, or secretions from an infected site on the body such as abscesses, wound infections, and burns not included in a category that requires another technique. A private room is not required; however, a protective gown is worn if soiling or contact with the drainage or secretion is possible. Gloves are required for touching infection sites or material from those sites, but masks are not indicated. Any dressing or other infected items are bagged and labeled before being sent for disinfection or resterilization or are discarded. Hands are washed for 2 minutes after touching the infected patient.

Enteric precautions

Enteric precautions are used to prevent infection transmitted by direct or indirect contact with fecal material. A private room is required if the patient's hygenic practices are not reliable. Protective gowns are worn if soiling is possible, as are gloves, if infective material may be touched. Masks are not worn. A bathroom should not be shared with other patients. Items used for patient care should be bagged and labeled contaminated if sent for disinfection or resterilization, and all other materials should be discarded.

Diseases requiring this isolation category are amoebic dysentery; cholera; coxsackievirus disease; diarrhea of suspected infectious etiology; encephalitis; gastroenteritis caused by *Giardia lamblia,* Salmonella species, and Shigella species; hepatitis A; viral meningitis; poliomyelitis; and typhoid fever.

AFB isolation

AFB isolation is used for patients with pulmonary tuberculosis who currently have a positive sputum culture for acid-fast bacilli or a chest x-ray that reflects active disease. The letters AFB are used rather than the actual name of the disease to protect the patient's right to confidentiality.

Isolation in this category requires a mask if the patient is not reliable about covering his mouth when coughing. Gowns are required only if gross contamination is possible, and gloves are not required. Generally this type of isolation is not required for infants and young children with active tuberculosis because they rarely cough and their bronchial secretions contain very few acid-fast bacilli.

Respiratory isolation

Diseases requiring *respiratory isolation* are spread by droplet contact as the patient talks, coughs, or sneezes. Masks are indicated for close contact with the patient. Gown and gloves are not indicated.

Some of the diseases spread by this route are bacterial meningococcal and hemophilus influenzae meningitis, measles, mumps, meningococcal and hemophilus influenzae pneumonia, and pertussis (whooping cough).

Contact isolation

Contact isolation is used for diseases spread by close or direct contact. Masks are required for anyone who comes close to the patient. Gowns are worn if soiling is possible, and gloves are worn if infective material might be touched. A private room or a room shared by a patient with the same infection is required.

Diseases in this category include acute respiratory infections in infants and young children (croup, colds, bronchitis); gonococcal conjunctivitis in newborns; diptheria; severe disseminated primary or neonatal herpes simplex; impetigo; influenza in infants and young children; multiply resistant bacterial infections such as *Staphylococcus aureus,* Pneumococcus, *Hemophilus influenzae,* or any resistant bacterial infections listed by the infection control team; pediculosis; viral Staphylococcus and group A streptococcal pneumonia; rabies; scabies, and any major skin, wound, or burn infected and draining with *Staphylococcus aureus* or group A streptococcus.

Blood and body fluid precautions

Blood and body fluid precautions are recommended for use by The Centers for Disease Control by healthcare workers when caring for all patients. The new emphasis on this category of precautions is called "universal blood and body fluid precautions" (MMWR, August 1987, 3S). It is the result of an effort to protect both patients and health workers from the diseases spread by infected blood and body fluids. Cautious handling of blood, blood-contaminated instruments, dressings, any bloodstained object, or needles used for injection of patients with these diseases is required. Blood spills should be removed immediately with 5.25% sodium hypochlorite diluted to a 1:10 strength with water.

Gowns are indicated if there is a possibility of clothing becoming contaminated. Gloves are worn if blood or body fluids may be touched, and eye protectors and masks are required if spattering of blood or body fluids is possible. Needle stick injuries must be avoided. Hands must be washed with antiseptic soap if contamination or suspected contamination occurs. If there is skin preparation for a special procedure that involves shaving, the razor must be a single-use type and discarded after use in the contaminated waste area. Gloves must be worn for skin preparation that involves shaving.

Although these precautions are to be used for all patient care, special emphasis must be placed on the need for them in the emergency care setting when the infectious status of the patient is not known. The diseases requiring blood and body fluid precautions are acquired immunodeficiency syndrome (AIDS) and AIDS-related complex; Creutzfeldt-Jakob disease; hepatitis B (including HBSAg antigen carrier); hepatitis non-A, non-B; leptospirosis; malaria; and syphilis (both primary and secondary with skin and mucous membrane lesions). A private room is required for patients who have the diseases listed in this category and who have poor hygenic habits such as failing to wash hands following contact with blood and body fluids and sharing contaminated materials with other patients, thereby contaminating the environment.

Strict isolation

Strict isolation procedure is used for patients with diseases transported by airborne or contact route. Microorganisms isolated by this means are highly infectious and their spread difficult to control.

Mask, gown, and gloves are worn by all persons entering a strict isolation unit. Hand-washing and decontamination of materials used for patient care are as described for other isolation categories. A private room or a room shared with another patient with the same disease is indicated.

Diseases requiring strict isolation are pharyngeal diptheria, Lassa fever, pneumonic plague, varicella (chickenpox), and herpes zoster (localized in immunocompromised patients or disseminated in any patient).

Strict isolation technique is also used on some occasions for patients who are themselves at high risk for infection because of a debilitated state, for immunosuppressed patients, for patients with severe burns, and for high-risk infants. This category was previously called *protective* or *reverse isolation.*

ENTERING AND LEAVING THE STRICT ISOLATION UNIT

The strict isolation category generally encompasses the procedures needed for all category-specific isolation. If the RT learns to enter and leave this type of isolation unit, he will be able to maintain the requirements of the other categories with little difficulty.

In order to enter and leave a strict isolation unit, the RT will need the assistance of another RT or a member of the nursing team who is caring for the patient in the unit. Remember that the patient who is in a strict isolation unit may feel alone and rejected. These patients are forced to remain in solitude for long periods of time and are often treated by visitors and hospital personnel as if they are undesirable. It is possible to carry out strict isolation procedure and treat the patient as a human being with dignity and worth. Before beginning your work with the patient, spend a few moments explaining the radiologic procedure to him. When the procedure is complete, allow a few moments for discussion and respond in a therapeutic manner to any questions that the patient may have.

When a patient is placed in a strict isolation unit in the hospital setting, a special room is set aside for this purpose. At the entrance to the room there is a sink for hand-washing, a stack of paper or cloth gowns, a container for masks and caps, and a box filled with clean, disposable gloves. Many items in the isolation unit that are used for patient care remain in the unit until the patient leaves it.

Before entering the isolation room, the RT must have the portable radiographic machine prepared with as many cassettes as are necessary. A protective plastic case must cover the cassettes and protect them from contamination. Have your assistant available and then proceed using the following step-by-step directions.

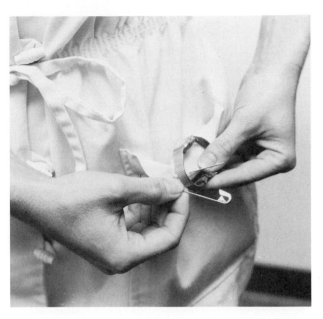

Figure 2-21

1. Push the portable radiographic machine into the room.

2. Stop at the area where you will don your protective clothing. Remove any jewelry that you are wearing, and pin it into your uniform pocket so it will not be lost (Fig. 2-21).

3. If your hair touches your collar, a cap must be put on (Fig. 2-22).

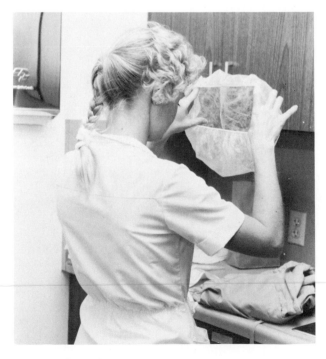

Figure 2-22

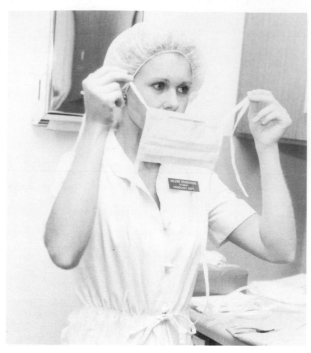

Figure 2-23

4. Remove a mask from the container and put it on (Fig. 2-23).

5. Wash your hands.

6. Take a gown from the stack. Hold it at the neck, and allow it to unfold. Put both arms into the sleeves of the gown, and work it on. Do not touch the outside of the gown (Fig. 2-24).

7. Tie the gown in back. Be certain that the gown is covering your clothing (Fig. 2-25).

8. Put gloves on, making certain that they cover the cuffs of the gown (Fig. 2-26).

9. Place an extra pair of gloves on the portable machine for later use.

10. Approach the patient, introduce yourself, and explain the procedure. Make necessary adjustments in the machine at this time because once you have touched the patient, you may not touch the machine again without changing gloves.

11. Place the cassette for the exposure (Fig. 2-27).

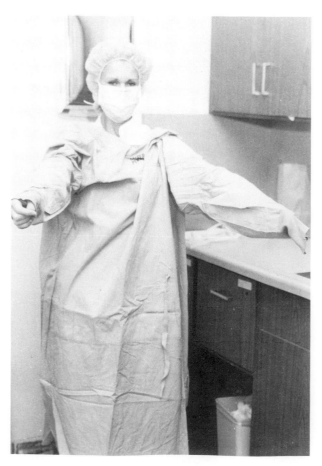

Figure 2-24

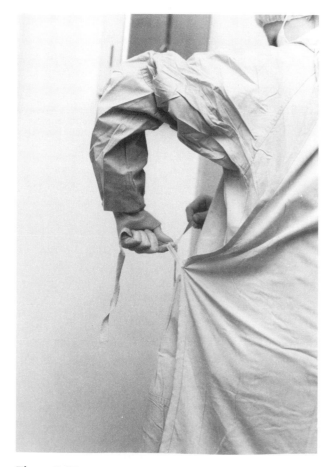

Figure 2-25

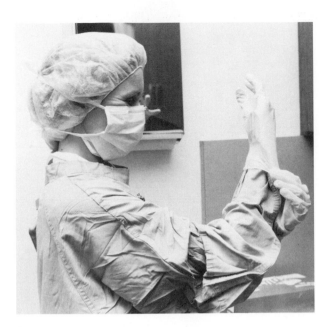

Figure 2-26

12. Remove contaminated gloves as described earlier in this chapter, and drop them into a waste receptacle.

13. Put on the clean gloves that you had placed on the machine.

14. Make the exposure. If additional exposures are necessary, it may be necessary to change gloves again. Do not allow your machine to become contaminated.

15. When the exposure is completed, remove the covered case and take it to the door of the unit where your assistant is waiting. Slide the plastic covering back from the cassette, and allow the assistant to remove it (Fig. 2-28).

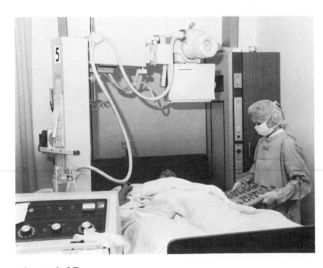

Figure 2-27

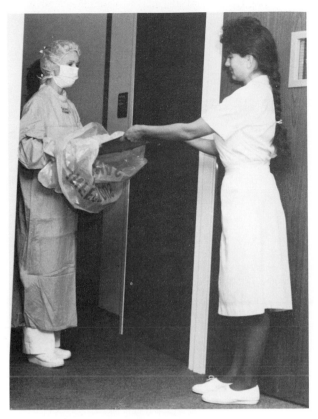

Figure 2-28

16. Return to the patient, and make him comfortable. Push the radiographic machine from the room. Then prepare to leave the unit.

17. Untie the waist tie of the gown before removing gloves (Fig. 2-29).

18. Remove gloves according to the procedure for removing contaminated gloves, and place them in the waste receptacle.

19. Wash your hands for 30 seconds. Dry them and then untie the top gown tie and mask ties. Do not touch any part of the mask except the ties (Fig. 2-30).

20. Remove the first sleeve of the gown by placing your fingers under the cuff of the sleeve and pulling it over the hand (Fig. 2-31).

21. Remove the other sleeve with your hand protected inside the sleeve of the gown.

22. Slip out of the gown and fold it forward so that the inside of the gown is facing outside (Fig. 2-32). If a cap has been worn, remove it without touching your hair, and dispose of it (Fig. 2-32).

23. Drop the soiled gown into the receptacle prepared for it.

24. Rewash your hands and dry them thoroughly.

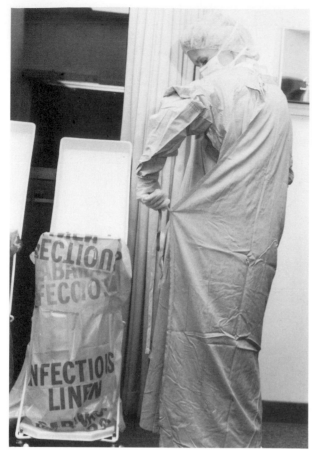

Figure 2-29

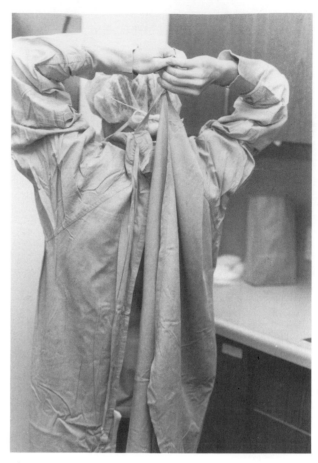

Figure 2-30

Do not touch faucet handles with bare hands. Use paper towels.

25. Leave the room. Cleanse the portable radiographic machine thoroughly with a disinfectant solution.

26. Wash your hands once again.

Transferring the patient with a communicable disease

Occasionally it is necessary for a patient with a communicable disease to come to the radiology department for radiographs or treatment. Precautions must be taken to prevent infecting anyone else and also to prevent contaminating a room or the equipment.

The patient must be transported by wheelchair or by gurney. If he has a disease that may be transmitted by droplet, airborne, or contact route, place a mask properly on his face and wear a gown and mask to protect yourself.

Place a sheet on the gurney or wheelchair, then cover it completely with a cotton blanket. Transfer the patient and wrap the cotton blanket around him (Fig. 2-33).

When the patient arrives at his destination, open the blanket without touching the inside. Place a protective sheet on the radiographic table, transfer the patient to the table, and place a draw sheet over him. Make the necessary exposures. Arrange your work so that the patient does not have to spend any more time than necessary in the department. Return the patient to the wheelchair or gurney. Wrap the cotton blanket around him and return him to his room. Notify the ward personnel that he has returned.

Once in the patient's room, dispose of the soiled sheet and blanket and wash your hands. Untie your gown and remove it as described. Cleanse the wheelchair or gurney with disinfectant, then rewash your hands.

Return to the radiology department and clean the table and all of the equipment that was used. Again, wash your hands.

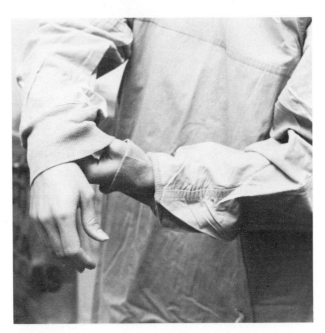

Figure 2-31

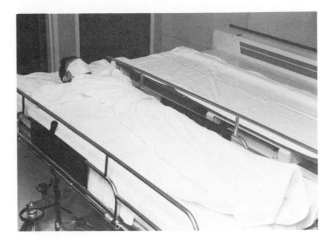

Figure 2-33

Summary

Infection control is the obligation of all persons entering a health-care institution. This includes hospital personnel, patients, and their visitors. All health workers must learn the concepts and procedures for infection control before beginning to work in their chosen specialty area, because it is their ethical obligation to carry out these practices in all health-care situations in order to prevent nosocomial infections.

Nosocomial infections are caused by four basic types of microorganisms: bacteria, fungi, viruses, and protozoa. Various forms of these microbes produce hospital infections, which are becoming increasingly difficult to control in spite of the body's own defenses against disease and the drugs used to control them.

The elements needed to produce infection are a source, a host, and a means of transmission. It is the RT's duty in his daily work to adhere strictly to infection-control techniques in order to break the cycle of infection. This can be done by careful hand-washing, correct disposal of waste material, maintaining a personal health-care regimen that includes adequate rest and meticulous hygenic practices, and adhering to techniques that protect the patient while in the RT's care.

Chapter 2, pre-post test

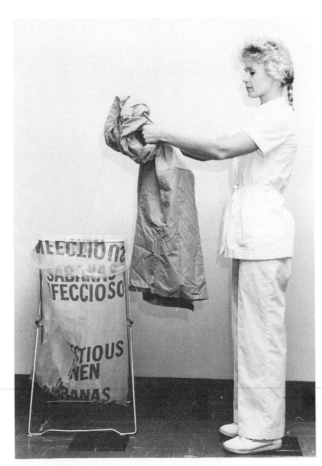

Figure 2-32

_____ 1. The chief purpose of hospital infection control is to prevent
  a. Contagion
  b. Urinary tract infections
  c. AIDS
  d. Nosocomial infections

_____ 2. Microorganisms that need a host cell to reproduce and are virtually unresponsive to antimicrobial drugs are
   a. Bacteria
   b. Fungi
   c. Protozoa
   d. Viruses

_____ 3. When one is in the incubation period of the disease process, the RT has no control over its tranmission.
   a. True
   b. False

_____ 4. The RT must use strict infection-control measures that include blood and body fluid precautions
   a. For every patient who enters the diagnostic imaging department
   b. For patients who have known communicable diseases
   c. Only for patients who have AIDS and hepatitis B
   d. For patients who seem ill

_____ 5. Blood and body fluid precautions include
   a. Use of clean, disposable gloves for sick persons
   b. Use of clean, disposable gloves for contact of the hands with blood or body fluids, a mask and goggles if blood or body fluids may spray on your face, and a gown if the blood and body fluids may touch your clothing, for any patient care that may involve contact with blood or body fluids
   c. Clean, disposable gloves as necessary
   d. Gown, gloves, mask and goggles for all patient care

_____ 6. The RT should always dress for the workplace with infection control in mind. This means that
   a. Clothing must be washable; fingernails must be kept short; shoes must be comfortable and have closed toes; and no jewelry must be worn except a wrist watch and wedding band
   b. The RT must look unattractive, because anything that looks good spreads infection
   c. A scrub suit be worn at all times
   d. The rules are to be followed when the infection-control officer is coming to the department

_____ 7. The most common means of spreading infection are
   a. Soiled instruments
   b. Infected patients
   c. The human hands
   d. Domestic animals

_____ 8. When leaving a strict isolation unit, the correct procedure to follow is to
   a. Untie your mask and top gown ties, remove your gloves, wash your hands, untie the waist gown tie, and remove the gown
   b. Untie all gown ties, remove your gloves, wash your hands, remove your mask, and then your gown
   c. Remove your gloves, untie the waist gown tie, wash your hands, then untie the top gown tie and mask ties
   d. Untie the waist gown tie, remove your gloves, wash your hands, and then untie the top gown tie and mask ties

_____ 9. The elements needed to produce an infection are a source, a host, and a means of transmission. An example of a source of infection might be
   a. An RT student who has a cold and comes to work
   b. A visitor in the hospital who has a "fever blister" on her mouth
   c. A patient who develops pneumonia
   d. A, b, and c

_____ 10. A safety precaution that must be taken when disposing of used hypodermic needles and syringes is:
   a. To place the needles in a waste basket as soon as possible
   b. To recap the needle and dispose of it quickly
   c. To place the syringe with the uncapped needle attached directly into the contaminated waste receptacle provided for them immediately after use
   d. To detach the needle from the syringe and place only the needle in the contaminated waste receptacle

_____ 11. Match the following means of transmitting infection with the correct definition:
   a. Direct contact
   b. Indirect contact
   c. Droplet contact
   d. Vehicle contact
   e. Airborne contact
      1. Touching objects that have been contaminated with disease-producing microbes
      2. Ingesting contaminated water, food, drugs or blood
      3. Inhaling air contaminated with infectious microbes
      4. Contact with secretions transferred by sneezing, coughing, or talking
      5. Touching contaminated material with hands

_____ 12. List and define the seven categories of isolation.

Laboratory reinforcement

1. In the school laboratory, demonstrate the proper method of hand-washing for medical asepsis.

2. In the school laboratory, remove linens from a radiographic table that has been used for a patient with an infectious disease and demonstrate the proper method of cleaning the equipment and the table.

3. Mrs. Gray is in an isolation ward unit on Ward 4. She has staphylococcal pneumonia. Her physician has or-

dered radiographs of her chest. She is too ill to be transferred to the radiology department. You are the RT who is given this assignment. Demonstrate in the school laboratory how you will manage to make these exposures.

4. In the school laboratory, demonstrate transferring a patient who has a communicable respiratory disease to and from the radiology department.

Chapter Three
Basic Patient Care in Diagnostic Imaging

Goal of this chapter:

The radiologic technology student will be able to explain how to admit patients for diagnostic imaging procedures and care for their basic needs in a safe and effective manner.

Behavioral objectives:

When the student has completed this chapter, he will be able to do the following:
1. Give clear verbal instructions to ambulatory patients about the correct manner of dressing or undressing for a diagnostic imaging procedure, and assess the need for assistance
2. Give a written explanation of what is to be done with the patient's belongings while he is being cared for in the diagnostic imaging department
3. Demonstrate the correct manner of moving, transferring, and positioning patients to prevent injury to himself and to the patient
4. Demonstrate the correct method of assisting the disabled patient with dressing or undressing for a diagnostic examination
5. List three safety measures that must be taken when transferring a patient from a hospital ward to the diagnostic imaging department and returning him to the ward
6. List three situations in the diagnostic imaging department that might result in damage to the patient's skin, and explain how to prevent them
7. Demonstrate the correct method of moving a patient who is wearing a plaster cast
8. List four signs of circulatory impairment that the RT must recognize in a patient who is wearing a plaster cast
9. Demonstrate the correct manner of assisting a patient with a bedpan or urinal

Glossary

Abrasion scraping away of a portion of skin

Adduction movement of a limb toward the body

Atrophy decrease in size of organ or tissue

Contracture a permanent tightening of a joint or muscle caused by disease or degeneration of muscle or bony tissue, which shortens the muscle

Defecation evacuation or elimination of fecal matter from rectum

Distal that part farthest away from the source or point of attachment

Decubitus ulcer bedsore that is open; often infected on bony prominences

Fasted patient has gone without food or drink for a long period of time for a particular reason

Incontinent unable to retain urine,

feces because of the loss of sphincter control or through cranial or spinal nerve damage
Perineal area external region between vulva and anus in women or

between scrotum and anus in men
Plantar flexion extension of foot so toes are pointing downward with respect to normal position
Posterior toward the back of the body

Tissue necrosis small areas of outer skin surrounded by healthy tissue that have died because of injury or lack of circulation

When a patient comes to the radiology department from outside the hospital, he is frequently required to remove all or some items of clothing before a radiographic examination can be performed. The RT will usually be the person who receives the patient and informs him which items of clothing are to be removed. The patient's discomfort or embarrassment can be lessened if the RT will approach this situation in a courteous and professional manner.

When the patient arrives for his examination, he should be taken to the specific place where he is expected to disrobe. The RT shows him how to close the dressing room door or draw the curtain of the cubicle while he is undressing. The RT should clearly explain how the patient is to don the examining gown and where he is to go for the examination once he is dressed. Doing this will take only a few moments and will make the patient feel more relaxed. Remember that everyone does not know that some types of examining gowns open at the back rather than at the front—it helps to be given an explanation.

The patient should be supplied with hangers for his clothing. If it is permissible for him to leave his clothing in the dressing room, this fact should be explained by the RT. If it is not, the patient should be shown where he may leave his clothing. Purses, jewelry, and other valuables should be treated with special care.

The RT, as a member of the health team, has the responsibility of protecting himself and his patients from injury in every way possible. Health workers are often injured while moving and lifting patients, yet almost all of these injuries can be prevented if the RT will practice good body mechanics at all times.

Patients are also the victims of injuries caused when they are improperly moved or lifted, and most of these injuries can also be prevented.

The RT must also protect the patient's skin from injury, which is a problem particularly when the patient is unable to move himself. The RT must be aware of how skin damage may occur in order to take the precautions necessary to prevent it.

Care of valuables

Many patients bring jewelry, a purse, or other valuables to the radiology department. The dressing rooms in most radiology departments are not safe

places to leave these items, and the patient will feel justifiably uneasy about leaving them there. Again, the RT should consider the patient's concerns and explain what must be done with them.

Metal items such as necklaces, rings, and watches are not to be worn for certain radiographic examinations and must be removed before the examination is begun. An envelope large enough to accommodate all such items should be offered to the patient. The envelope may be kept in the patient's purse or pocket, or in a secure place in the radiology department. If billfolds and purses are not carried by the patient, identifying information should be written on a receipt, and all items should be tagged and placed in a designated safety area by the RT. This procedure will prevent losses that may result in inconvenience and expense to both the patient and the department. The RT should never place value on a patient's belongings—an item that may seen insignificant to the RT may be the patient's most treasured belonging. Every article of clothing or jewelry or other personal effects that a patient brings to the radiology department should be treated as valuable.

Body mechanics

Constant abuse of the spine from moving and lifting patients is the leading cause of injuries to health-care personnel in all health-care institutions. The RT will be less fatigued and will avoid injury to himself and his patients if he employs the rules of correct body mechanics. These rules are based on the laws of gravity.

Gravity is the force that pulls objects toward the center of the earth. Any movement made requires an expenditure of energy to overcome the force of gravity. When an object is balanced, it is firm and stable. If it is off balance, it will fall because of the pull of gravity. The center of gravity is the point at which the mass of any body is centered. When a person is standing, his center of gravity is at the center of the pelvis (Fig. 3-1).

Safe body mechanics require good posture. Good posture means that the body is in alignment with all parts in balance. This permits the musculoskeletal system (the bones and joints) to work at maximal efficiency with a minimal amount of strain on joints, tendons, ligaments, and muscles. Good posture also

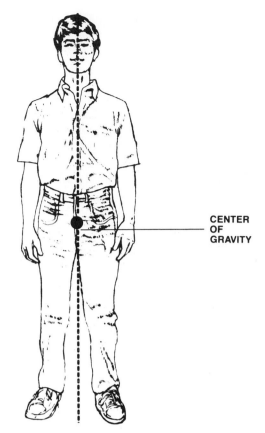

CENTER
OF
GRAVITY

Figure 3-1

aids other body systems to work efficiently. For instance, if the chest is held up and out (the musculoskeletal system), the lungs (the respiratory system) can work at maximal efficiency.

Rules for correct upright posture are as follows:

The chest should be held up and slightly forward with the waist extended. This allows the lungs to expand properly and fill to capacity.

The head should be held erect with the chin held in. This puts the spine in proper alignment, and there is no curve in the neck.

Stand with the feet parallel and at right angles to the lower legs. The feet should be 4 to 8 inches apart. Keep body weight equally distributed on both feet.

Keep the knees slightly bent. They act as a ''shock absorber'' for the body.

Keep the buttocks in and the abdomen up and in. This prevents strain on the back and abdominal muscles.

When you move and lift objects or persons, you must overcome the forces of weight and friction. The center of gravity must be determined and a plan made to surmount the weight of the object or person. This can be done by keeping the heaviest part close to your own body. If this is not possible, another person or persons should assist with moving or lifting the load.

The force of friction opposes movement. When you move or transfer a patient, friction must be reduced to the minimum to facilitate movement. This can be done by reducing the surface area to be moved or, in the case of patients, employing some of the patient's own strength to assist with the move if possible. If the patient is unable to assist, you should reduce friction by placing his arms across his chest to reduce the surface area. Pulling rather than pushing also reduces friction. A pull sheet placed under the immobile patient will also work to reduce friction during a move. Directions for the use of a pull sheet will be presented later in this chapter.

The RT should always remember to protect himself by keeping the body's line of balance close to the center of gravity, which is at, or just below, the waistline. When picking up an object from the floor, bend the knees and lower your body. Do not bend from the waist. The biceps muscles are the strongest arm muscles and are effective in pulling; therefore, pull the weight—do not push it (Fig. 3-2).

When a patient must be lifted, balance the weight over both feet. Hold the patient close to your body, bend your knees, and set your spine to support the load. Use your arms and leg muscles to lift. The spine must always be protected. Instead of twisting your body to move with a load, change foot positions. Always keep your body balanced over your feet, which are spread to provide a firm base of support. Make certain that the floor area where the work is being done is clear of all objects.

Moving and transferring patients

The RT will occasionally be called on to transfer a patient to or from a hospital ward, or he may have to direct a porter to do this. Several precautions must be taken when this is to be done, in order to be certain that the *right* patient is transported at the *right* time for the *right* procedure and that he is moved in as safe a manner as possible.

After being informed of the patient's name, room number, and the radiographic examination to be done, the RT or the porter should go to the nurse's station on the ward where the patient is. The nurse in charge should be told which patient is wanted and for what procedure. She will hand the RT the patient's chart. The RT should ask about specific precautions to be followed for the patient at this time. Then the RT proceeds to the patient's room, greets him, and checks his identifying name band with his

Figure 3-2

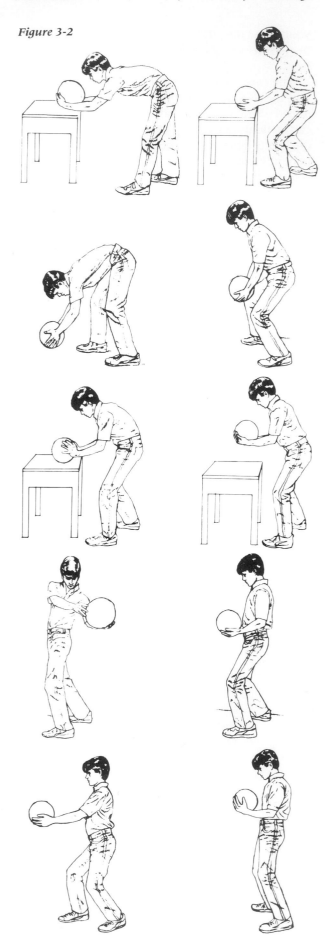

chart. When you are certain that he is the correct patient, proceed with the transfer.

When returning a patient to his hospital room, stop at the appropriate nurse's station, return the chart, and inform the ward personnel that the patient is being returned to his room. If help is needed to return the patient to his bed, request it at this time. The RT or a porter must never attempt to transfer a patient from a gurney to a hospital bed without assistance. Before you leave the patient's room, be certain that he is safe. Always place the side rails on the hospital bed up. If the bed has been raised to a higher position to facilitate moving the patient, be certain that the bed is returned to the lowest possible position before you leave the room.

Assessing the patient's mobility

Before the RT begins to move a patient, he must assess the patient's ability to aid in the process. This assessment can take place with the patient sitting, lying, or standing.

The RT must identify any abnormalities in the patient's body alignment. If there are one or more abnormalities, he must determine the reasons for the problem. Deviations from correct body alignment may result from poor posture, trauma, muscle damage, or dysfunction of the nervous system. Other factors that contribute to body misalignment are malnutrition, fatigue, and emotional disturbance. If abnormalities of body alignment are not correctable, they must be considered; support blocks, pillows, or sandbags must be on hand to support the patient. The RT can then assess the patient's mobility and limitations in his range of joint motion. Any stiffness, instability, swelling, inflammation, pain, limitation of movement, or atrophy of muscle mass surrounding each joint must be noted because these abnormalities will need to be considered if the diagnostic imaging procedure planned involves frequent position changes.

The patient's ability to walk (his gait) must be assessed so that the RT knows how much assistance the patient will need as he moves on and off the diagnostic imaging table. Gait includes the rhythm, speed, cadence, and any other mannerisms of walking that may signal a problem with balance, posture, or independence of movement.

Mobility is also affected by the patient's cardiovascular, respiratory, metabolic, and musculoskeletal systems. The RT is not expected to make extensive diagnosis of problems with these systems; however, he must be able to assess patients with obvious respiratory or cardiac distress or a severe endocrine problem because these will need special considerations during diagnostic examinations or radiologic treatment. Assessment and care of patients with these types of systemic problems are discussed in Chapter 4.

The RT must ask himself the following questions before he begins to move or transfer a patient:

The patient's general condition: how well or how poorly is he functioning?

The patient's mobility: are his motions restricted in any way?

The patient's strength and endurance: will he become fatigued and be unable to complete the transfer without assistance?

The patient's ability to maintain his balance: can he sit or stand for as long a period as is required?

The patient's ability to understand what is expected of him during the transfer: is he responsive and alert?

The patient's acceptance of the move: does he fear or resent the transfer? Will the transfer increase his pain, or does he feel that it is unnecessary?

The RT must then decide how the patient can be transferred the most safely and most comfortably, by gurney or by wheelchair. Hospitalized patients are rarely allowed to walk to and from the diagnostic imaging department for reasons of safety. If there is any question about what the patient can do for himself, the nurse in charge of the patient must be consulted. Assistants to negotiate the move safely must be on hand. A patient must never be moved without adequate help; to do so may cause injury to the patient or to the RT. Rules to remember when moving patients are the following:

Give only the assistance that the patient needs for comfort and safety.

Always transfer a patient across the shortest distance.

Lock all wheels on beds, gurneys, and wheelchairs.

Generally, it is better to move a patient toward his strong side while the RT assists at his weak side.

The patient should wear shoes for standing transfers, but slippery bedroom slippers should not be worn.

The patient must be informed of the plan of the move, and his help should be encouraged.

The patient should be given short, simple commands, and the RT must help the patient to carry them out.

Methods of transfer

There are essentially three ways of transferring patients: by gurney, by wheelchair, and by ambulation.

BY GURNEY

When a patient is moved from a gurney to a radiographic table, or the reverse, great care must be exercised in order to prevent injury. If the patient is unconscious or unable to cooperate in the move, his spine, head, and extremities must be well supported. One convenient way to do this is to place a sheet under him, which may be used to slide him from one surface to another.

Using a sheet for transfer   To place a sheet under a patient, use the following procedure: Obtain a heavy draw sheet, or use a full bed sheet and fold it in half. If an assistant is needed, there should be one person on each side of the bed or table. Turn the patient onto his side and move him to the distal side of the bed or table. Place the sheet on the table or bed and then roll one half of the sheet as close to the patient's back as possible (Fig. 3-3). Tell the patient that he will be turned back toward you and that he will be moving over the rolled sheet. Then turn him across the sheet roll and have your assistant straighten the sheet on the distal side. The patient may then be returned to a supine position, and the transfer may begin.

If the patient is an adult, three or four people should participate in the maneuver. One person stands at the patient's head to guide and support it during the move, another should be at the side of the surface to which the patient will be moved, and the third person should be at the side of the surface on which the patient is lying. If there are four people,

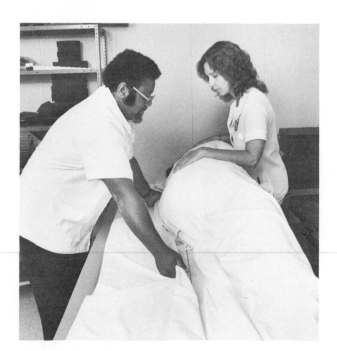

Figure 3-3.   Pull sheet.

two may stand at each side. The sheet is rolled at the side of the patient so that the RT can easily grasp it in his hands close to the patient's body. In unison (usually on the count of three), the team transfers the patient to the other surface (Figs. 3-4 and 3-5).

If the radiographic table is a stationary cradle type, extra padding should be placed over the metal parts of the table's edge to protect the patient from being bruised as he is moved (Fig. 3-6). Some cradle tables have a floating top. In this case, the top should be moved forward, close to the edge of the gurney. Conscious patients should be cautioned that the center part of these tables is lower than the surface, so that they are not frightened when lowered into it.

Tube housing above radiographic tables should be moved out of the way when patients are being moved, in order to protect both patient and RT from bumping into them. To avoid bumping into a stationary device such as a fluoroscopic unit, the patient should be warned not to sit up, and the RT must also be careful not to injure himself.

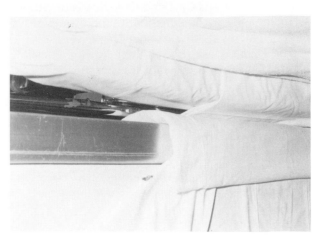

Figure 3-6

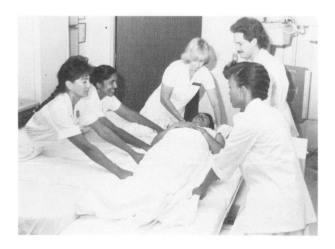

Figure 3-4

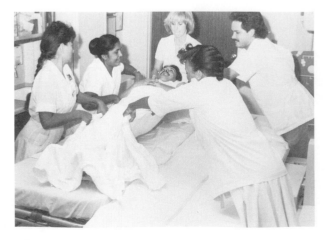

Figure 3-5

Three-carrier lift   A three-carrier lift can be used to move a patient from one place to another. This lift, if properly performed, can be accomplished without injury to patient or RT. Begin by sliding the patient to the edge of the area from which he is to be lifted. Have the gurney at a right angle to the end of the radiographic table with the wheels locked. All three persons who are going to lift the patient then go to that side of the table; one stands at the patient's head and neck, one at the buttocks, and one at the legs and ankles. Cross the patient's arms over his chest. The lifters all place their bodies against the area on which the patient is lying and place their arms under the part of the patient that they are going to lift (Fig. 3-7).

At the signal, the movers roll the patient off of the table and onto their chests (Fig. 3-8). All three pivot and place the patient onto the area to which he is being moved (Fig. 3-9).

Log roll   Occasionally it is necessary to turn a patient without flexing his neck or back. This type of move is called a log roll. Five persons are necessary to negotiate this patient move safely, so the RT must call for four assistants. Two persons stand at each side of the table or bed on which the turn will take place. One person keeps the head and neck immobile by placing his hands flat against the sides of the patient's face with palms held firmly at the angle of his jaw. Two assist with maintaining alignment of the torso and two with the legs. Use the sheet that is under the patient as a turn sheet.

Place the patient's arms across his chest and ask him to hold himself rigid if he is able to assist. Place a pillow or support bolster between the patient's knees in order to prevent pressure and to assist with maintenance of body alignment as he is turned. Place another bolster in the place where the patient's head

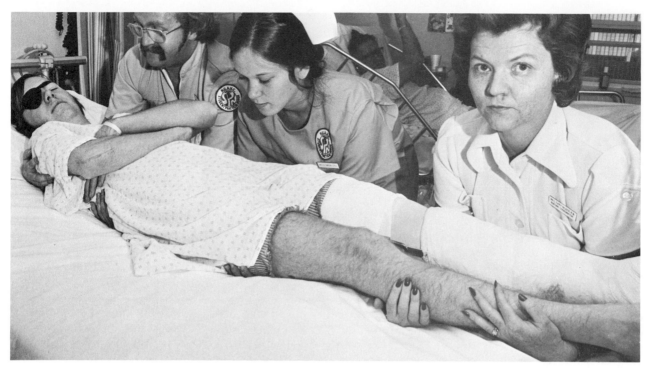

Figure 3-7

will rest when the turn is complete to support the head and neck in alignment.

When the patient is prepared and each member of the team understands his duty as the patient is turned, begin the move. The sheet is brought up over the patient's distal side and grasped by the two persons on that side close to the patient's body. The person in charge of the head and neck stands at the head

of the table or at the top side of the table and positions his hands for firm support. The fourth member of the team assists with maintainance of the patient's torso alignment. In unison, the team rolls the patient to the desired side as if he were a log keeping his head, neck, and torso immobile during the move (Fig. 3-10). When the turn is complete, the patient's head should be resting on the bolster positioned before the

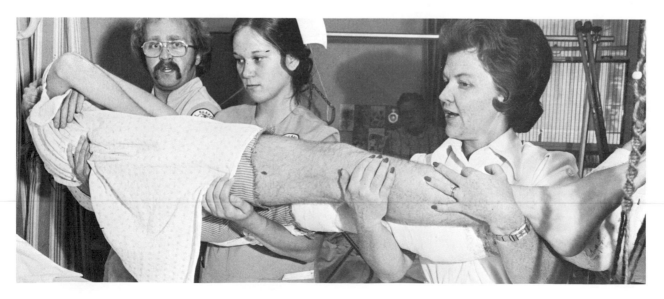

Figure 3-8

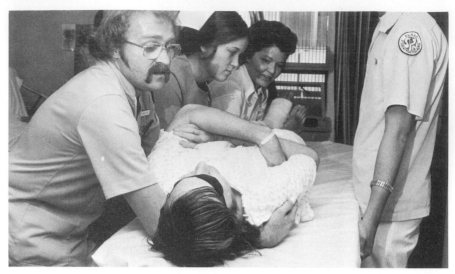

Figure 3-9

move began. The back must be firmly supported with bolsters or pillows. The upper leg may be flexed after the move is completed.

BY WHEELCHAIR

If a patient must be moved from a bed or radiographic table to a wheelchair, or the reverse, he must be helped. The RT should never allow a patient to get off of a table or into a wheelchair without some assistance. The patient is often not as strong as he believes himself to be. The sudden movement may cause dizziness, and the patient may fall.

If the patient has been in a supine position and is to be helped to a sitting position, the RT should have him turn to his side with his knees flexed. The RT then places himself in front of the patient with one arm under his shoulders and the other across his knees. If the patient can assist, instruct him to push up with his upper arm when told to do so (Fig. 3-11). Then, on the count of three, move the patient or help him to move to a sitting position at the edge of the table. Before helping the patient to stand, allow him to sit for a moment and regain his sense of balance. Then, if the patient needs further assistance, the RT may stand in front of him and place his arms across the RT's shoulders (Fig. 3-12). If firm support is necessary, put your knees around the patient's knees. Help him to stand and pivot, and then lower him onto the chair, bending your knees and keeping your back straight as you do so (Fig. 3-13). If the patient needs only minimal assistance, the RT may stand at his side and take his arm in order to help him off the table.

If the radiographic table is high, the RT should never allow a patient to step down without providing

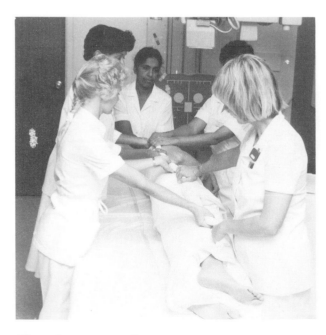

Figure 3-10.   Log roll.

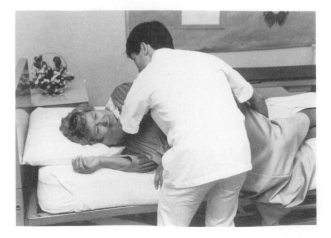

Figure 3-11

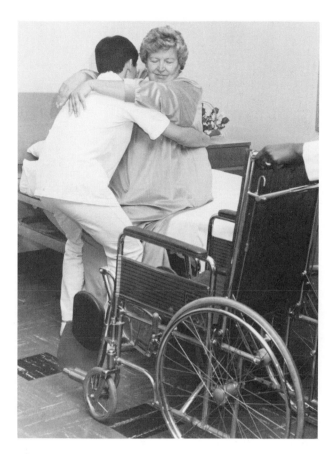

Figure 3-12

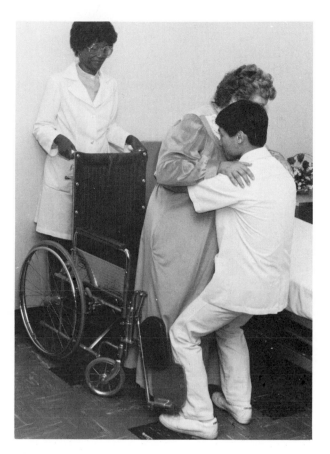

Figure 3-13

a secure stepping stool. The RT should always stay at the patient's side in order to assist him.

The wheelchair must be close enough so that the patient can be seated in the chair with one pivot. Have the foot supports of the chair up and the wheels locked. The RT should stand in front of the patient, spread his feet for a broad base of support, flex his knees, support the patient at his sides, pivot with the patient and seat him in the chair. The footrests on the wheelchair should then be put down and the wheels unlocked. A safety belt should be put across an unsteady patient.

The patient must be kept covered as much as possible during any move or transfer. He should never be transferred by gurney or wheelchair without being covered with a sheet or blanket. When he is placed on a radiographic table, he must be covered with a protective sheet. He must not be allowed to become chilled if it is at all possible to prevent this. A confused, disoriented, or unconscious person or a child must never be left alone on a radiographic table or a gurney. If the patient's behavior cannot be predicted, or if he is in a wheelchair, he should be carefully observed. A soft restraint belt should be placed over any patient left on a gurney. The side rails of the gurney should be up (Fig. 3-14).

Positioning the patient for diagnostic imaging examinations

When a patient must spend long periods of time in the diagnostic imaging department, it will be the RT's duty to assist him to maintain his body in normal alignment for comfort and to maintain normal physiologic functioning. There are several protective po-

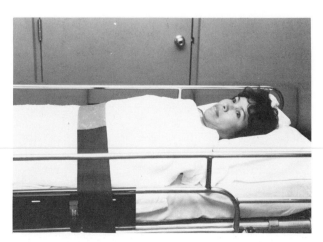

Figure 3-14

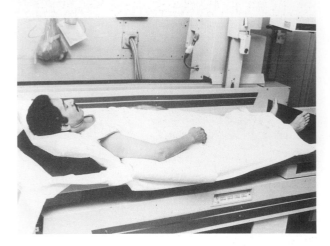

Figure 3-15.   Supine position.

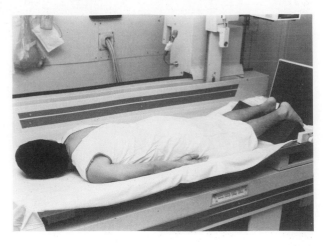

Figure 3-17

sitions that the body may assume or be assisted to assume for comfort. There are also several positions that the patient may be requested to assume to facilitate diagnosis or treatment. The RT must familiarize himself with all these positions and the problems that may be encountered with each in order to assist the patient as the need arises. The positions are as follows:

> Supine position—*patient is flat on his back. The feet and the neck will need to be protected when the patient is lying in this position. A pillow may be placed under the head to tilt it forward. The feet should be supported to prevent plantar flexion or footdrop (Fig. 3-15).*

> Protective side-lying position—*patient lies on either side with a pillow for support under the head and neck and another pillow under the arm and one or two to support the leg. This position prevents lateral flexion of the neck, inward rotation of the arm, and internal rotation and adduction of the femur (Fig. 3-16).*

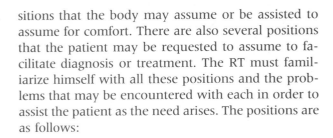

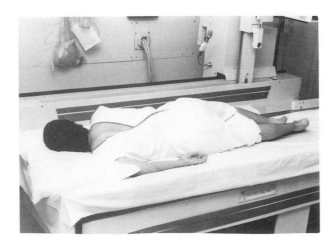

Figure 3-16

Protective prone position—*patient lies face down. A small pillow should support the head to prevent flexion of the cervical spine. The patient may be moved down on the table so that his feet drop over the edge, or a pillow may be placed under the lower legs at the ankles to prevent footdrop (Fig. 3-17).*

Fowler's position—*patient semisits with his head raised from a 45- to 60-degree angle.*

Semi-Fowler's position— *patient's head is raised from a 15- to 30-degree angle. The arms must be supported to prevent pull on the shoulders, and the feet must be supported to prevent plantar flexion or footdrop. In this position, the abdominal organs drop and provide more space for respiratory excursion; therefore, these are therapeutic positions for patients in respiratory distress (Fig. 3-18).*

Sims' position—*patient lies on either his left or right side with the forward arm flexed and the posterior arm extended behind his body. The body is inclined slightly forward with the top knee bent sharply and the bottom knee slightly bent. This position is frequently used for diagnostic imaging of the lower bowel (Fig. 3-19).*

Trendelenburg position—*the table or bed is inclined with the patient's head lower than the rest of the body. Patients are occasionally placed in this position during diagnostic imaging procedures and for promotion of venous return in patients with inadequate peripheral perfusion caused by disease.*

Assisting the patient to dress and undress

The patient may arrive in the radiology department alone if he comes from outside the hospital. As the RT is making an initial assessment of the patient's

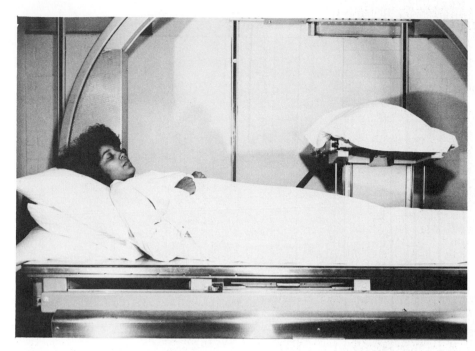

Figure 3-18. Semi-Fowler's position.

condition, he may observe that the patient will need help in removing his clothing. This assistance may be necessary if the patient is in a cast or a brace, is very young, or is in too weakened a condition to help himself. He may have a contracture of an extremity. His eyesight may be poor. Whatever the problem, if the RT senses that the patient will have difficulty undressing if left alone, he should offer assistance and stay near the dressing room in order to provide help when it is needed.

Occasionally the patient is brought to the radiology department as an emergency case. Removing his clothing in the conventional way may cause further injury or pain. The RT might consider cutting the garments away, but except in extreme emergencies he must not cut any item of clothing without gaining

the patient's consent. If the patient is unable to give consent, a member of his family should do so in writing for the RT's protection.

If the patient is very young and is accompanied by a familiar adult, he will be more relaxed and cooperative if the adult helps him to dress and undress. Explain to the adult how the child should be dressed for the examination, arrange a meeting place, and leave them alone.

If the RT must assist a patient who has a disability of the lower extremities, the clothing should be removed from the top part of the body first. Then place a long examining gown on the patient. Instruct him to loosen belt buckles, buttons, or hooks around the waist and slip his trousers over his hips. If he cannot do this for himself, the RT must reach under the gown and pull the trousers down over the hips. Then have the patient sit down. The RT can squat in front of the patient and gently pull the clothing over his legs and feet to remove it (Fig. 3-20). If the patient is not able to help, an assistant should be called.

Some dresses may be removed in the same way. But if this method is not practical, and the dress must be pulled over the woman's head, the RT should place a draw sheet over the patient and then help her to remove her slip and brassiere. Help her to put on an examining gown, then remove the draw sheet.

To redress a patient with a paralyzed leg, a leg injury, a cast, or a brace, slide the clothing (pants or skirt) over the feet or legs as far as the hips while the patient is sitting and still wearing an examining gown. Then have him stand, and pull the clothing over the hips if he can tolerate it. If the patient is not able to pull his clothing over his hips by himself, the

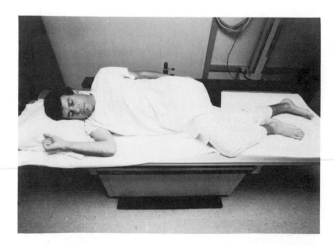

Figure 3-19

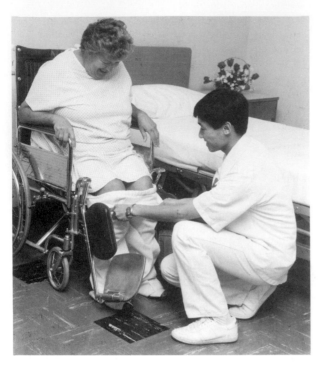

Figure 3-20

RT should have an assistant raise him off the chair so that the clothing may be slipped over the hips and waist by the RT. Then remove the patient's arms from the sleeves of the gown. Have him hold the gown over his chest, and carefully pull the shirt over his head, or put it on him one sleeve at a time. When the outside items of clothing are on the patient, remove the gown from under the clothes.

The disabled patient

If a patient is on a gurney or the radiographic table and the RT must change his clothing, this will be most easily accomplished with the patient in a supine position. Cover him with a draw sheet and have an examining gown ready. Explain what is to be done and ask the patient to help if he is able. If he is paralyzed or unconscious, summon help before beginning the procedure.

Remove the clothing from the less affected side first. Then remove the clothing from the more affected side and place the clean gown on that side, making sure to keep the patient covered with the draw sheet. Next place the clean gown on the unaffected side and tie the gown at the back, if practical (Fig. 3-21).

If the patient is wearing an article of clothing that must be pulled over his head, roll the garment up above the waist. Then remove the patient's arms from the clothing, first from the unaffected side and then from the affected side. Next, gently lift the clothing

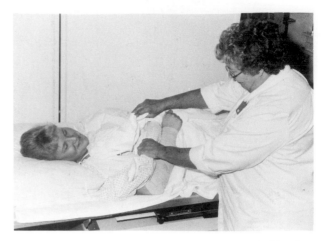

Figure 3-21.   Remove clothing from uninjured side, then injured side.

over the patient's head. One person alone should not attempt to undress a disabled patient; to do so may cause further injury or discomfort.

To remove trousers, loosen buckles and buttons and have the patient raise his buttocks as you slip the trousers over the hips. If the patient is unable to help, have an assistant stand at the opposite side of the table. After the trousers have been loosened, have the assistant pull the patient toward him, then slide the trousers off one side of the hip. Next, draw the patient toward yourself and have the assistant slide the trousers off of the other hip. Then, together, slip the trousers below the knees and off (Fig. 3-22).

Fold the clothing and place it in a paper bag on which the patient's name has been printed. If the patient is accompanied by a relative or a friend, ask that person to keep the patient's clothing. If the patient is alone, the RT will be responsible for caring for the clothing.

When a patient's gown becomes wet or soiled in the radiology department, it is the RT's duty to change it. If a patient is allowed to remain in a wet or soiled gown, his skin may become damaged, or he may become chilled.

When changing the gown of a patient who has an injury or is paralyzed on one side, remove the gown from the unaffected side first. Then, with the patient covered by the soiled gown, place the clean gown first on the affected side and then on the unaffected side. Pull the soiled gown from under the clean one.

The patient with an intravenous infusion

Frequently patients are taken to the diagnostic imaging department with an IV infusion in place. If the patient's gown must be changed, the clothing should

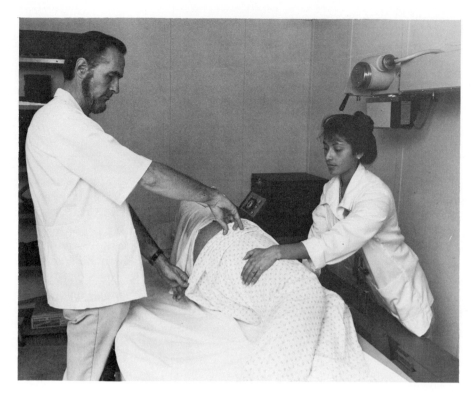

Figure 3-22.   *Removing the trousers.*

be slipped off the unaffected side first. Next, carefully slide the sleeve of the unaffected side over the IV tubing and catheter, then over the container of fluid. For this step, the container must be removed from the standard. When replacing the soiled gown with a clean one, first place the sleeve on the affected side over the container of fluid, then over the tubing and onto the arm with the venous catheter in place (Fig. 3-23). Rehang the bottle of fluid and complete the change. When moving the arm of a patient who has

an IV catheter in place, support the arm firmly so that the catheter does not become dislodged. Remember to keep the bottle of fluid above the infusion site in order to prevent blood from flowing into the tubing.

If the intravenous infusion is being controlled by a pump and the patient's gown becomes wet or soiled and must be changed, the RT should not attempt to disengage the IV tubing from the pump. Remove the gown from the unaffected arm, and place the soiled gown to one side of the table until the nurse in charge

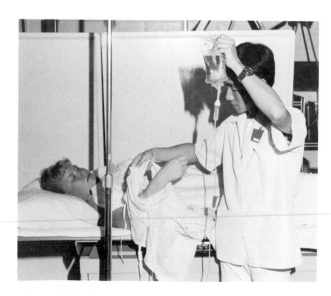

Figure 3-23

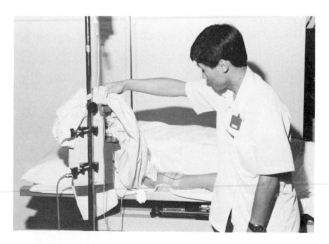

Figure 3-24.   *Place the soiled gown to one side of the table or on top of the I.V. pump. Do not disengage the tubing from the I.V. pump.*

of monitoring the infusion can remove it. Then replace the soiled gown with a clean gown over the unaffected side and the chest only (Fig. 3-24).

Skin care

The RT is responsible for the care of his patient's skin or integumentary system while he is in the diagnostic imaging department. Skin breakdown can occur in a brief period of time (1 to 2 hours) and result in a decubitus ulcer that may take weeks or months to heal. Mechanical factors that may predispose the skin to break down are immobility, pressure, and shearing force.

Immobilizing a patient in one position for an extended period of time creates pressure on the skin bearing the patient's weight. This in turn restricts capillary blood flow to that area and can result in tissue necrosis.

Moving a patient to or from a diagnostic imaging table from a wheelchair or gurney too rapidly or without adequately protecting his skin during the move may damage the external skin or the underlying tissues as they are pulled over each other creating a shearing force. This too may lead to tissue necrosis.

Another factor that contributes to skin breakdown is friction caused by movement back and forth on a rough or uneven surface such as a wrinkled bed sheet. Allowing a patient to lie on a damp sheet or remain in a wet gown may lead to skin damage. Similarly, urine or fecal material that is allowed to remain on the skin acts as an irritant and is damaging to the skin.

Early signs that indicate imminent skin breakdown are blanching and a feeling of coldness over pressure areas. This condition is called *ischemia*. Ischemia is followed by heat and redness in the area as the blood rushes there in an attempt to provide the traumatized skin with nourishment. This process is called *reactive hyperemia*. If, at the time of reactive hyperemia, the pressure on the threatened area is not relieved, the tissues begin to necrose, and a small ulceration is soon visible. Ischemia and reactive hyperemia are difficult to visualize in patients who are dark skinned. In these cases, the RT must feel the skin to assess for threat of skin damage.

A shearing injury to the skin may cause it to appear bluish and bruised. If such an area is not cared for, necrosis and ulceration will also occur.

Persons who are most prone to skin breakdown are the malnourished, the elderly, and the chronically ill. A patient who is elderly or who is in poor health may have dehydrated skin, an accumulation of fluid in the tissues (edema), increased or decreased skin temperature, or a loss of subcutaneous fat that acts to protect the skin. Any of these factors will contribute to the potential for skin breakdown, and the RT must be particularly cautious when moving or caring for this type of patient.

Prevention of decubitus ulcers

Skin care must always be a consideration when caring for patients in the diagnostic imaging department. The tables on which the patients must be placed for care are hard, and often the surface is unprotected. The areas most susceptible to decubitus ulcers are the scapulae, the sacrum, the trochanters, the knees, and the heels of the feet.

The RT should assist the patient who is on a gurney or diagnostic imaging table for long periods of time to change his position or change it for him if he is unable to do so. Pressure should be kept off hips, knees, and heels. This can be done by placing a pillow or soft blanket under the patient or by turning him to a different position whenever possible. This is done in the usual hospital situation every 2 hours. If the patient is lying on a hard surface, it should be done every 30 minutes. If a patient is perspiring profusely or is incontinent of urine or feces, the RT should make certain that he is kept clean and dry, and precautions must be taken when moving the patient to prevent skin abrasions.

Special precautions should be taken to protect the patient's feet and lower legs during a position change or transfer. The feet should be protected by shoes and care taken to prevent bruising as the move is made. Circulatory impairment in the lower extremities is common, and the slightest bump may be the beginning of an ulceration.

Casts

Patients will often come to the diagnostic imaging department in a plaster cast. A fresh cast still contains water and can accidentally be compressed. Compression of a cast may produce pressure on the patient's skin, which may lead to the formation of a decubitus ulcer under the cast. A cast that becomes too tight may cause circulatory impairment or compression of a nerve. To prevent these kinds of complications, the RT must be able to assess the patient for circulatory impairment and move the cast with care.

When moving a patient who has a fresh plaster cast that is still wet (a green cast), the RT should slide his opened, flattened hands under the cast.

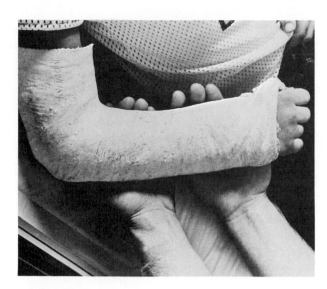

Figure 3-25

Avoid grasping it with your fingers, because this may produce indentations (Fig. 3-25). Support the cast at the joints when moving it, and move the casted extremity as a whole unit (Fig. 3-26).

In order to position a patient who is in a cast, have bolsters or sandbags on hand so that the cast can be well supported. If a cast is allowed to put pressure on the skin in any area, it may impede circulation or damage underlying nerves.

A patient with a plaster cast who is in the diagnostic imaging department for any length of time should be observed for signs of impaired circulation or nerve compression every 15 minutes. A cast applied to an arm may cause a circulatory disturbance in the hand; a leg or body cast may adversely affect the feet, toes, or lower leg. Signs of impaired circulation or nerve compression that the RT may easily

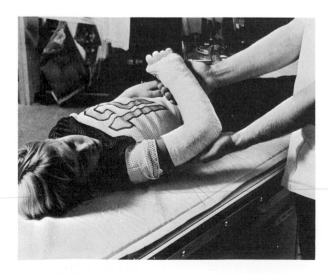

Figure 3-26

detect are pain, coldness, numbness, burning or tingling of fingers or toes, swelling, color changes (to a pale or bluish color), or inability to move fingers or toes. If a patient complains of any of these symptoms, or if the RT can see or feel any of these changes, he should change the patient's position in an attempt to relieve the pressure, and notify the radiologist immediately.

Assisting the patient with a bedpan or urinal

A patient may spend several hours in the radiology department; often he is not able to postpone urination or defecation. He may be embarrassed about making the required request and will wait until the last possible moment to do so. When such a request is made, the RT should respond quickly yet treat it in a manner-of-fact manner.

If possible, help the patient to reach the lavatory near his examining room; this is the most desirable way to handle the situation. However, do not allow the patient to go to the toilet without assistance. Help him to put on his slippers or shoes, and wrap the draw sheet around him if no robe is available. Help him off the radiographic table or out of his wheelchair, and lead him to the lavatory. A patient may have been fasting, or he may have been given drugs that make him very unsteady; therefore, it is not safe to leave him unattended. If the patient can help himself in the lavatory, close the door and tell him that you will be just outside in case he needs you. Each lavatory should be equipped with an emergency call button, and the RT should explain its use to the patient. If there is no emergency call button, the RT should check on the patient at frequent intervals in order to be certain that his condition is stable.

After the patient has finished using the lavatory, help him to wash his hands if he cannot do so himself. Then accompany him back to the examination area. Cover him and make him comfortable. Return to the lavatory and make certain that it is clean. Then wash your hands.

The bedpan

The patient who is unable to get to the lavatory must be offered a bedpan or urinal. In the radiology department, clean bedpans and urinals are usually stored in a specific place. Be certain that the bedpan or urinal to be used has been sterilized between uses.

There are two types of bedpans. The standard bedpan is made of metal or plastic and is approxi-

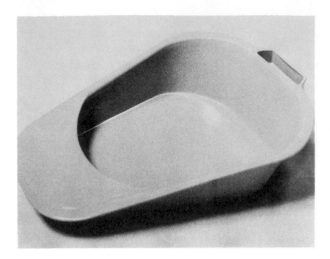

Figure 3-27

mately 4 inches high. It can be used by most patients. However, a patient may have a fracture or another disability that makes it impossible for him to use a pan of this height. For these patients, the fracture pan is used. All diagnostic imaging departments should have these pans available (Fig. 3-27).

Before assisting the patient, the RT must wash his hands and then obtain tissue and a bedpan with a cover. If the pan is cold, run warm water over it, then dry it. If possible, close the examining-room door, or screen the patient to ensure privacy. Always place a sheet over the patient while helping him onto the bedpan.

Next, approach the patient. Remove the bedpan cover, and place it at the end of the table. If the patient is able to move himself, place one hand under his lower back, and ask him to raise his hips. Place the pan under the hips (Fig. 3-28). Be sure he is covered with a sheet. If he is able to sit up, assist him

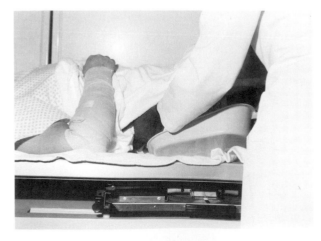

Figure 3-28.   Place one hand under the patient's lower back and ask him to raise his hips so you may place the pan.

to a sitting position. Do not leave a patient sitting on a bedpan—he is poorly balanced and may fall. If you cannot stay with the patient, or if the patient is not able to sit up, place two or three pillows behind his shoulders and head so that he is comfortable. Leave the toilet tissue where he can reach it. Let the patient alone, but remain nearby so that when he has finished you are on hand to assist him.

When the patient has finished using the bedpan, don clean, disposable gloves and help him off the pan. Have the patient lie back, place one of your hands under the lumbar area, and have him raise his hips. Then remove the pan, cover it, and empty it in the designated area. Then rinse it clean with cold water and return it to the area where used equipment is placed. Offer the patient a wet paper towel or washcloth to wash his hands and a dry paper towel to dry them. Then remove your gloves as described in Chapter 2 and wash your hands.

If a patient is unable to assist in getting himself onto and off a bedpan, do not attempt to help him alone. Enlist the aid of another team member. Have that person stand at the opposite side of the table. With the assistance of the second RT, turn the patient to a side-lying position. Place the pan against the patient's hips, then turn him back to a supine position while holding the pan in place. Be certain that his hips are in good alignment on the pan. Place pillows under the patient's shoulders and head and stay nearby. When he has finished using the pan, put on clean gloves and reverse the procedure in order to remove the pan.

If the patient is not able to clean the perineal area himself, the RT will have to assist him. Wear clean, disposable gloves to do this. Take several thicknesses of tissue and fold them into a pad. Wipe the patient's perineum from front to back, then drop the tissue into the pan; if necessary, repeat the procedure until the perineum is clean and dry. Cover the pan and empty it and place it in the soiled equipment area for resterilization. Remove your gloves correctly and wash your hands.

If a patient has difficulty in moving or adjusting to the height of a regular bedpan, follow the same procedure using the fracture pan. The end with the lip is the back of the pan.

The male urinal

The male urinal is made of plastic or metal and is so shaped that it can be used by a patient who is supine, lying on his right or left side, or in Fowler's position (Fig. 3-29). The urinal may be offered to the male patient who is unable to get off of the gurney or examining table to go to the lavatory.

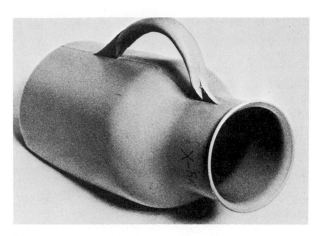

Figure 3-29.   Male urinal.

If the patient is unable to help himself, simply hand him an aseptic urinal and allow him to use it, providing privacy whenever possible. When he has finished, put on clean, disposable gloves, remove the urinal, empty it, and rinse it with cold water. Then place it with the soiled supplies to be resterilized. Offer the patient a washcloth with which to cleanse his hands. Remove gloves and wash your own hands.

If a patient is unable to assist himself in using the urinal, the RT must position the urinal for him. Don clean, disposable gloves, raise the cover sheet sufficiently to permit adequate visibility, but do not expose the patient unduly. Spread the patient's legs and put the urinal between them. Put the penis into the urinal far enough so that it does not slip out, and hold the urinal in place by the handle until the patient finishes voiding. Remove the urinal, empty it, replace it, remove your gloves, and wash your hands.

Summary

When a patient from outside the hospital arrives in the diagnostic imaging department, it is often necessary that he undress entirely or partially for the diagnostic examination or treatment. The RT should always show the patient where and how to do so in a sensitive manner in order to spare the patient embarrassment.

It is also the RT's responsibility to provide the patient with a safe place for his personal belongings. Remember that an article that may not seem valuable to the RT may be treasured by the patient. Everything that belongs to the patient must be treated as if it were of value.

RTs must always use correct body mechanics, beginning with good posture. When moving or lifting objects or patients in the workplace, keep the weight close to your body and maintain a firm base of body support. This is accomplished by having the feet slightly spread and the knees flexed. Never twist the body or bend at the waist when lifting a heavy load. Weight should be pulled, not pushed. Arm and leg muscles, not the spine, should be used for lifting.

The three ways of moving patients are by gurney, by wheelchair, or by ambulation. When moving and lifting patients, the RT must assess the patient and resolve potential problems before beginning the transfer. The plan for moving the patient should be explained to him, and his help should be enlisted before beginning. The RT must always notify the ward personnel when taking a patient to or from his room in the hospital.

When a patient is on the radiographic table or on a gurney in the diagnostic imaging department, his body must be in good alignment. If he is moved to a particular position for an examination, correct body alignment must be restored as soon as possible.

Care must be taken to prevent the patient's skin from being damaged while he is being cared for in the diagnostic imaging department. This can be done by preventing injury that may come from immobility, pressure, shearing force, or friction. Patients most vulnerable for skin breakdown are the malnourished, the elderly, and the chronically ill. Special care must be taken to protect these patients from injuries to their integumentary system, because it may result in a decubitus ulcer that can take months to heal.

The RT must also take extra precautions when caring for a patient who is wearing a plaster cast. The extremities must be observed for evidence of neurocirculatory impairment that may result from the pressure of a cast on the skin. Some symptoms of neurocirculatory impairment that are easily detected are pain, coldness, numbness, burning or tingling of fingers or toes, swelling, color changes of the skin, or an inability to move fingers or toes. If these symptoms are noted, the RT must change the patient's position and report the problem to the radiologist immediately.

If a patient cannot help himself to undress, the RT must offer assistance. This assistance should be given in a matter-of-fact manner that does not violate the patient's privacy.

Patients must be kept clean and dry while in the diagnostic imaging department. It will be the RT's duty to change the disabled patient's gown and covering if they become wet or soiled. This must be done in a prescribed manner to ensure privacy, safety, and comfort.

Some examinations done in the diagnostic imaging department are long and tedious. They often stimulate peristalsis and a need to defecate or urinate. Meeting these needs cannot be postponed. The RT must be prepared to assist with the bedpan or urinal if necessary. This should be done in a way that assures the patient as much privacy as possible.

Infection-control measures must be taken by the RT as he assists with bedpans or urinals. These items must be used for one patient only and then taken to an area for resterilization. The RT must don clean, disposable gloves when assisting with the patient's elimination needs, and he must wash hands following removal of the gloves.

The patient must never be left unattended while on a bedpan, a gurney, or a diagnostic imaging table. Patients are often weak because of illness or fasting prior to an examination. They must also be carefully attended as they are taken to a lavatory or a dressing area following an examination or treatment.

Chapter 3, pre-post test

____ 1. When admitting a patient to the diagnostic imaging department, the RT should
   a. Take the patient to the dressing area and explain in some detail how the patient should dress (or undress) for the procedure
   b. Give the patient directions concerning how to care for purses or valuables brought to the department with her
   c. Assist any patient who appears to need assistance with preparation for an examination
   d. a and b
   e. a, b, and c

____ 2. The most effective means of reducing friction when moving a patient is by
   a. Placing the patient's arms across his chest and using a pull sheet
   b. Pushing rather than pulling the patient
   c. Rolling the patient to a prone position
   d. Asking the patient to cooperate with you

____ 3. When transporting a patient back to his hospital room, some safety measures to be used are
   a. Place the side rails up and the bed in "low" position
   b. Inform the nurse in charge of the patient that the patient has been returned to his room
   c. Give the patient something to eat or drink
   d. a and b
   e. a, b, and c

____ 4. The following procedure(s) must be observed when assisting a patient with a bedpan:
   a. The patient's privacy must be respected
   b. Assistance should be sought for an immobile patient
   c. Clean gloves are worn to remove the bedpan
   d. a and c
   e. a, b, and c

____ 5. When it is necessary to log roll a patient, one must have in assistance
   a. two persons
   b. three persons
   c. four persons
   d. five persons

____ 6. Match the following patient positions with the correct definition:
   a. Fowler's position
   b. Supine position
   c. Semi-Fowler's position
   d. Trendelenburg position
   e. Sims' position

   1. Patient on side with forward arm flexed and top knee flexed
   2. Semisitting with head raised 45 to 60 degrees
   3. Patient lying flat on back
   4. Patient on back with head lower than extremities
   5. Patient on back with head raised 15 to 30 degrees

____ 7. Contributing factor(s) to skin breakdown are
   a. Turning every 1 to 2 hours
   b. Friction and pressure
   c. Frequent diagnostic imaging procedures
   d. An unstable environment

____ 8. When caring for a patient who has a new cast applied to an extremity, the RT must remember to
   a. Hold the cast firmly at a position between the joints when moving it
   b. Observe for signs of impaired circulation
   c. Support the cast with bolsters and sandbags
   d. a, b, and c
   e. b and c

____ 9. When caring for a patient who is disabled and difficult to move, the RT must remember that it is essential to
   a. Keep the patient as quiet as possible
   b. Work quickly
   c. Obtain as much help as necessary to avoid injury to the patient and the RT
   d. Move the patient by gurney

10. List four signs of circulatory impairment if a patient is wearing a plaster cast.

____ 11. The leading cause of work-related injuries in the field of health care is (are)
   a. Bumping into misplaced equipment
   b. Overexposure to radiation
   c. Poor hand-washing techniques
   d. Abuse of the spine when moving and lifting patients

____ 12. List five general rules for correct upright posture.

____ 13. The body's center of gravity is
   a. At or just below the waistline
   b. In the pelvis
   c. At chest level
   d. In the shoulders and arms

14. When lifting, the _____ and _____ muscles should be used.

15. When moving a heavy object, the RT should _____ the weight, not _____ it.

16. List six rules to remember when moving patients.

17. List three methods of transferring patients.

____ 18. When moving a patient into an unnatural position for a radiographic examination, the patient should maintain that position
   a. Until he asks to be moved
   b. Until the firm is developed and approved by the radiologist
   c. Only for the time it takes to make the exposure
   d. a and b
   e. b and c

19. List the four areas of the body that are most susceptible to skin breakdown.

20. List four signs of circulatory impairment.

Laboratory reinforcement

1. A patient who is totally paralyzed on her right side comes to the radiology department from a hospital ward. Her gown has become wet and must be changed. Demonstrate, in the school laboratory, how you will perform this task.

2. The paralyzed patient in situation 1 must use the bedpan for urination. Demonstrate in the laboratory the proper way to assist her.

3. In the school laboratory, using a fellow student as a patient, demonstrate the following:

   A. A sheet transfer from a hospital bed to a gurney

   B. A log-roll move

   C. The proper method of assisting a disabled patient from the radiographic table to a wheelchair

   D. The proper method of positioning a patient in the prone position

   E. The proper method of assisting a patient from a supine position to a sitting position

Chapter Four
Vital Signs and Oxygen Administration

Goal of this chapter:

The radiologic technology student will be able to monitor vital signs accurately and be prepared to assist with oxygen administration.

Behavioral objectives:

When the student has completed this chapter, he will be able to do the following:
1. Define vital signs and explain when the RT is responsible for their assessment
2. Correctly read a clinical thermometer
3. Accurately monitor pulse rate
4. Accurately monitor respirations
5. Correctly monitor blood pressure
6. List the rates of temperature, pulse, respiration, and blood pressure that are considered within normal limits for an adult male or female
7. Identify various types of oxygen administration equipment
8. List the precautions that the RT must take when oxygen is being administered in a patient's room or in the diagnostic imaging department

Glossary

Alveolar air cells in the lungs where gases are exchanged

Cardiovascular pertains to heart and blood vessels

Doppler a device used to measure heart sounds or other sounds using frequency of sound waves and distances

Dyspnea difficult breathing resulting from insufficient air flow to lungs

Enzymatic organic substances produced by living cells of complex proteins (enzymes) capable of inducing chemical changes in other substances found in mouth, stomach, intestines, blood, and lungs

Hypoxia reduction in the amount of cellular oxygen

Hypercapnia increased amount of carbon dioxide in the blood

Hemoglobin iron-containing pigment of red blood cells that carry oxygen from lungs to the tissues

Hemorrhoids enlarged veins in the anal canal that bleed easily and often are painful

Invasive procedure an exam or surgical procedure that accomplishes a desired result but must enter or invade the body

Noninvasive procedures that do not require entering the body or puncturing the skin

Oral taken by mouth

Peripheral the outer part or surface of a body

Pulmonary involving the lungs

Viscosity the thickness or gumminess of a fluid

Volatile easily vaporized or evaporated; unstable; or of an explosive nature

Toxic poisonous; having the qualities of a poison

Taking a patient's vital signs (also called *cardinal signs*) is an important part of a physical assessment and includes measurement of body temperature, pulse, respiration, and blood pressure. The RT must know how to measure each vital sign, so that if he needs this skill in an emergency situation, he will be able to use it. It is also important to learn what your patient's vital signs are under normal circumstances because all persons have some variation of what is considered normal for their particular age group. Once the RT knows what the patient's usual or baseline vital signs are, he can judge whether his patient's vital signs are deviating from that baseline. Changes in vital signs can be an indication of a problem or a potential problem. If the patient does not come to the diagnostic imaging department with a chart where his baseline vital signs can be found, the RT will have to use accepted normal values for a patient in his patient's age group as baseline information.

Oxygen is an essential physiologic need for survival. It comes from the environment to the lungs, then is transported to the bloodstream and body tissues. The human brain cannot function for longer than 4 to 5 minutes without an adequate oxygen supply. It is occasionally necessary to administer oxygen in the diagnostic imaging department, and the RT may be expected to assist in its administration. A patient receiving oxygen therapy in his hospital room may be unable to leave the room to go to the diagnostic imaging department for necessary procedures. In these instances the RT will be required to make portable radiographic exposures at the bedside. Because oxygen is a potentially toxic and volatile substance, the RT must understand the precautions that are to be taken when assisting with its administration or when using radiographic equipment while oxygen is in use.

Measuring vital signs

A physician's order is not required for vital signs to be measured. The RT should take vital signs when a patient is admitted to the diagnostic imaging department for any invasive diagnostic treatment or procedure, before and after the patient receives medication, any time the patient's general condition suddenly changes, or if the patient reports nonspecific symptoms of physical distress such as simply not feeling well or feeling "different," unless there is a registered nurse present to do so.

Temperature

Body temperature must remain stable in order for the body's cellular and enzymatic activity to remain efficient. Body temperature is the physiologic balance between heat produced in the body tissues and heat lost to the environment. Heat is produced in the body by chemical processes that result from metabolic activity. When the body's metabolism is increased, more heat is produced. When it is decreased, less is produced.

When a patient's body temperature is elevated above normal limits, we say that he has a *fever*. Fever indicates a disturbance in the heat-regulating center of the body. Both normal and abnormal conditions of the body can produce changes in body temperature. Environmental temperature, time of day, age, weight, physical exercise, disease, and injury are some of the factors that might influence body temperature.

A body temperature of 37° C or 98.6° F is considered to be average or normal. A variation of 1 degree above or below average is not considered abnormal; if a person's temperature is 36° or 38° C, or 97.6° or 99° F, the reading would be considered within normal limits. The normal body temperature of infants and children up to 13 years of age varies somewhat from these readings. Average body temperature in well children from ages 3 months to 3 years is from 99° F (37.2° C) to 99.7° F (37.7° C). From 5 years of age to 13 years the normal temperature is from 97.8° F (36.7° C) to 98.6° F (37° C). Symptoms of a fever are increased pulse and respiratory rate, general discomfort or aching, flushed dry skin that feels hot to the touch, chills (occasionally), and loss of appetite. Fevers that are allowed to remain very high for a prolonged period of time can cause irreparable damage to the central nervous system.

Measurement

There are three areas of the body in which temperature can be measured: the mouth, the axilla, and the rectum. The reading will vary depending on where it is measured. Because of this, the area of the body where the temperature was measured must be specified when the reading is reported. Temperature readings are reported in most institutions as follows:

A rectal temperature of 99.6° is written 99.6 R;

An oral temperature of 98.6° is written 98.6 O;

An axillary temperature of 97.6° is written 97.6 Ax *(Fig. 4-1).*

Oral temperature is taken by mouth, under the tongue; the average temperature reading here is 37° C (98.6° F). The axillary temperature is taken in the axilla or armpit. The average temperature here is 36.4° C to 36.7° C (97.6° F to 98° F). Rectal tem-

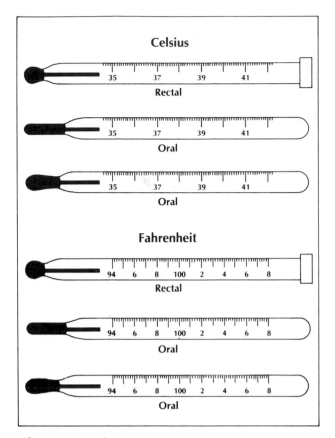

Figure 4-1. Glass clinical thermometers. (Top) These three thermometers are calibrated to measure degrees Celsius. (Bottom) These three measure in the Fahrenheit scale. Those with blunt bulbs are rectal thermometers.

perature is taken at the anal opening to the rectum. The average temperature here is 37.5° C (99.6° F).

THE CLINICAL THERMOMETER

The instrument most commonly used to measure body temperature is the clinical thermometer, a tube-shaped glass instrument that contains mercury in a bulb at one end. The end with the bulb is placed into the mouth, rectum, or armpit. When the mercury is exposed to heat, it rises in the tube. Numbers inscribed on the tube indicate the amount of heat in the body at that location. The RT must be certain that the thermometer used to measure a patient's temperature has been properly sterilized. A thermometer must never be wiped clean and reused for a different person but must be resterilized for each patient.

OTHER INSTRUMENTS

Another instrument used to measure body temperature is the electronic thermometer, which measures body temperature accurately within seconds by means of a probe that is covered by a separate plastic sheath for each patient. The reading is flashed digitally or may be read from a needle (Fig. 4-2).

There are also disposable disks or tapes that are heat-sensitive. They may be used if glass thermometers are a hazard for the patient or if resterilization is inconvenient (Fig. 4-3).

Taking an oral temperature The mouth is the most accessible and often the most convenient site for measuring body temperature. This site should not be used if the patient is apt to be injured during the procedure by biting down on the glass thermometer, or if he is unable to hold the instrument under his tongue for the specified period of time with lips closed. This would include patients who have had facial injuries or oral surgery, or those with a history of convulsions, those unable to breathe with their mouths closed, and young children.

When measuring oral temperature with a clinical thermometer, obtain an oral thermometer that has an elongated tip. Shake the thermometer down to a mercury reading of 35° C (96° F). Wash your hands, approach the patient, and place the thermometer under his tongue. Have the patient close his lips over the tip of the thermometer, and leave it in place for 3 to 5 minutes. Then remove it, wipe it with a tissue, and read it.

When reading a thermometer, hold it at eye level by the blunt end and turn it until the mercury column can be seen. Observe where on the marked scale the mercury stops; this is the temperature to be recorded. Each long line on the thermometer represents one full degree of body temperature and is numbered accordingly. The short lines each represent two tenths of one degree of body temperature, and these lines are not numbered. After the thermometer has been read, place it with the soiled thermometers, and wash your hands. Report the temperature reading to the patient's physician if it is abnormal, and record it on the patient's chart.

Taking an axillary temperature This is the least accurate but the safest method of measuring body temperature because it is a noninvasive procedure. When it is necessary to take an axillary temperature, an oral thermometer with a rounded tip will be used. Wash your hands and shake the thermometer down. Dry the patient's armpit with a paper towel or a dry washcloth. Lift the patient's arm and place the thermometer into the center of the armpit. Place the arm down tightly over the thermometer with the arm crossed over the patient's chest. Leave the thermometer in place for 5 to 10 minutes. Then remove it, read it, wipe it, and put it in its proper place. A child's arm must be gently held in place until the thermometer has registered.

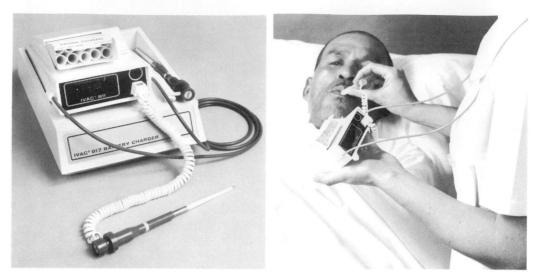

Figure 4-2. **(Left)** *An electric thermometer. There are interchangeable oral and rectal probes. The cylindrical objects near the top of this model are disposable plastic probe covers.* **(Right)** *The RT reads the thermometer on the clock-like face when the thermometer signals that peak temperature has been reached.*

Taking a rectal temperature This site is considered to provide the most reliable measurement of body temperature, because factors that can alter the results are minimized. It is also in close proximity to the pelvic viscera or the "core" temperature of the body. Body temperature should not be measured rectally if the patient is a restless adult or a restless child or if the patient has rectal pathology such as tumors or hemorrhoids.

In order to take a rectal temperature, a thermometer with a blunt tip must be used. Do not use an oral thermometer to take a rectal temperature. Wash your hands and don clean gloves. Have the patient turn on his side to assume the Sims' position. Expose the patient only as much as is necessary for clearly viewing the rectal area. Lubricate the tip of the thermometer with a lubricating jelly. Gently insert the tip of the thermometer into the rectum about 1½ inches and hold it in place for 2 to 3 minutes. Do

not leave a patient who has a rectal thermometer in place; the thermometer must be held. When enough time has passed, remove the thermometer. Return the patient to a comfortable position and wipe the thermometer with a tissue. Read it and place it with the soiled rectal thermometers. Remove your gloves in the specified manner and wash your hands.

Pulse

As the heart beats, blood is pumped in a pulsating fashion into the arteries. This results in a throb, or pulsation, of the artery. At areas of the body where arteries are superficial, the pulse can be felt by holding the artery beneath the skin against a solid surface such as bone. The pulse can be detected most easily in the following areas of the body:

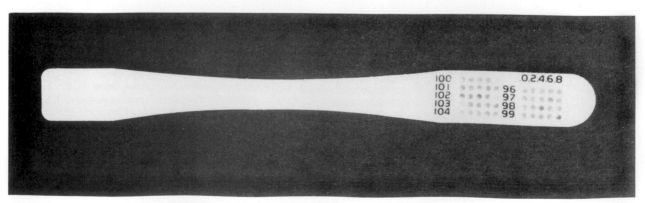

Figure 4-3. Disposable thermometer.

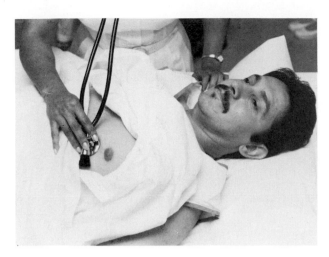

Figure 4-4.   Apical pulse.

The apical pulse—over the apex of the heart (heard with a stethoscope) (Fig. 4-4)

The radial pulse—over the radial artery at the wrist, at the base of the thumb (Fig. 4-5)

The carotid pulse—over the carotid artery, at the front of the neck (Fig. 4-6)

The femoral pulse—over the femoral artery, in the groin (Fig. 4-7)

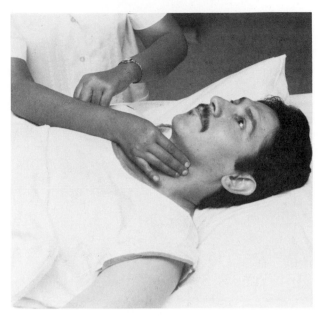

Figure 4-6.   Carotid pulse.

The popliteal pulse—at the posterior surface of the knee (Fig. 4-8)

The temporal pulse—over the temporal artery in front of the ear (Fig. 4-9)

The dorsalis pedis pulse—at the top of the feet in line with the groove between the extensor tendons of the great and first toe (may be congenitally absent) (Fig. 4-10)

The posterior tibial pulse—on the inner side of the ankles (Fig. 4-11)

The brachial pulse—in the groove between the biceps and triceps muscles above the elbow at the antecubital fossa (Fig. 4-12)

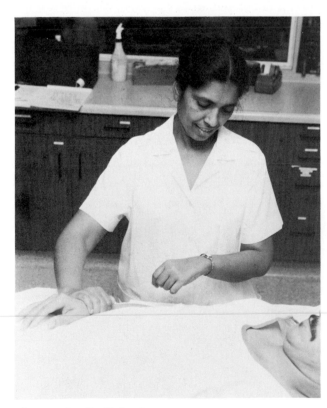

Figure 4-5.   Radial pulse.

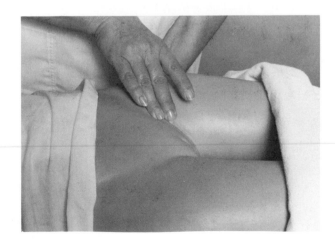

Figure 4-7.   Femoral pulse.

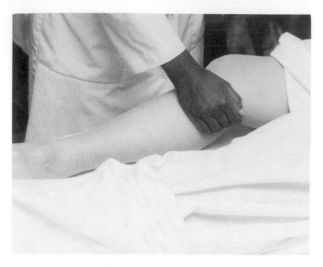

Figure 4-8.   Popliteal pulse.

Usually the pulse rate is rapid if the blood pressure is low and slower if the blood pressure is high. The patient who is losing blood has an unusually rapid pulse rate and a very low blood pressure. The average pulse rate in an adult man or woman is between 60 and 90 beats/min in a resting state. The average pulse rate for an infant is 120 beats/min. A child from 4 to 10 years of age has an average pulse rate of from 90 to 100 beats/min.

Assessment of the pulse

The pulse rate is a rapid and relatively efficient means of assessing cardiovascular function. *Tachycardia* is the

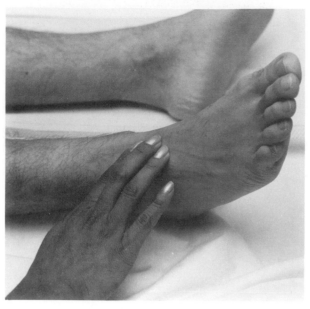

Figure 4-10.   Dorsalis pedis pulse.

term used to describe an abnormally rapid heart rate (over 100 beats/min), and *bradycardia* is the term used to describe an abnormally slow heart rate (below 60 beats/min). The RT must be prepared to make this assessment prior to any invasive diagnostic imaging procedure to establish a baseline reading and then reassess it frequently until the procedure is complete and the patient leaves the department, if a registered nurse is not present to do so. The radial pulse is usually the most accessible and can be taken most conveniently on an adult patient. It should be counted wherever it is taken, for one full minute. If there is

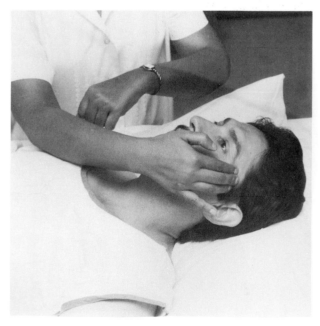

Figure 4-9.   Temporal pulse.

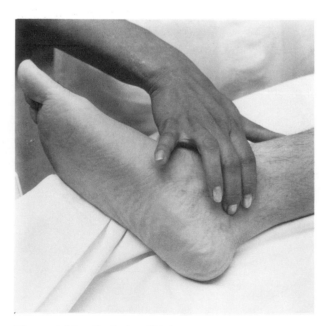

Figure 4-11.   Posterior tibial pulse.

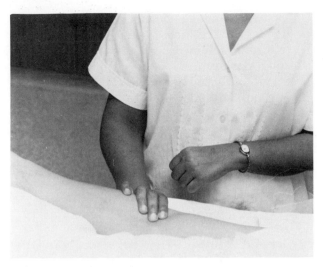

Figure 4-12. Brachial pulse.

any irregularity of this pulse rate, the apical pulse must be taken. The apical pulse is also monitored if the radial pulse is inaccessible.

For infants and children, the apical pulse is the most accurate for cardiovascular assessment. The femoral, popliteal, and pedal pulses are assessed bilaterally if peripheral blood flow is to be assessed.

When pulse rate is being assessed, the strength and regularity of the beat as well as the number of beats per minute must be reported. The normal rhythm of the pulse beat is regular, with equal time intervals between beats. The pulse should not be obliterated by the pressure of the fingers. When it is, it is reported as weak or thready. If the beat is irregular, unusually rapid, unusually slow, or unusually weak, it must be reported to the physician in charge of the patient immediately. Changes in pulse rate during a procedure must also be reported.

In order to assess the pulse, one needs a watch with a second hand and a pad and pencil to record the findings. For monitoring apical pulse, a stethoscope is necessary, along with alcohol sponges for wiping the earpieces and the bladder of the instrument.

To assess radial, femoral, carotid, popliteal, pedal, and temporal pulses, wash your hands, approach the patient, and lightly place your index finger and middle finger flat over the artery chosen for assessment. Do not press too hard, or your fingers will compress the artery and the beat will not be felt. When the throbbing of the artery is felt, count the throbs for 1 minute. Do not use the thumb when counting the pulse rate, because it too has a pulse that may be mistaken for the patient's pulse.

To assess the apical pulse, wash your hands, and wipe the earpieces and bladder of the stethoscope with alcohol. Approach the patient and place him in

a comfortable sitting or supine position. Drape the patient so that the lower chest area is exposed. Place the bladder of the stethoscope at the fifth intercostal space 5 cm from the left sternal margin (the nipple of the breast can be used as a landmark for 5 cm). If the beat cannot be heard, move the stethoscope slightly in every direction until you can hear it. Count the beats for 1 minute. Assess the beats for regular rate and rhythm. Then remove the stethoscope, wipe the earpieces and bladder with alcohol, cover the patient, and make him comfortable. Wash your hands, and record the pulse rate. Report any irregularities to the patient's physician.

Respiration

The function of the respiratory system is to exchange oxygen and carbon dioxide between the external environment and the blood circulating in the body. Oxygen is taken into the lungs during inspiration. It passes through the bronchi, into the bronchioles, and then into the gas-exchange units of the lungs, the alveoli. Oxygen is transported to the body tissues by the arterial blood. Deoxygenated blood is returned to the right side of the heart through the venous system. It is then pumped into the right and left pulmonary arteries and reoxygenated by passing through the capillary network on the alveolar surfaces. The blood is then returned to the left side of the heart through the pulmonary veins for recirculation. During this process, carbon dioxide is also deposited in the alveoli and exhaled from the lungs during expiration.

The average rate of respiration (one inspiration and one expiration) for an adult man or woman is 10 to 20 breaths/min, and for an infant, 30 to 60 breaths/min. Respirations of fewer than 10 breaths/min for an adult may result in cyanosis, apprehension, restlessness, and a change in level of consciousness, because the supply of oxygen is inadequate to meet the needs of the body.

Normal respirations are quiet, effortless, and uniform. Medication, illness, exercise, or age may increase or decrease respirations, depending on the body's metabolic need for oxygen. When a patient is using more than the normal effort to breathe, he may be described as dyspneic or to be having dyspnea.

Assessment of respiration

As with other vital signs, it is important to establish a baseline respiratory rate, because changes in respiration are often an early sign of a threatened physiologic state. When one assesses respiration, the rate, depth, quality, and pattern should be observed. The chest wall should be observed for symmetrical movement. There should be an even rise and fall of the chest with no involvement of muscles other than the diaphragm. Abdominal, intercostal, or neck muscle involvement in breathing is a sign of respiratory distress and should be noted. In the adult patient, a need to assume a sitting position in order to breathe easily or to lean forward and place the arms up over the back of a chair or on the knees also indicates respiratory distress. Infants with respiratory distress will have retractions of the intercostal spaces of the ribs, sternal and substernal retractions, nasal flaring, and cyanosis.

The RT should also observe skin color during respiratory assessment. Cyanosis or bluish discoloration is easily observed around the mouth, in the gums, in the nail beds, and in the earlobes and may be a sign of respiratory distress. Noisy respirations should also be noted.

Abnormal respiratory patterns would be described as rapid, shallow, labored, regular, or irregular. Noisy respirations may simply be described as noisy, or they may be more specifically described as crackles and wheezes.

The patient should be in a sitting or supine position when respirations are counted. He should be in a quiet state and should remain unaware that his respirations are being assessed. When a patient suspects that his respirations are being observed, he may consciously or unconsciously cause the rate and quality to change. The most convenient time to count respirations is immediately following the pulse count. The RT may appear to be continuing to count the pulse rate but may be observing the respirations instead. The respirations are counted by observing the rise and fall of the patient's chest. Respiration should be observed and counted for one full minute.

When recording pulse and respiration, use the abbreviations *P* for pulse and *R* for respiration. For example, P 80 equals a pulse rate of 80 beats/min and R 20 equals 20 respirations/min. Should abnormalities be noted, they should be recorded as in the following example: P 96, weak and irregular; R 26, labored and noisy. Any abnormalities that the RT observes in vital signs should be reported to the physician in charge of the patient immediately following their observation.

Blood pressure

Blood pressure (BP) is the force exerted by the blood on the walls of the vessels as it is pumped by the heart. The instrument used to measure blood pressure is called a sphygmomanometer. Two numbers, read in millimeters of mercury (mm Hg), are recorded when reporting blood pressure: systolic pressure and diastolic pressure. The systolic reading is the highest point reached during contraction of the left ventricle of the heart as it pumps blood into the aorta. The diastolic pressure is the lowest point to which the pressure drops during relaxation of the ventricles and indicates the minimal pressure exerted against the arterial walls continuously. Pulse pressure is the difference between the systolic and diastolic blood pressure.

Blood pressure readings vary with age, sex, physical development, and health status. The normal systolic pressure in men and women ranges from 110 mm Hg to 140 mm Hg, and the normal diastolic, from 60 mm Hg to 80 mm Hg. Physiologic factors that may increase blood pressure are increased cardiac output, increased peripheral vascular resistance, increased blood volume, increased blood viscosity, and decreased arterial elasticity. Physiologic factors that decrease blood pressure are decreased cardiac output, decreased peripheral vascular resistance, decreased blood volume, decreased blood viscosity, and increased arterial elasticity.

The RT must have a baseline blood pressure reading so that he may evaluate his patient's blood pressure effectively if necessary. A patient is considered to be hypertensive if his systolic blood pressure is consistently greater than 140 mm Hg and his diastolic blood pressure is consistently greater than 90 mm Hg. A patient is considered to be hypotensive if his systolic blood pressure is less than 90 mm Hg.

Equipment needed to measure blood pressure

There are two types of sphygmomanometers, a mercury manometer and an aneroid manometer (Fig. 4-13). They are composed of a cloth cuff, which comes in a variety of sizes. Within the cuff is an inflatable bladder, which should be nearly long enough to encircle the arm. There are a pressure manometer, a thumb screw valve to maintain or release the pressure, a pressure bulb to inflate the bladder, and rubber tubings that lead to the gauge and to the pressure bulb. The bulb and the tubing must be free of leaks.

The mercury manometer is the more accurate of the two but less convenient to use. The aneroid manometer needle should point to zero before the bladder of the cuff is inflated, and its calibration should be checked for accuracy and recalibrated by means of a perfectly accurate mercury manometer at least once each year.

The blood pressure cuff should be selected according to patient size. A cuff that is too large or too

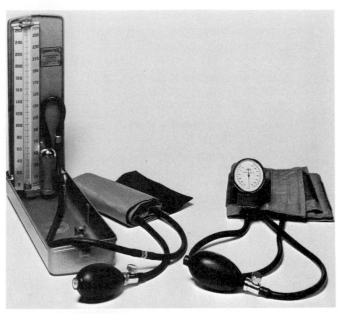

Figure 4-13. Two types of sphygmomanometers. (Left) A mercury manometer. (Right) An aneroid manometer with self-securing cuffs. There are several varieties of aneroid manometers.

small for the patient's arm will give an incorrect reading.

A stethoscope that has a bladder and a bell, strong plastic or rubber tubing 12 to 18 inches in length (30 to 40 cm) that leads to firm but flexible binaurals (the metal tubings leading to the earpieces) and earpieces that fit snugly and securely into the ears should be chosen. Either the bladder or the bell of the stethoscope may be used for assessing blood pressure. The bell transmits low sounds and should be held lightly against the skin; the diaphragm transmits high-pitched sounds and is held firmly against the skin (Fig. 4-14).

There are many types of dopplers and electronic blood pressure monitoring devices used in clinical practice. Their methods of operation vary and will not be discussed in this chapter.

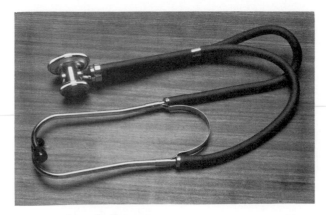

Figure 4-14. Stethoscope.

Measuring blood pressure

The patient should be sitting in a chair with his arm supported or in a reclining supine position. Frequently during a physical assessment, blood pressure is measured in reclining, sitting, and standing positions; however, for the RT's purposes this is not indicated. The room should be as quiet as possible to facilitate hearing the pulsations. There should be no clothing between the BP cuff and the skin. The bladder and bell of the stethoscope and the earpieces should be cleansed with alcohol sponges prior to and following each use to prevent passing infection from one person to another by this indirect means.

Place the deflated sphygmomanometer cuff evenly around the patient's upper arm above the elbow, and place the bell or bladder of the stethoscope over the brachial artery. This artery is located at the center of the anterior elbow and may be identified by feeling its pulsations (Fig. 4-15). Place the gauge of the sphygmomanometer on a flat surface so that it can be read easily. Secure the cuff of the sphygmomanometer so that it will not work loose. Do not allow the stethoscope to touch the patient's clothing or the tubing. Place the earpieces of the stethoscope in your ears, tighten the thumbscrew of the pressure bulb, and pump the bulb until it reaches 180 mm Hg or until you are no longer able to hear the pulse beat (Fig. 4-16). Open the valve slowly and allow the mercury to fall. Listen carefully for the pulse beat to begin, and take the reading at the level of mercury, or on the gauge, where it is first heard. This first reading will be the systolic reading. Continue to listen until the pulsation becomes soft or quiet, or where

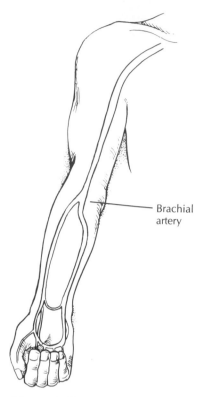

Brachial
artery

Figure 4-15

the sound changes from loud to very soft. This is the diastolic reading.

Frequently, as you listen for the diastolic pressure, there is a change in intensity of the sound before the sound is completely muffled. The point at which this softer sound is heard should be noted, and then the point at which there is no pulsation heard should be noted. This reading is a more accurate indication of intraarterial diastolic pressure. Both readings should be recorded, with the first, softer sound recorded first.

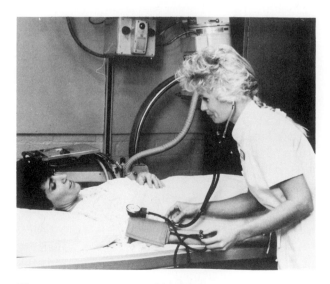

Figure 4-16. Measuring blood pressure.

Blood pressure is recorded in the following manner: if the systolic reading is 120 and the diastolic reading is 80, it is written *BP 120/80* and is read "one twenty over eighty." If the diastolic reading is soft at 80 and then completely muffled at 60, it should be written *120/80/60.*

Blood pressure measurement for infants and small children is a more complex procedure. It should be performed by a physician or nurse educated in this skill. Usually a nurse is on hand when invasive diagnostic imaging procedures are to be done for patients in this age group, and she will monitor the child.

Oxygen therapy

An adequate oxygen supply is essential to life. Because oxygen cannot be stored in the body, the supply from the external environment must be constant. When a human being's oxygen supply is suddenly interrupted or interfered with in any manner, it becomes an emergency that must be dealt with immediately to prevent a life-threatening situation. This type of emergency may occur in the diagnostic imaging department; therefore, the RT may be the first person to observe a problem. It will be his responsibility to ensure that the equipment needed to administer oxygen is available and in functioning condition in his work area at all times and to assist with oxygen administration in emergency situations. He must also become acquainted with the methods of oxygen administration that he may encounter in other areas of patient care.

The lungs supply oxygen and remove carbon dioxide from the body. Oxygen and carbon dioxide are carried to and from the various body systems in the blood. Only small amounts of oxygen are carried in solution in the blood. The major supply of oxygen is carried in chemical combination with hemoglobin. The oxygen capacity of the blood is expressed in percentage of the volume. The amount of oxygen in either air or blood is called the oxygen tension (partial pressure) and is written PO_2. Carbon dioxide is described similarly as PCO_2.

Carbon dioxide diffuses into the plasma of systemic capillary blood, but the major part enters the red blood cells. Carbon dioxide also is carried in combination with hemoglobin, which assists with its removal from the body. When there is an excessive build-up of carbon dioxide in the bloodstream, the pH (acidity or alkalinity) of the blood is changed, often with dire physiologic effects. Prevention of excessive acidity of the blood is prevented by the presence of a bicarbonate (HCO_3) buffer in the bloodstream.

The effectiveness of pulmonary function (the lungs' ability to exchange oxygen and carbon dioxide efficiently) is most accurately measured by laboratory testing of arterial blood for the concentrations of oxygen, carbon dioxide, bicarbonate, acidity, and the saturation of hemoglobin with oxygen (Sa O_2). Laboratory values (called *arterial blood gases*) considered within normal limits are as follows:

pH: 7.35 to 7.45

Pa CO_2: 35 to 45 mm Hg

Pa O_2: 80 to 100 mm Hg

HCO_3: 18 to 25 mEq/l

Sa O_2: 97%

When pulmonary function is disturbed, the level of oxygen in the arterial blood becomes inadequate to meet the patient's physiologic needs. This condition is referred to as hypoxemia. Carbon dioxide may be retained in the arterial blood, which results in a condition called hypercapnea. When the Pa O_2 is below 60 mm Hg or the hemoglobin saturation is less than 90%, it can be assumed that adequate oxygenation of the blood is not taking place. The RT will usually rely on observation of physical symptoms of this problem, which will be discussed in Chapter 5, as this condition occasionally occurs with little warning, and there is no time for laboratory analysis of arterial blood gases.

Oxygen is administered by artificial means when the patient is unable to obtain adequate amounts from the atmosphere to supply the needs of his body. Oxygen therapy must be ordered by a physician, and the order will specify the method of administration and the concentration desired.

Hazards of oxygen administration

Oxygen supports combustion; therefore, care must be taken to prevent sparks or flames where oxygen is being administered. Smoking is prohibited in rooms where oxygen is in use, and anything that may produce sparks or flames must be used with extreme caution. The RT must take precautions when his equipment is to be used in the presence of pure oxygen to be certain that it will not produce sparks.

Varying degrees of oxygen toxicity may result from inhalation of 100% oxygen for longer than a few hours. Mild oxygen toxicity may produce reversible tracheobronchitis. Severe oxygen toxicity may cause irreversible parenchymal lung injury. Because of this potential complication, oxygen should always be administered at the lowest possible dose that achieves

desirable results. Special care must be taken when oxygen is administered to patients with chronic respiratory disease. The respiratory stimulus in these patients is a decrease in blood oxygen rather than in exhaled carbon dioxide as is normally the case. The RT must be aware of this, and if oxygen is being administered in his department to patients with respiratory disease, he must keep in mind that excessive oxygen in the blood may depress the patient's respiratory drive and increase the CO_2 in the blood so severely that the patient might die.

Oxygen delivery systems

During oxygen therapy, oxygen is delivered to the respiratory tract under pressure by artificial means. When the flow rate (liters per minute—LPM) is high, the oxygen is humidified to prevent excessive drying of the mucous membranes. This can be done by passing the oxygen through distilled water, because it is only slightly soluble in water. The procedure for moisturizing oxygen varies somewhat from one institution to another, but often the receptacle for distilled water is able to be attached at the wall outlet, and the oxygen passes through the water and then into the delivery system.

In most hospitals the oxygen is piped into hospital rooms, postanesthesia areas, emergency suites, and the diagnostic imaging department. Wall outlets make it readily available. Oxygen supplied in this fashion comes through pipes from a central source at 60 to 80 pounds of pressure per square inch. A flowmeter is attached to each wall outlet to regulate flow (Fig. 4-17).

If oxygen is not piped in through wall outlets, it is available compressed and dispensed in tanks of varying sizes. A full tank contains 2000 pounds per square inch of pressure. These tanks have two regulator valves, one of which indicates how much oxygen is in the tank and the other, the rate of flow. If the RT must use this type of system, care must be taken not to allow the tank to fall or the regulator to become cracked (Fig. 4-18).

Twenty-one percent of the air we breathe normally is composed of oxygen. This is often abbreviated as $F_1 O_2$. This percentage of oxygen may need to be increased if a patient is in respiratory distress and unable to inspire enough room air to fulfill his body's oxygen needs.

There are two basic types of oxygen delivery systems that transport the oxygen from wall outlets or tanks, high-flow and low-flow. The low-flow systems provide only part of the gas inspired; the remainder is room air. High-flow systems deliver a controlled amount of premixed room air and oxygen. When the RT is called upon to assist with oxygen administra-

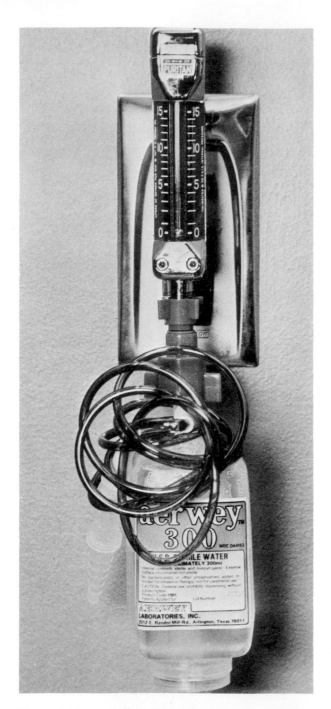

Figure 4-17. A wall oxygen outlet. The container above the outlet contains sterile water for humidifying the oxygen. The flowmeter is located below the container.

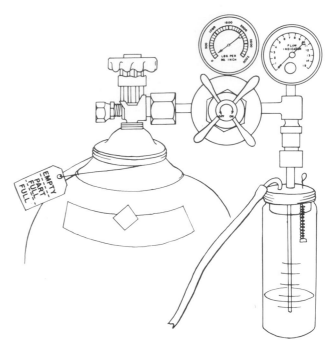

Figure 4-18. An oxygen tank. The regulator valve on top of the tank allows the oxygen to flow out of the tank. The valve to the right of the tank regulates the flow. The gauge on the left indicates the amount of oxygen in the tank; the one on the right indicates the rate of flow. The container to the right of the tank is a humidifier.

tion, it is generally a low-flow system with which he will be dealing.

LOW-FLOW SYSTEMS

Low-flow delivery systems utilize oxygen mixed with room air to deliver the prescribed concentration of oxygen needed by the patient. The devices used to administer this concentration of oxygen will vary as the patient's breathing varies. The concentration of inspired oxygen varies with the patient's rate and depth of respiration. The amount that the patient needs and the type of delivery device needed are determined by the physician. The flow rate of oxygen is measured in liters per minute (LPM). There are several methods of low-flow delivery.

Nasal cannula The nasal cannula is a disposable plastic device with two hollow prongs that deliver oxygen into the nostrils (Fig. 4-19). The other end of the cannula is attached to the oxygen supply, which may or may not pass through a humidifier, and has a flowmeter attached. The cannula is held in place by an elastic strap that fits over the ears and behind the patient's head.

The concentration of oxygen delivered by this method varies wih the amount of room air inspired by the patient and can vary from 21% to 60%. Oxygen delivery by nasal cannula is indicated for patients whose breathing rate and depth are normal and even. With this method, 1 to 6 liters/min (LPM) of oxygen is usually prescribed for adults. For children, the rate is much lower (¼ to ½ LPM).

The RT must remember to have the oxygen turned on and flowing at the desired rate before placing any low-flow device on a patient. The nasal prongs must be kept in place in both nostrils.

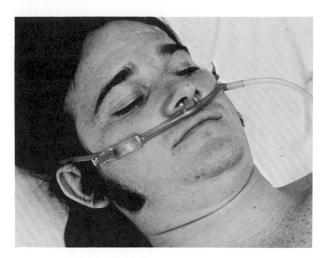

Figure 4-19.   Nasal cannula.

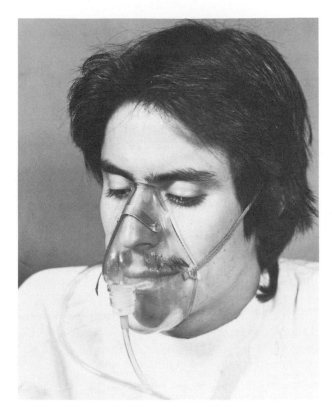

Figure 4-20.   Simple oxygen face mask.

Nasal catheter   A nasal catheter is another means of low-flow delivery of oxygen. In this system, a French-tipped catheter is inserted into one nostril until it reaches the oral pharynx. It is used to deliver a moderate to high concentration of oxygen. As with the nasal cannula, the other end of the catheter is attached to the oxygen supply with a flowmeter attached. The prescribed flow rate for this method of delivery is usually 1 to 6 liter/min. The hazards of oxygen delivery by nasal catheter are that oxygen may be misdirected into the stomach, causing gastric distention, and that the mucous membranes may become dry, causing a sore throat. This method of oxygen delivery is used infrequently.

Face mask   A simple face mask is used to deliver oxygen for short periods of time. It too is attached to an oxygen supply and a flowmeter. The mask is placed over the nose and mouth and attached over the ears and behind the head with an elastic band (Fig. 4-20). A mask is uncomfortable for long periods because the patient is unable to eat, drink, or talk with it in place. Moreover, the percentage of oxygen is so variable with the face mask that it is not the method of choice for long periods. When this type of delivery system is used, it should be run at no less than 5 liter/min. This rate is needed in order to flush the CO_2 from the mask.

HIGH-FLOW SYSTEMS

Face masks are usually used to administer high-flow concentrations of oxygen. There are several masks available at present, and the physician will prescribe the one best suited to the patient's needs. The high-flow masks include a nonrebreathing mask, which, if correctly used, may supply 100% oxygen; a partial rebreathing mask, which may deliver 60 to 90% oxygen; a venturi mask, which limits oxygen to 24 to 50%; and an aerosol mask, which provides 60 to 80% oxygen. If the high-flow mask has a reservoir bag attached, the bag fills with oxygen to provide a constant supply of oxygen. A valve prevents the exhaled gases from entering the reservoir bag and prevents rebreathing of exhaled gases (Fig. 4-21).

Patients in acute respiratory failure are often placed on mechanical ventilators that control or partially

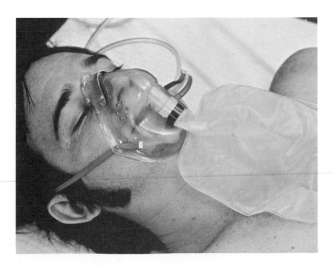

Figure 4-21.   Re-breather mask.

control inspiration and expiration and $F_1 O_2$. The RT will usually encounter these patients in the critical care units of the hospital. Before working with any patient who is on high-flow oxygen therapy or a mechanical ventilator, the RT must consult with the nurse in charge of the patient and plan his work carefully before beginning.

Oxygen tent   Oxygen tents are used when there is a need for humidity and a higher concentration of oxygen than is present in the natural environment of the hospital room (Fig. 4-22). This method of delivery is rarely used for adults, but the RT may be called to the pediatric unit to attend a child in a tent. If this is the case, the RT may request that the oxygen be turned off for brief periods while he makes the required exposures. When finished, he must replace the tent, raise the side rails, and request that the nurse restart the oxygen and mist at the required concentration. The hazard of fire is especially great with a tent. Smoking is not permitted, nor is the use of any equipment that might generate sparks.

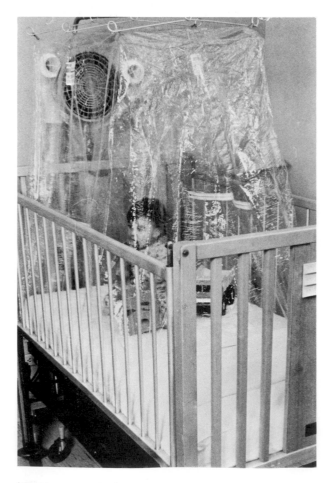

Figure 4-22.   Oxygen tent.

Summary

Fever indicates a disturbance in the heat-regulating centers of the body. It can be detected by an elevation in body temperature, which can be measured by a clinical thermometer or another device if a glass thermometer is not safe or practical to use. The body temperature of a normal adult man or woman is 36.7° C (97.6° F) axillary, 37° C (98.6° F) oral, and 38° C (99.6° F) rectal. These readings vary somewhat in infants and children. Time of day, age, exercise, environmental temperature, and disease alter body temperature.

The pulse is a reflection of the heartbeat, which sends blood to the arteries and causes them to throb. The areas where pulse can be measured best are at the radial artery (radial pulse), the temporal artery (temporal pulse), the carotid artery (carotid pulse), the femoral artery (femoral pulse), the apex of the heart (apical pulse), the dorsalis pedis artery (pedal pulse), the posterior tibial artery (posterior tibial pulse), and the popliteal artery (popliteal pulse). The apical pulse is measured by listening to it through a stethoscope. The average adult man or woman has a pulse rate of 60 to 90 beats/min. This rate varies with infants and children. The rate changes with age, exercise, time, and physiologic disturbances.

The exchange of oxygen and carbon dioxide between the atmosphere and the circulating blood is accomplished by respiration, which involves the inspiration of air containing oxygen and the expiration of air containing carbon dioxide. The rate of respiration for a normal adult male or female is from 12 to 20 pr breaths/min. This varies in infants and small children. Exercise, medication, age, or disease may change the respiratory rate.

Blood pressure is the pressure exerted by the blood on the walls of the blood vessels during the expulsion of blood from the heart and during the resting phase of the heart. It is measured with a sphygmomanometer and a stethoscope or with an electronic device. The most practical place to measure blood pressure is at the brachial artery, located at the center of the anterior elbow.

To record blood pressure, two or three readings are noted. The systolic reading is the highest point of pressure reached during a heart contraction. The diastolic reading is the lowest point to which the pressure drops during the relaxation of the ventricles and indicates the minimal pressure exerted against the arterial walls continuously. The diastolic reading may be heard first as a softening and then as a disappearance of sound, in which case both readings are recorded. Blood pressure readings are influenced by age, exercise, medication, disease, and time of day.

In order to determine critical changes in a patient's vital signs, the RT must know what the patient's usual or baseline vital sign readings are. If these are not available, he will have to rely on established norms to detect critical changes in his patient's vital signs.

Life could not continue without oxygen, yet oxygen cannot be stored in the human body. When a disease that prevents the body from taking in enough oxygen is present, the necessary oxygen must be supplied by artificial means. Oxygen may be administered in the radiology department in emergency situations and is frequently administered on hospital wards. Pure oxygen is a hazardous substance to be used only when prescribed by a physician. It supports combustion, so precautions must be taken when it is in use. No flames or machinery that might produce sparks may be used when oxygen therapy is in prog-

ress. It may also be toxic to lung tissues and produce other harmful physiologic effects if not cautiously used. No radiographic exposures should be made without consulting the nurse in charge of the patient first if a patient is receiving oxygen.

There are basically two types of oxygen delivery systems: high-flow and low-flow. Low-flow systems include nasal cannulas, catheters, and low-flow masks. High-flow delivery systems include nonrebreather and partial rebreathing masks. High-flow systems deliver a controlled amount of oxygen mixed with room air. Low-flow systems deliver only part of the gas inspired; the remainder is room air.

The RT may be responsible for assisting with low-flow oxygen administration or for monitoring vital signs in emergency situations in the diagnostic imaging department and must become proficient in these skills.

Chapter 4, pre-post test

_____ 1. An essential part of the initial assessment of a patient who is in the diagnostic imaging department for an invasive procedure is measuring vital signs. Why is this initial assessment of vital signs important?
   a. It establishes a baseline for further assessments.
   b. It allows the RT to become acquainted with the patient.
   c. It allows the RT to know if the patient is hypertensive.
   d. It assists the physician.

_____ 2. Systolic blood pressure can be defined as
   a. The lowest point to which the blood pressure drops during relaxation of the ventricles
   b. The highest point reached during contraction of the left ventricle
   c. The difference between the systolic and diastolic blood pressure
   d. The pressure in the pulmonary vein

_____ 3. What range of breaths/min is the normal adult respiratory rate?
   a. 20 to 30
   b. 80 to 90
   c. 10 to 20
   d. 8 to 10

_____ 4. An adult patient is considered to be hypertensive or to have hypertension if his systolic blood pressure and diastolic blood pressure are consistently greater than
   a. 120 systolic and 80 diastolic
   b. 130 systolic and 86 diastolic
   c. 100 systolic and 60 diastolic
   d. 140 systolic and 90 diastolic

_____ 5. Oxygen can be toxic to patients if it is incorrectly used. What must the RT remember?
   a. Oxygen can be administered prn.
   b. Oxygen administration must be ordered by the patient's physician.
   c. Oxygen is a vasodilator.
   d. Oxygen is inflammable.

_____ 6. One may say that the patient has tachycardia if his pulse rate is higher than
   a. 80 beats/min
   b. 90 beats/min
   c. 60 beats/min
   d. 120 beats/min

_____ 7. Low-flow oxygen delivery systems provide all of the gas needed for human inspiration.
   a. True
   b. False

_____ 8. Supplemental oxygen is part of many emergency treatment measures. It is within the scope of the RT's practice to begin oxygen administration on his own volition if he feels that it is called for.
   a. True
   b. False

_____ 9. The normal body temperature of a man or woman when taken orally is
   a. 96.6° F
   b. 38° C or 99.6° F
   c. 37° C or 98.6° F
   d. 37.7° C or 97.6° F

_____ 10. Match the following:
   1. Sphygmomanometer
   2. Clinical thermometer

3. Stethoscope
4. Brachial artery
5. Radial artery
a. Point where the blood pressure is most often measured
b. Used to measure apical pulse
c. Used to measure blood pressure
d. Used to measure body temperature

e. Point where the pulse is most often measured

—— 11. List four devices that might be used to deliver oxygen by the low-flow method.

—— 12. List two hazards of which the RT must be aware when assisting with oxygen administration.

Laboratory reinforcement

1. In the school laboratory measure the temperature, pulse, and respiration of several fellow students. Record the measurements on a sheet of paper. List other observations made when measuring pulse and respiration. Your instructor will check your readings.

2. In the school laboratory measure the blood pressure of several fellow students. Then, with a double stethoscope, have your instructor check the blood pressure with you.

3. Demonstrate how to prepare for administering oxygen by mask with a wall attachment and with a tank attachment. If this equipment is not available in the school laboratory, do this in the radiology department of a hospital, with your instructor observing the demonstration.

Chapter Five
Medical Emergencies in Diagnostic Imaging

Goal of this chapter:

The radiologic technology student will be able to recognize life-threatening emergencies and initiate appropriate medical action.

Behavioral objectives:

When the student has completed this chapter, he will be able to do the following:
1. List the visible symptoms of shock
2. List the visible symptoms of an anaphylactic reaction
3. List the observable symptoms of diabetic ketoacidosis, hypoglycemia, and hyperosmolar coma and describe the actions the RT must take if he observes these symptoms in his patient
4. List the early symptoms of a cerebral vascular accident and describe the action the RT should take if these symptoms are observed
5. List the symptoms of respiratory failure and describe the action that an RT must take if this emergency occurs in his department
6. List the symptoms of cardiac failure and describe the actions that the RT must take if this emergency occurs
7. List the symptoms of mechanical airway obstruction and describe the action an RT should take if this emergency occurs
8. List the emergency action that the RT must take if a patient is having a convulsion or is fainting

Glossary

Angioneurotic edema or angioedema a benign, allergic reaction characterized by rapid development of edematous areas of skin (round and swollen elevations of skin area)
Antidiuretic a drug that is used to decrease urine secretion
Anuria no urine formation taking place
Apathetic indifferent, without interest

Ataxia defective muscular coordination especially when voluntary muscular movements are attempted
Cardiac arrest sudden cessation of circulatory function of the heart
Cardiogenic originating within the heart
Cerebral pertains to the brain
Comatose an abnormal deep stupor occurring as a result of illness or an injury

Diaphoresis profuse sweating; heavy perspiration
Eclampsia convulsive seizures between 20th week of pregnancy and the end of the 1st week postpartum (after delivery); cause is not known
Edema local or generalized condition in which body tissues contain an excessive amount of fluid
Fainting temporary loss of consciousness caused by inadequate

blood flow to the brain; contributing factors include fatigue, pain, dehydration, hunger, anemia, poor ventilation

Histamine a substance normally present in the body; released by the tissues in response to allergic reactions; constricts bronchial muscles in lungs

Infarct an area of dying tissue in an organ or artery caused by obstruction of the blood vessels normally supplying the part

Lethargy a condition of indifference or suppression of emotions

Myocardial infarction cardiac muscle undergoing necrosis (tissue death) following cessation of blood supply

Neurogenic originating from nervous tissue or from nervous impulses

Oliguria diminished amount of urine formation

Pallor absence or lack of skin color; paleness

Productive cough activity that expels mucus or phlegm from the respiratory tract (throat and lungs)

Psychic trauma a painful emotional experience that may cause anxiety, fear, or shock

Pulmonary embolus undissolved matter, solid, liquid, or gaseous, in the artery carrying the venous blood from heart to lungs

Respiratory arrest complete cessation of lung ventilation; can be due to respiratory failure

Seizure sudden attack of pain, symptoms, or disease occurring periodically as involuntary muscular spasms

Sputum substance from the respiratory tract expelled by coughing or clearing the throat; contains saliva and material from bronchi and throat

Tissue perfusion passage of blood and fluids through small blood vessels in body tissues

Umbilicus the scar that marks the former attachment of the umbilical cord to the fetus found as a depression in middle of abdomen

Uremia a toxic condition caused by the presence in the blood of waste products normally eliminated in the urine and resulting from failure of kidneys to secrete urine

Urticaria giant hives accompanied by severe itching resulting from allergy

Vasodilatation dilation of blood vessels and arterioles

Wheezing a whistling sound while breathing

Many patients come to the diagnostic imaging department in poor physical condition. This may be due to illness, injury, or because of necessary preparation for the examination that they are scheduled to undergo while in the department. When a person is in a weakened physical condition, his physiologic reactions may be abnormal. Many of these reactions occur quickly, with little or no warning, and they are often life-threatening if not recognized and treated immediately.

The medical emergencies most likely to occur in diagnostic imaging not necessarily related to trauma are shock, anaphylaxis, diabetic reactions, cerebral vascular accidents, cardiac and respiratory failure, fainting, and convulsions. The RT may be the first member of the health team to observe these reactions; therefore, he must be able to recognize them and initiate the correct action.

In most cases, the first action an RT will take in a life-threatening emergency is to call the hospital emergency team, the physician conducting the procedure, and his colleagues for assistance. He must learn the correct procedure in the institution in which he works for calling the hospital emergency team. In many hospitals this is termed *calling a CODE*. The RT must have the telephone number memorized and be prepared to explain the exact location of the emergency and the problem.

All diagnostic imaging departments have an emergency cart that contains medications and equipment needed when a patient's condition becomes suddenly critical. This is often called a *crash cart*. The RT must know where to obtain this cart quickly. Care must be taken to keep all medications

and equipment that are part of this cart up-to-date and in working condition. He must also familiarize himself with the oxygen administration equipment so that he can assist with its administration with no delays.

Shock

Shock is a physiologic reaction to illness or trauma in which there is a disturbance of blood flow to the vital organs or a decreased ability of the body tissues to use oxygen and other nutrients needed to maintain them in a healthy state. It is most frequently seen in the very young, the elderly, and the generally debilitated and may be caused by injury, disease, or an intense emotional reaction. Shock may occur quickly and without warning. For this reason, the RT caring for a seriously injured or ill patient must observe closely for visible signs and symptoms of shock.

General symptoms

General signs and symptoms of shock include decreased temperature; a weak, thready pulse; a rapid heartbeat; rapid, shallow respirations; hypotension; skin pallor; cyanosis; and increased thirst. If the patient is dark-skinned, observe for cyanosis by pressing lightly on his fingernails or earlobes. If he is cyanotic, the color will not return to the compressed area in the usual 1-second interval. A bluish discoloration of the tongue and soft palate of the mouth is also indicative of cyanosis.

Because of an inadequate supply of oxygen to the brain, the patient will also generally display signs of restlessness, confusion, and anxiety in the early stages of shock. Later, if the problem is allowed to progress, the patient will become apathetic, confused, and comatose. It is important for the RT to know his patient's baseline vital signs so that he can detect changes that may indicate early stages of shock.

Shock may be classified in many ways. For the RT's purposes, it will be presented in the following categories: hypovolemic, septic, cardiogenic, neurogenic, and anaphylactic.

Types

HYPOVOLEMIC SHOCK

Hypovolemic shock is caused by an abnormally low volume of circulating blood in the body. It may be due to internal or external hemorrhage, loss of plasma because of burns, fluid loss from prolonged vomiting or diarrhea, heat prostration, or insufficient release of antidiuretic hormone (ADH).

Signs and symptoms

Restlessness; thirst; cold, clammy skin

Pallor, sweating

Falling blood pressure; weak, thready pulse and rapid respirations; extreme weakness; lethargy

Cold extremities, semiconsciousness, coma

Systolic blood pressure lower than 60 mm Hg

Oliguria to anuria

RT actions

Cardiac and respiratory failure will follow if this condition is allowed to continue.

Stop the radiographic examination; place the patient in a flat, supine position and allow him to rest.

Notify the physician in charge of the patient immediately and call for assistance.

Make certain that the patient is able to breathe without obstruction that may be due to positioning or blood or mucus in his airway.

Note any visible discharge of bodily fluids such as blood, vomitus, feces, or urine.

If there are body fluids visible, put on gloves and wipe them away.

Keep any visible blood out of patient's view.

If there is blood loss from an open wound, don gloves and apply pressure directly to the wound with a dry, sterile dressing.

Be prepared to assist with administration of oxygen, intravenous fluids, or medications. Keep the patient warm and dry; check blood pressure, pulse, and respirations every 10 minutes. Do not overheat patients suffering from hypovolemic shock; to do so will increase body metabolism and the need for oxygen.

Observe the patient's skin color and body temperature; report any changes to the physician.

Maintain a nonstressful environment.

Do not offer food or fluids.

Do not leave the patient unattended.

SEPTIC SHOCK

Septic shock is caused by severe systemic infections and bacteremia (bacterial endotoxins released in the bloodstream). Symptoms progress somewhat differently from those of other types of shock.

Signs and symptoms

In early stages, the skin is warm, dry, and flushed.

Urine output may be normal or excessive.

The patient may have chills.

As the shock progresses, there may be an abrupt personality change or a decrease in the level of consciousness.

There is an increase in pulse and respiration and a decrease in urinary output.

The skin becomes cold and clammy.

Seizures, circulatory collapse, and cardiorespiratory failure will follow if the course is not reversed.

RT actions

Stop the procedure, notify the physician in charge of the patient, and call for assistance.

Place the patient in a flat, supine position and keep him quiet. Do not leave him unattended. If the patient's skin is very warm, cover him only with a sheet.

Take the vital signs every 10 minutes.

Prepare to assist with administration of oxygen, intravenous fluids, and medications.

CARDIOGENIC SHOCK

Cardiogenic shock is caused by a failure of the heart to pump an adequate amount of blood to the vital organs. This causes inadequate tissue perfusion. The onset of cardiogenic shock is sudden and often occurs in patients hospitalized for acute myocardial infarction, cardiac tamponade, or pulmonary embolus. It may follow cardiac surgery.

Signs and symptoms

Restlessness, anxiety, falling blood pressure, and falling pulse pressure

Weak, rapid pulse and shallow, labored respirations

Decreased urinary output

Cool, clammy skin

Possible semiconsciousness or coma

RT actions

Summon emergency assistance and place the emergency cart nearby.

Notify the physician in charge of the patient.

Place the patient in a semi-Fowler's position or a position of comfort.

Keep the patient warm and quiet.

Take the vital signs every 5 to 10 minutes.

Do not give the patient anything to eat or drink.

Do not leave the patient alone.

Be prepared to assist with oxygen and intravenous fluids, and medication administration.

Be prepared to begin CPR.

NEUROGENIC SHOCK

Neurogenic shock occurs when concussion, spinal cord injury, psychic trauma, or spinal anesthesia causes abnormal dilatation of the peripheral blood vessels. This dilatation in turn causes a fall in blood pressure as blood pools in the veins. This leads to reduced cardiac output.

Signs and symptoms

Hypotension and bradycardia

Warm, dry skin and subnormal body temperature

Initial alertness unless the patient is unconscious because of head injury

Initially good, but deteriorating, tissue perfusion

Visible signs of poor tissue perfusion—coolness of extremities and diminishing peripheral pulses

RT actions

Notify the physician in charge of the patient.

Summon assistance and stay with the patient.

Keep the patient flat, and monitor vital signs every 10 minutes.

Do not move the patient if there is a possible spinal cord injury.

Prepare to assist with oxygen, intravenous fluid, and medication administration.

ANAPHYLACTIC SHOCK

Anaphylactic shock is often classified with neurogenic shock because of the physiologic similarities. In this text it will be discussed separately because it is the type of shock seen most often in diagnostic imaging, and the RT must be able to recognize it at the onset to prevent life-threatening consequences.

Anaphylactic shock (anaphylaxis) is the result of an exaggerated hypersensitivity reaction (allergic reaction) to an antigen that was previously encountered by the body's immune system. When this occurs, vasodilator substances (histamine and histaminelike compounds), which may produce massive vasodilatation and peripheral pooling of blood, are released in the body. This reaction is accompanied by contraction of nonvascular smooth muscles, particularly the smooth muscles of the respiratory system. This reaction can produce shock, respiratory failure, and death within minutes following exposure to the agent that produces the reaction. The more abrupt the onset of symptoms, the more severe the reaction tends to become.

The common causes of anaphylaxis are drugs, iodinated contrast agents, chemotherapeutic agents, anesthetics, certain foods, and insect venoms entering the body. The path of entry may be through the skin, the respiratory tract, or the gastrointestinal tract.

When iodinated contrast agents are being used for diagnostic procedures, the RT must observe the patient continuously for any sign of allergic reaction. If early symptoms of anaphylaxis are observed, the RT must act quickly, because death may follow in a few moments.

Early signs and symptoms

Itching at the site of a medication injection or around the eyes and nose

Sneezing and coughing

Apprehensiveness; a feeling of doom

Nausea, vomiting, and diarrhea; usually accompanies a reaction to food

Later symptoms

Angioneurotic edema of the face, hands, and other body parts; urticaria

Choking, wheezing, or dyspnea and cyanosis

Hypotension; weak, rapid pulse; and dilated pupils

RT actions

Keep the emergency cart readily available and correctly prepared whenever an iodinated contrast medium is being administered.

Before starting any procedure that involves the use of iodinated contrast medium, ask the patient the following questions:

> *"Are you allergic to any food or medicine?"*
> *If the answer is yes, ask, "Which ones?"*
> *"Do you have asthma or hay fever?"*
> *"Have you ever had hives or other allergic skin reactions?"*
> *"Have you ever had an x-ray examination that involved the use of contrast medium? If so, did you have a reaction during or following that examination?"*

If any of the questions elicit a positive response, this should be reported to the radiologist before the contrast agent is administered. If the patient has a long history of allergic responses to food and drugs, the examination may have to be cancelled. However, a patient who has no history of allergy may also have an anaphylactic reaction.

Never leave a patient who is receiving an iodinated contrast agent unattended. If he complains of itching, if swelling or redness of the skin is noted, or if the patient seems unduly anxious, stop the infusion or injection immediately and notify the radiologist. Monitor the vital signs, and observe for respiratory distress. Do not leave the patient alone. If the patient is in anaphylactic shock, call the emergency team; place the patient in a semi-Fowler's or sitting position if this is possible. Prepare to assist with the administration of oxygen, intravenous fluids, and medications.

Medications usually given are epinephrine, diphenhydramine, hydrocortisone, and aminophylline. If the patient stops breathing, begin pulmonary resuscitation. If the patient becomes both breathless and pulseless, administer CPR.

Diabetic emergencies

Diabetes melitus is a chronic disease involving a disorder of carbohydrate, protein, and fat metabolism, which also affects the structure and function of the blood vessels. The underlying cause is a disturbance in the production, action, or utilization of insulin, a hormone normally secreted by the islands of Langerhans located in the pancreas. Medical treatment consists of diet therapy, insulin injections, or use of oral hypoglycemic drugs.

There are two major classifications of diabetes melitus: type I, insulin-dependent form; and type II, noninsulin-dependent form. Persons who have insulin-dependent diabetes melitus (IDDM) have fewer islands of Langerhans cells and produce practically no insulin. These persons are totally dependent on outside sources of insulin for their entire lives.

The majority of persons who develop IDDM are quite young, frequently in their early teenage years. Patients who have IDDM often wear bracelets that identify their condition and their need for insulin so that, if they are in a situation in which they cannot help themselves, their need for insulin can be identified. These persons are most likely to develop ketoacidosis.

Persons with noninsulin-dependent diabetes melitus (NIDDM) produce less insulin than is necessary or the insulin does not have the desired effect on the body. The majority of persons with this type of diabetes melitus are overweight and middle-aged. Diabetes melitus is diagnosed by laboratory measurement of blood glucose levels. A normal adult blood glucose level should range from 80 to 115 mg/dl.

There are three acute complications that the RT must consider if his patient has diabetes melitus. They are hypoglycemia, diabetic ketoacidosis, and nonketotic hyperosmolar, hyperglycemic nonketotic coma (HHNK or hyperosmolar coma). The RT must remember that persons who have diabetes melitus are extremely susceptible to infections, and therefore he must take extra skin care and infection-control precautions when caring for patients with this disease.

Hypoglycemia

Hypoglycemia (insulin reaction) occurs when patients who have diabetes melitus have an access amount of insulin in their bloodstream, an increased rate of glucose utilization, or an inadequate diet to utilize the insulin. A patient who has diabetes melitus may come to the diagnostic imaging department after he has taken insulin or some other hypoglycemic agent, but before his body has had sufficient nourishment to utilize the medication. The result may be a hypoglycemic reaction. The onset of symptoms is rapid, and immediate action is necessary in order to prevent coma.

Signs and symptoms

Shaking, nervousness, and irritability

Dizziness and hunger; may complain of headache

Profuse perspiration; cold, clammy skin

Blurred vision

Tremor, numbness of lips or tongue, slurred speech

Impaired motor function; convulsions

Diminishing level of consciousness; quick lapse into coma

RT actions

If the patient is conscious and complains of the above symptoms or says that he is a diabetic and says that he has not eaten and feels "shaky," notify the radiologist and administer some type of sugar immediately.

If there is nothing else available, the packets of sugar kept in the coffee room for coffee or tea or a carbonated beverage sweetened with sugar is acceptable. If you offer orange juice, put three or four packets or teaspoonsful of sugar in it and have the patient drink it immediately. Check his chart or look for a bracelet which identifies the patient as a diabetic.

If the patient is unconscious or is having trouble swallowing, place granulated sugar, corn syrup, or jelly into his mouth under his tongue. It will be absorbed through the mucous membranes. Stop the diagnostic imaging procedure immediately. Notify the radiologist. Do not leave the patient unattended.

Call for help; monitor the vital signs.

Prepare to assist with administration of oxygen, intravenous fluids, and medications.

Usually, in this type of coma, 20 to 50 ml of 50% glucose in solution is administered intravenously.

Another form of emergency treatment is to administer glucagon intramuscularly followed by IV glucose solution.

Hypoglycemia must be treated immediately because it interferes with the oxygen supply to nerve tissue and may result in brain damage.

Diabetic ketoacidosis

When a diabetic patient has insufficient insulin available to metabolize the glucose that is present, his body begins to mobilize fatty acids, and the result is an acidotic state called diabetic ketoacidosis. In this condition, acid and ketone bodies accumulate in the blood. If this accumulation is not corrected quickly, the patient will become comatose and may die. Ketoacidosis occurs more slowly than hypoglycemia but may result if a diabetic is detained for too long in the diagnostic imaging department and misses an insulin injection.

Signs and symptoms

Weakness, drowsiness, and dull headache

Sweet odor to the breath, hypotension

Warm, dry skin; parched tongue; dry mucous membranes; extreme thirst

General weakness, lethargy, and fatigue

Flushed face, deep and rapid respirations

Tachycardia, weak, thready pulse and, ultimately, coma

RT actions

Check patient chart or look for a bracelet identifying him as a diabetic.

Stop treatment, and notify the physician.

Call for assistance.

Do not leave patient unattended.

Monitor vital signs.

Give fluids by mouth if possible.

Prepare to assist with administration of intravenous fluids, medications, and oxygen.

Hyperosmolar coma

Hyperosmolar coma (hyperglycemic, nonketotic coma [HHNK]) is a complication of diabetes melitus that usually occurs in the elderly diabetic patient. It is frequently mistaken for a stroke or drunkeness and is an extremely serious, life-threatening problem. Factors that precipitate this reaction are often diagnostic procedures that require changes in diet, especially a nothing-by-mouth status, as is frequently the case for diagnostic imaging procedures. Other causes for this condition are hyperglycemic-inducing agents and resistance to insulin. The blood glucose level in patients with this problem is greater than 600 ml/dl; there is little or no ketosis and the plasma is hyperosmolar.

Signs and symptoms

Extreme patient dehydration; dry skin, sunken eyes

Increased body temperature; polyuria; extreme thirst

Muscle twitching; difficult, slurred speech

Mental confusion; convulsion

Coma

RT actions

Call for assistance; do not leave patient unattended.

Notify the physician in charge of the patient and stop the diagnostic procedure.

Monitor vital signs, prepare to administer intravenous fluids, medication, and oxygen.

Respiratory failure, cardiac failure, and airway obstruction

There are three components of the basic life support process: maintenance of airway, breathing, and circulation. The RT must have the ability to assess problems in these areas and initiate emergency care when they occur in his work area. Respiratory failure, cardiac failure (cardiac arrest), or an airway obstruction may occur in the diagnostic imaging department without any warning and when least expected. The human brain can survive without oxygen for only 2 to 4 minutes. This means that there is little time to ponder the situation before acting.

The information in this text concerning treatment of these emergencies was obtained from the Standards and Guidelines for Cardiopulmonary Resuscitation (CPR) and Emergency Cardiac Care (ECC), *Journal of the American Medical Association,* June 6, 1986. All hospital employees including RTs are required to be prepared to perform basic cardiopulmonary resuscitation and life support. Many hospitals have classes for their employees on a regular basis to teach and keep them current in these procedures. Others require that the employee obtain this training at classes offered in the community. The American Red Cross and the American Heart Association provide basic CPR classes regularly for the general public. The techniques must be demonstrated by a licensed instructor, and return demonstrations must be given by the student until he is proficient. The RT must understand that the brief explanation of CPR and life support methods that follows does not prepare him to administer these techniques. The explanations and directions are not complete because it is not within the scope of this text to make them so. It is the RT's obligation to his patient to receive adequate training in basic CPR. Note that basic life support for an infant requires special consideration and will only be addressed briefly.

Respiratory failure or cardiac arrest

Respiratory failure or severe respiratory dysfunction may result from airway obstruction caused by the patient's position, the tongue, a foreign object, vomitus lodged in the throat, disease, drug overdose, injury, or coma. Whatever the cause, gas exchange is no longer adequate to maintain normal arterial blood gases.

Symptoms of a partially obstructed airway include labored, noisy breathing; wheezing; use of accessory muscles of the neck, abdomen, or chest for breathing; neck-vein distention; diaphoresis; anxiety; cyanosis of the lips and nail beds; and possibly a productive cough with pink-tinged, frothy sputum. If the patient displays symptoms of dyspnea, the RT should call for help and assist the patient to a sitting or semi-Fowler's position. Attempt to relieve the patient's anxiety by staying with him. Prepare to assist with oxygen administration and have the emergency cart at hand.

If the patient lapses into complete respiratory failure, his pulse will continue to beat for a brief period of time; however, the pulse quickly becomes weak and then ceases. Chest movement stops and no air can be detected moving through the patient's nose or mouth. Immediate intervention in respiratory arrest may prevent cardiac arrest.

RT ACTION: NUMBER ONE = AIRWAY

If you suspect that your patient has had respiratory or cardiac arrest, the first consideration is an open airway. Check the larynx and trachea to make certain that the patient's tongue, epiglottis, or a foreign body is not blocking his airway. The tongue is the most common obstruction to breathing in an unconscious person.

Next, tilt the head by placing one hand on the patient's forehead and applying firm backward pressure with the palm to tilt the head back. Then place the fingers of the other hand under the lower jaw near the chin and lift so that the chin is brought forward and the teeth are almost together. Do not use your thumbs, because they may press too firmly and occlude respiration. The lips should remain apart (Fig. 5-1). If the patient has dentures that do not stay in place, remove them. For a child, tilt the head and lift the chin only slightly.

If a neck or cervical spine injury is suspected, a jaw thrust maneuver must be used rather than tilting the head as described above. The head should be well supported without tilting it or turning the patient. Thrust the jaw down by placing your fingers under the angle of the jaw and your thumb on the chin. Then pull the jaw downward with your index finger, and sweep the mouth to remove any vomitus or foreign material that may be present. If the patient does not resume breathing following these actions, rescue breathing must be begun.

RT ACTION: NUMBER TWO = BREATHING

Rescue breathing by means of the mouth-to-mouth technique provides adequate oxygen from the rescuer's exhaled air to support life if the patient's lungs are adequately inflated with each breath. If you suspect that a patient has had respiratory or cardiac arrest, shake him, call him by name, and ask if he is all right. If there is no response, call for help and have your helper summon the hospital emergency team. Move the patient to a supine position, log rolling him into position with assistance if you suspect a spinal cord injury.

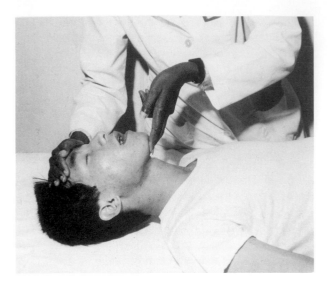

Figure 5-1

Check the patient's respiration by observing for the chest movement that is present in normal respiration. If no chest movement is seen, put your ear close to the patient's mouth and nose, and listen and feel for expiration of air. If the chest is not moving and you do not feel air, check the carotid pulse. If you are able to palpate the carotid pulse, begin mouth-to-mouth breathing (pulmonary resuscitation) only.

Keep the patient's airway open by maintaining the head tilt, chin lift, or the jaw thrust position. If the patient is an adult, squeeze the nostrils together and cover his mouth tightly with yours, being careful not to allow air to escape. If the patient is an infant or a very small child, both mouth and nose are covered with your mouth. Inflate the patient's lungs by giving two full breaths in succession into his mouth. Allow the patient time to exhale these breaths as you inhale between each. If this is correctly done, the patient's chest will rise as you breathe into his mouth. If you are not successful in getting the chest to rise and fall, reposition the head and repeat. If still not successful, there is a possibility that the airway is obstructed, and airway obstruction procedure must be begun. Discussion of this follows in a later paragraph.

After these first steps, recheck the carotid pulse; if present, continue pulmonary resuscitation by breathing into the patient's mouth at the rate of 12 breaths per minute. Check the carotid pulse each minute to be certain that it is still present. If the pulse is absent, cardiac compression must be started immediately.

RT ACTION: THREE = CIRCULATION

External cardiac compression is effective only if the patient is lying on a firm surface. If he is on a radio-

graphic table, kneel on the table beside the patient because these tables have hard surfaces. If the patient is lying on a soft surface, either he should be moved to the floor or a cardiac board may be placed under his chest.

Take an adequate amount of time to determine pulselessness (5 to 10 seconds). Performing cardiac compressions on a person whose heart is functioning is extremely dangerous to the patient. Once compressions have started, do not interrupt them for more than 7 seconds at a time.

The RT must be certain that his hands are positioned carefully to prevent internal injury as the chest is compressed. The way to determine this is by moving your fingers up the lower margin of the rib cage to the area where the ribs and the sternum meet. When you have located this area, place your index finger above this area and place the heel of your hand beside the index finger with the second hand on top of it (Fig. 5-2). Be certain that your hand is in the midline of the sternum above the xiphoid process. Pressure on the xiphoid may cause internal injuries. For children, the landmarks are the same, but only one hand is used to prevent excessive pressure. For infants the area of compression is at the midline of

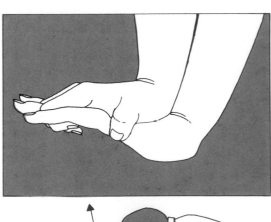

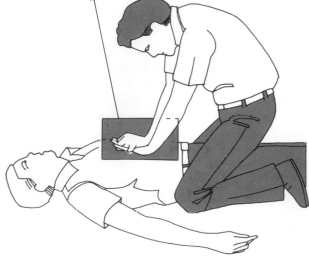

Figure 5-2. External cardiac compression.

the chest slightly below the nipples, and only two or three fingers are used for compression.

For adult cardiac compression, the lower half of the sternum is compressed. Compress the sternum 1½ to 2 inches directly downward and then release the compression completely. Do not apply pressure on the rib cage itself. Keep your elbows straight and give 15 compressions in a smooth, even rhythm. Then inflate the patient's lungs two more times. Next, give 15 more compressions, then two more inflations. This rhythm must be maintained until help arrives. Following the initial cycles of compressions and ventilations, pause to reassess the pulse and breathlessness. If the patient remains breathless and pulseless, continue the cycle of two ventilations and 15 compressions, maintaining 80 to 100 external chest compressions per minute.

When the emergency team arrives, the RT allows them to take over at a time specified for the change. The RT remains on the scene to assist with oxygen and drug administration if it is necessary or to render service in any way possible.

Cardiopulmonary resuscitation rates for infants and children vary according to their weight and size and must be learned from an instructor certified to teach this. Two-person CPR will not be discussed in this text, as it also demands actual demonstration to be useful.

To prevent becoming infected by a patient with a communicable disease during mouth-to-mouth ventilation, a manual resuscitation bag may be used if it is available and the RT has been instructed in its use. There are several types on the market, and special demonstration of their use must be received before they can be used safely and effectively for patients in respiratory failure.

Airway obstruction

A foreign body such as a piece of chewing gum or food may lodge in a patient's throat and produce respiratory arrest. This type of accident occurs most often in the elderly, the very young, or the intoxicated while they are eating. However, it must be considered by the RT in any case of respiratory arrest.

Signs and symptoms

When airway obstruction caused by a foreign object occurs, the patient usually appears to be quite normal, then suddenly begins to choke.

He grabs his throat and is unable to speak.

If no one is present to observe this, the patient eventually loses consciousness.

Unless the early signs are observed, it is impossible to know the cause of the unconscious state.

Airway obstruction may occur with the patient sitting, standing, or lying down and must be dealt with initially in that position.

RT actions

If the patient does not respond, and breathlessness is established as described in the preceding paragraphs, seal the nose and mouth and ventilate the patient as in the initial steps of pulmonary resuscitation.

If you see the patient's chest rise and fall, you proceed as for basic CPR.

If the chest does not rise and fall, reposition the head using the head tilt, chin lift, or jaw thrust as indicated. Then attempt to ventilate again.

If this is unsuccessful, assume that the airway is obstructed and use the Heimlich maneuver (also called the subdiaphragmatic abdominal thrust or simply the abdominal thrust) to attempt to remove the obstruction.

ABDOMINAL THRUST: PATIENT STANDING OR SITTING

The RT stands behind the patient and grasps him with both hands above the umbilicus and below the xiphoid process of the sternum. The lower hand is positioned with the thumb inward; the other hand firmly grips the lower hand. Then make a rapid upward movement that forces the abdomen inward, and thrust upward against the diaphragm (Fig. 5-3). This maneuver forces air up through the trachea and dislodges the foreign object. The RT must never attempt to practice this maneuver on a person not in distress because he may cause serious injury. The hands must be placed so that the xiphoid process is avoided to prevent internal injury.

ABDOMINAL THRUST: PATIENT IN SUPINE POSITION

Place the patient lying in a supine position with face up. Kneel astride the patient's thighs, and place the heel of one hand against the patient's abdomen above the navel and below the tip of the xiphoid process. Place your second hand over the first, and press the abdomen quickly upward. Be certain to direct the thrust directly up, and do not deviate to left or right. This maneuver acts the same as it does when the patient is sitting or standing (Fig. 5-4).

CHEST THRUST: PATIENT SITTING OR STANDING

This position is used to dislodge a foreign object only if the patient is in advanced stages of pregnancy or if excessively obese, and the abdominal thrust cannot be used effectively.

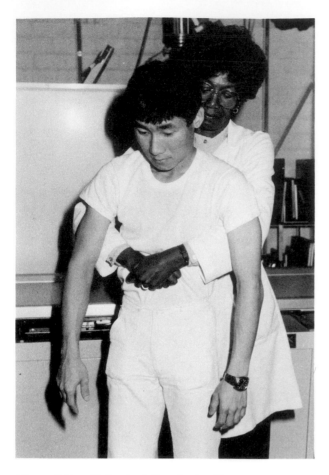

Figure 5-3.   Abdominal thrust, standing.

The RT stands behind the patient and puts his arms under the patient's armpits and around his chest. Place the thumb side of your fist in the middle of the sternum avoiding the xiphoid process and the margins of the rib cage. Place the other hand on top and thrust backward. Repeat this maneuver until the object is dislodged.

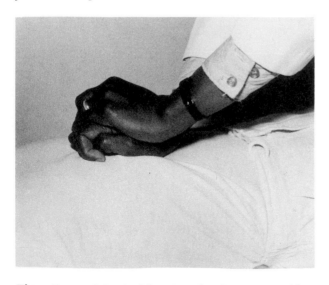

Figure 5-4.   Abdominal thrust, patient in supine position.

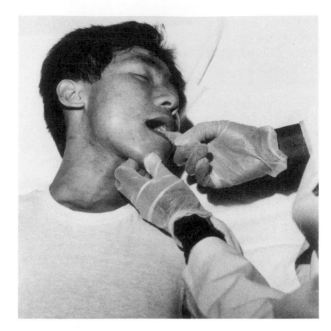

Figure 5-5.   Finger sweep.

If the patient is an infant and an airway obstruction is suspected, place him face down over your forearm with legs straddling your elbow. Support the head and neck on your hand between the thumb and index finger with the head lower than the chest but not straight down. Administer four sharp blows on the back between the shoulder blades. If this is not successful, chest thrusts with two or three fingers on the midsternum are applied at about one each second.

The method of dealing with foreign body airway obstruction for infants and children also varies with their weight, age, and size.

CHEST THRUST: PATIENT LYING SUPINE AND
UNCONSCIOUS

Determine breathlessness in the prescribed manner; attempt ventilation. If this is not successful, and the patient is in the advanced stages of pregnancy or is excessively obese, use the chest thrust to attempt to dislodge the foreign object.

Kneel beside the patient and place the hands in the same position as that used for external cardiac compression. Thrust slowly and firmly as many times as is necessary to relieve the obstruction.

FINGER SWEEP

This maneuver is to be used only on an unconscious patient with the patient lying in a supine position, face up. Open the patient's mouth by grasping the tongue and lower jaw between the thumb and fingers. Lift the mandible. This is done to move the tongue away from a foreign body that may be lodged behind it. Next insert the index finger of the other hand along the base of the tongue using a hooking motion to dislodge and remove the object (Fig. 5-5). This must be done with extreme care so that a foreign object is not forced further into the airway.

Reminder: The methods described in this text to remove airway obstructions for adult, child, or infant patients are taught in basic CPR classes, and all RT students must have formal instruction in this type of treatment. The foregoing descriptions do not render the RT competent to perform these maneuvers.

Cerebral vascular accident (stroke)

Cerebral vascular accidents (CVA) are caused by occlusion or rupture of the cerebral arteries directly into the brain tissue or into the subarachnoid space. This is commonly called a stroke. Strokes vary in severity from a mild transischemic attack (TIA) to severe life-threatening situations. CVAs occur most frequently with little or no warning and may possibly occur in the diagnostic imaging department during a stressful procedure. The RT must be familiar with the warning signs and symptoms of this medical crisis and be prepared to initiate emergency care.

Signs and symptoms
Possible severe headache

Muscle weakness or flaccidity of face or extremities; usually one-sided

Eye deviation, usually one-sided; may lose vision

Dizziness or stupor

Difficult speech (dysphasia) or no speech (aphasia)

Ataxia

May complain of stiff neck

Nausea or vomiting may occur

Loss of consciousness

RT actions
Call for emergency aid. Do not leave patient alone.

Put patient in resting position with head slightly elevated.

Monitor vital signs every 10 minutes and report to the physician in charge of the patient.

Prepare to administer intravenous medications, fluids, and oxygen.

Prepare to administer CPR if the patient becomes breathless or pulseless.

Fainting and convulsive seizures

Fainting and convulsive seizures are medical emergencies that can occur in the diagnostic imaging department. Both require immediate action in order to prevent injury to the patient.

Fainting

Fainting is caused by an insufficiency in the supply of blood to the brain. Heart disease, hunger, poor ventilation, fatigue, and emotional shock are all causes. For example, patients are frequently instructed not to eat breakfast before coming to the diagnostic imaging department from their homes or hospital rooms. Often they are ill, and lack of nourishment may increase the likelihood of fainting. The patient cannot choose the ''proper'' place in which to faint, so he may fall and injure himself. The RT must be able to recognize and watch for the symptoms that indicate that a patient is about to faint.

Signs and symptoms
Pallor, dizziness, and possibly nausea

Cold, clammy skin

RT actions
Have the patient lie down, if possible. Position his head so it is level with or somewhat lower than his body.

If there is no convenient place where the patient can lie down, do not try to keep him standing, but support and assist him to the floor in a manner that will prevent serious injury. As soon as the patient is in a safe position, summon medical assistance.

Convulsive seizures

Convulsive seizures may be associated with many physical disorders, including uremia, eclampsia, tetanus, infections characterized by high body temperature, poisoning, and increased intracranial pressure caused by a brain tumor. Epilepsy is the most common cause of convulsive seizures. Children are more susceptible than adults to seizures of all types.

Seizures, like fainting, often begin without warning. Although the seizure itself will not cause injury, the patient may be badly injured by falling or by violent body movement during the seizure.

There are several classifications of seizures. In one classification, the nomenclature includes the terms *grand mal* or *generalized* seizures, *partial* seizures, and *petit mal* or *absence* seizures. In a grand mal seizure, the person's whole body convulses, and he loses consciousness for a period of minutes. In a partial seizure one focal point is affected; the seizure may become generalized or may remain concentrated at the focal point.

Signs and symptoms (grand mal, or generalized, seizure)

May utter a sharp cry as air is rapidly exhaled.

Muscles become rigid, and eyes open wide (tonic phase).

May exhibit jerky body movements and rapid, irregular respirations (clonic phase).

May vomit.

May froth, and may have blood-streaked saliva caused by biting his lips or tongue.

May exhibit urinary or fecal incontinence.

Usually falls into a deep sleep following the seizure.

PETIT MAL

In petit mal, or absence, seizures the attack is so brief that an observer may not be aware that it has occurred. Though not as frightening to the observer, these seizures may be more difficult to control medically than the grand mal type. This type of seizure is rare in adults.

Signs and symptoms (petit mal)

A brief loss of awareness accompanied by a blank stare and then total return of consciousness.

There may be eye blinking, lip smacking, or mild body movements.

If the patient has been addressing someone, he may stop speaking, lower his head for a moment, and then resume speaking.

RT actions (grand mal and petit mal seizures)

The most important action is to prevent the patient from injuring himself during a seizure.

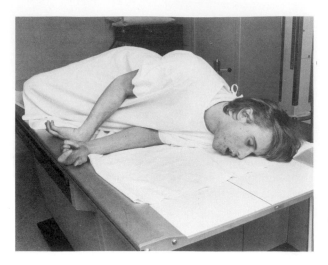

Figure 5-6

Do not attempt to insert hard objects into the patient's mouth during a seizure. Do not place your own fingers into a patient's mouth; they may be severely bitten. Stay with the patient; protect him from hitting his head or limbs against hard objects.

Restrain him gently.

If he is lying on the radiographic table, hold him. Restrain him gently to keep him from falling. Call for help but do not leave the patient.

After the seizure, position the patient to prevent choking or aspiration of secretion and vomitus.

Turn the patient onto his side or to a prone position. If on his side, put the head back and the face downward so that vomitus or secretions may drain out of the mouth (Fig. 5-6).

Prepare to assist in oxygen administration.

If possible, remove dentures or foreign objects from the mouth.

Note and report as much about the onset of the seizure as possible to the physician.

Summary

Medical emergencies occur frequently in the diagnostic imaging department. The RT may be the first or only person present at the onset of the problem, so it is important that he learn to recognize the symptoms of beginning problems and know what action to take.

Shock is a common medical emergency. There are many causes of physiologic shock. Blood loss, infection, and cardiac failure are among the most common. Anaphylactic shock is caused by allergic re-

action and is the type that the RT is most likely to see in diagnostic imaging. This is because iodinated contrast agents used for some procedures and examinations may produce severe anaphylactic shock. If early symptoms of this type of reaction are suspected, the RT must not wait, but must stop the administration of this agent immediately and initiate emergency action. Early symptoms of an anaphylactic reaction are apprehensiveness; sneezing; itching at injection site or around the eyes and nose; angioneurotic edema of face, hands, and other body parts; choking and shortness of breath; and ultimately, if the situation is not reversed, respiratory failure.

Diabetic ketoacidosis, hypoglycemia, and hyperosmolar coma are sometimes seen in the diagnostic imaging department because patients who have diabetes melitus may come for diagnostic imaging having taken antihypoglycemic medications, but not having eaten. This combination may induce a hypoglycemic reaction. Ketoacidosis occurs when a diabetic patient has not had sufficient insulin and his body is not able to metabolize the glucose present. Hyperosmolar coma occurs most frequently in elderly diabetic patients when they have dietary changes in preparation for diagnostic examinations or their bodies are unable to metabolize insulin. Any of these reactions constitutes a medical emergency that, if left untreated, will result in coma and death. Sugar in some form is the treatment for hypoglycemic reactions. For all these conditions, the physician in charge of the examination or treatment must be notified at once, and the RT must prepare to administer intravenous fluids and oxygen.

Cerebral vascular accidents are medical emergencies that must be recognized and dealt with immediately in order to prevent life-threatening consequences. The early signs and symptoms are often one-sided flaccidity of face and limbs, difficult or absent speech, eye deviation, dizziness, ataxia, possible neck stiffness, nausea, vomiting, and loss of consciousness.

Respiratory failure and cardiac failure should be differentiated by the RT. Respiratory failure can be recognized by a lack of chest movement, absence of breath sounds, a diminishing pulse rate, and loss of consciousness. Cardiac failure results in an immediate cessation of the pulse and respiration and a loss of consciousness. Both call for immediate action if the patient's life is to be saved.

Airway obstruction caused by a foreign object must be suspected if the patient is feeling well and suddenly begins to demonstrate respiratory distress, or if a patient is found unconscious and, when ventilation is attempted, the chest cannot be made to rise and fall as usual during mouth-to-mouth resuscitation. The Heimlich maneuver must be performed in the manner required for this emergency.

Fainting and convulsive seizures may occur with little or no warning. The RT should be able to recognize these problems and protect the patient from injuries caused by aspiration of saliva or vomitus, by falls, or by hitting his head or extremities against hard surfaces.

The RT must know where emergency drugs, oxygen, suction equipment, and other supplies are kept in the diagnostic imaging department. When the radiologist and the emergency medical personnel have come to the patient's assistance, the RT should stay close by to offer assistance as needed.

It is the RT's professional obligation to be prepared to administer basic life support procedures to adults and children. He must keep his classroom training current by taking a refresher course as recommended by specialists in this medical care.

Chapter 5, pre-post test

_____ 1. General signs and symptoms that the RT must learn to recognize as probable indicators that his patient is in shock area are the following:
   a. Strong, irregular pulse; hypertension; flushed face; noisy respirations
   b. Aggressive behavior, acetone breath, convulsions, and decreased temperature
   c. Decreased temperature; weak, thready pulse; rapid heartbeat; hypotension; and skin pallor
   d. Deep, shallow respirations; hot, flushed skin; confusion; and decreased pulse rate

_____ 2. For what reason is anaphylactic shock the type of shock most often seen in diagnostic imaging?
   a. Patients who come for diagnostic imaging procedures are weak and debilitated
   b. Iodinated contrast agents are frequently used
   c. Patients here have more allergies
   d. X-radiation causes this problem

_____ 3. Early signs and symptoms of anaphylactic reaction are
   a. Choking, dyspnea, and cyanosis
   b. Hypertension; pallor; a calm, relaxed facies
   c. Itching, sneezing, and apprehension
   d. Hypotension; weak, rapid pulse; dilated pupils

_____ 4. Myrtle Maywriter is a 43-year-old female who has come to diagnostic imaging this morning from her home for an upper GI series. After she has been in the room for a short time, she begins to complain of a severe headache. Shortly after that, you notice that she has cold, clammy skin and speaks in a slurred manner. You suspect that Ms. Maywriter is
   a. A diabetic and is having a ketoacidotic reaction
   b. Having a cardiac arrest
   c. An alcoholic and is drunk
   d. An epileptic and is having a seizure
   e. A diabetic and is having a hypoglycemic reaction

_____ 5. Your immediate emergency treatment of Ms. Maywriter's (question 4) problem would include
   a. To prepare for oxygen administration and call the emergency team
   b. Check for an identification of the patient as a diabetic, give her some form of concentrated sugar, and notify the physician in charge
   c. Place the patient in a supine position, keep her warm, and call the emergency team
   d. Continue with your work, do not leave the patient alone, and stop the IV

_____ 6. Symptoms of a partially obstructed airway may include
   a. Cold, clammy skin; pallor; weakness; anxiety
   b. Flushed, hot skin; hyperactivity; confusion; seizures
   c. Labored, noisy breathing; wheezing; use of neck muscles to assist
   d. Acetone breath, irregular pulse, noisy respirations, rapid heartbeat, flushed skin

_____ 7. A 16-year-old male patient comes into the diagnostic imaging department for a computerized tomography examination. He is lying on the table in a supine position. He suddenly seems to lose consciousness and begins to move violently, with jerking motions. You realize that he is having a grand mal seizure. The action that you must take is
   a. Go to the patient immediately and restrain him gently
   b. Call for help, but do not leave the patient
   c. Place the patient on the floor and begin CPR

   d. a and b
   e. a, b, and c

_____ 8. Fainting is a common medical emergency in the diagnostic imaging department. If a patient appears to be fainting, the first thing that the RT should do is
   a. Assist the patient to a safe position and then call for help
   b. Give smelling salts
   c. Get the emergency cart
   d. Prepare to administer oxygen

9. Match the following items:
   _e_ 1. Hypovolemic shock
   _H_ 2. Cerebral vascular accident
   _B_ 3. Airway obstruction
   _D_ 4. Cardiogenic shock
   _C_ 5. Anaphylactic shock

   a. Difficult speech; severe headache; one-sided, drooping eye and face; loss of consciousness
   b. Choking, inability to speak, eventual loss of consciousness
   c. Itching of eyes, apprehensiveness, wheezing, choking
   d. Loss of consciousness; decreased BP; weak, rapid pulse
   e. Pallor; thirst; cold, clammy skin; restlessness

10. List the questions that the RT must ask a patient prior to the patient's receiving an iodinated contrast agent.

11. Compare the symptoms of diabetic ketoacidosis, hyperosmolar coma, and hypoglycemia.

Laboratory reinforcement

All RT students must take a formal class in cardiopulmonary resuscitation and emergency treatment of airway obstruction. This will include laboratory practice of these emergency measures.

1. Using a fellow student or a mannequin as a patient, demonstrate the jaw-thrust method of clearing the airway.

2. Using a mannequin or a fellow student, demonstrate opening and clearing the mouth of foreign material before beginning CPR.

3. Demonstrate the position in which a patient should be placed following a convulsive seizure.

Chapter Six
Care of Patients with Special Problems

Goal of this chapter:

The RT student will be able to make the necessary modifications in his work when dealing with the patient who is very ill, severely injured, very young or very old, confused, agitated, or combative.

Behavioral objectives:

When the student has completed this chapter, he will be able to do the following:
1. List the special care considerations necessary in diagnostic imaging when the patient is an infant or child
2. Demonstrate safe methods of restraining a pediatric patient
3. List the special problems of the geriatric patient in diagnostic imaging and the special care required for them
4. List the precautions to be taken by the RT if the patient has a head injury
5. List the precautions to be taken by the RT if the patient has facial injuries
6. List the precautions to be taken by the RT if the patient has a possible spinal cord injury
7. List the precautions to be taken by the RT if the patient has a fracture or possible fracture
8. List the precautions to be taken by the RT if the patient is confused, agitated, or assaultive

Glossary

Asymmetrical lacks similarity of form or arrangement on either side of a dividing line or plane; not balanced or proportional

Buccal mucosa cheek membrane

Cerebrospinal fluid clear liquid surrounding the brain and spinal cord as protection from physical impact

Cholecystitis inflammation of the gallbladder

Conjunctival thin, transparent membrane lining eyelids

Ecchymosis an oozing of blood from a vessel into tissues, forming a discolored area of various sizes on the skin

Emesis sudden removal through the mouth of stomach contents; vomiting

Etiologies study of causes of diseases

Flaccid paralysis loss of muscle tone; atrophy and degeneration of muscle and loss of tendon reflexes; flabby and weak

Gait manner of moving or walking

Geriatrics the branch of medicine that deals with all aspects of aging including pathologic (diseases) and sociological problems of old age

Homeostasis automatic maintenance of normal, internal stability of the body by coordinated responses of all the systems

Hypovolemic diminished blood volume

Hypoxia decrease in the oxygen supplied to, or utilized by, the body

Pancreatitis an inflammation of the pancreas

Paresthesia abnormal sensation of numbness or prickling skin surfaces

Pediatric concerning the development and care of infants and children and with the treatment of their diseases

Priapism abnormal, painful, and continued erection of the penis caused by disease or spinal cord injury, usually without sexual desire

Psychosis a major mental disorder in which the person has lost contact

with reality; two types: functional or organic
Pulmonary congestion fluid filling the lungs

Trauma a physical injury or an emotional shock, either of which can be very painful
Ulcer an open sore or lesion of the skin or internal organ accompanied by sloughing of inflamed dead tissue

Visceral internal organs and their muscles contained within the body cavity, e.g., intestinal muscles

Pediatric patients range in age from infancy to 14 years of age. Children in this broad age group require special care, depending on their age and their ability to understand. In the RT's initial assessment of each child he must first determine the age of the child and then decide how he will be able to relate most successfully to that child.

The infant will often be accompanied by worried parents. They will be the persons to whom the examination or procedure should be explained. Older children, however, will need a personal explanation. In all cases, though, care of the pediatric patient in diagnostic imaging requires that the RT be honest and gentle, but firm.

The elderly patient also has special needs. As a person ages, there is a gradual decline of all bodily functions. This decline varies with each person, so the RT must assess the aged patient's abilities in order to determine what adaptations he will want to make to keep the patient safe and comfortable during the diagnostic procedure or treatment.

Occasionally the RT will be required to care for a patient who is confused, agitated, or combative. A patient with this kind of problem will require special consideration in order to protect both patient and RT from injury.

The patient may have a fracture, a spinal cord injury, facial injuries, or acute abdominal pain. Acutely ill or injured patients are usually first admitted to the emergency suite and are then sent to the diagnostic imaging department for emergency radiographs to determine the extent of the injury or to diagnose the illness. In such cases, the patient may not be able to be transferred, and the RT will then have to take the diagnostic radiographs right in the emergency suite. As a rule, the RT is taught to make perfect exposures, but in emergency situations such as these, such quality may not be possible. He must settle for the best exposures that the situation allows without extending the injury or causing the patient extreme pain and discomfort. The RT must exercise great care and understanding when dealing with patients suffering from traumatic injuries and with the critically ill.

The pediatric patient

Children of all ages respond in a positive manner to honesty and friendliness. A small child may be very frightened when he enters the diagnostic imaging department and sees the darkened rooms and the massive equipment. If the RT spends a few moments establishing rapport with the child and acquainting him with the new environment, he will save himself a great deal of time later. The work will proceed more smoothly, and the RT will have a more secure and content patient.

Children are resistant to immediate close contact with strangers. Therefore, it is best to talk at a comfortable distance and allow the child to become accustomed to your presence before you approach him. The RT must explain just what is going to occur during the procedure to the child who is old enough to understand. He should also tell how long the procedure will last and what will be expected of the patient. The child should be prepared for any discomfort that he may feel. If he is to receive medication, the method of administration should be explained. Explanations to children are most effective if they are brief, simple, and to the point. Do not give the child choices when this is not appropriate because this may be confusing to him.

Parents who accompany their child to diagnostic imaging will feel less anxious if they too are given an explanation of the treatment or procedure. Using the therapeutic communication techniques described in Chapter 1, allow the parent to voice concerns as you respond in a therapeutic manner. It may be of help to the RT and the child if the parent is enlisted to assist the RT. The small child is more responsive to a parent's request and will allow the parent to dress or hold him without feeling the anxiety that might be present if a stranger were to do so. However, in some departments regulations do not permit parents to participate so this will be out of the question.

Transporting infants and children

The RT will be responsible for transporting infants and children from place to place in the diagnostic imaging department and may be responsible for transporting them to the department from their hospital rooms. This must be done with care to prevent injuring the young patient.

The method of transfer will depend on the child's size and the nature of the illness or injury. Under most circumstances, it is safe to carry infants and very small children for short distances, *i.e.*, from one diagnostic imaging room to another. For longer distances, it will be necessary to place them in a crib

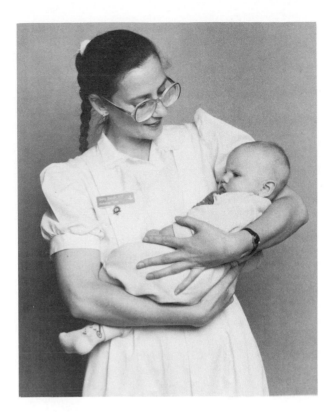

Figure 6-1

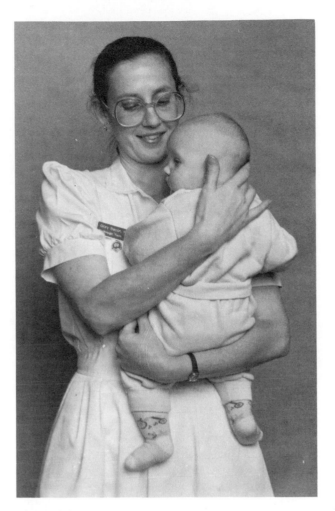

Figure 6-2

with all sides up and locked. Older children may be transported on a gurney with side rails up and locked and a safety belt attached. Some older children may prefer to be transported in a wheelchair. If this means of transportation is appropriate, the safety belt must be securely fastened for the entire time that they are seated in the wheelchair. Children must never be left alone while in diagnostic imaging. If they are placed on a radiographic table, an attendant must be at their side until the procedure is complete and they are taken from the procedure room.

It is necessary to provide back support for infants or small children if they are being held or carried. This may be done in a horizontal hold with the child supported against your body with the head supported on your arm at the elbow and your hand grasping the patient's thigh (Fig. 6-1). Another method of holding an infant or small child is upright with the buttocks resting on the RT's arm and the other arm around the infant supporting the back and head (Fig. 6-2).

Restraining the anxious child

Occasionally the very anxious child will not be able to stay quietly in one place long enough for a successful diagnostic procedure to be completed, and he will have to be restrained. In other situations, a child may not be able to be safely held in position for an examination and restraints will be necessary. Restraints should be used only when no other means are safe or logical and should be of a quality that will not cause injury to the patient.

There are several methods of restraining children. A restraint can be made by folding a sheet in a specified manner, or there are commercial restraints that are effective for certain procedures. The child may also be held in position by one or two assistants. Whatever type of restraint that is chosen, the child who is old enough must be made to understand before the restraint is applied that this is not a method of punishment. His parents must also be informed of the use of the restraint and the reason for it.

If a child is to be physically restrained by an assistant during an examination, the RT must instruct the assistant not to be too forceful in his hold. Care should be taken not to pinch or bruise the skin or to interfere with circulation. It is better to use a sheet or mechanical restraint than to have the assistant use force, because the former is less frightening to a child. In order to prevent a small child from rolling his head from side to side, the person holding the child should stand at the head of the table and support the child's head between his hands, making sure that there is no pressure on the ears or on the fontanels. Any person who holds a child during a radiographic examination must wear a protective lead covering.

SHEET RESTRAINTS

Sheet restraints are effective and can easily be formed into any size or fashion desired. To make a sheet restraint, take a large sheet and fold it lengthwise. Place the top of the sheet at the child's shoulders and the bottom at his feet. Leave the greater portion of the sheet at one side of the child. Bring the longer side back over the arm and under the body and other arm. Next, bring the sheet back over the exposed arm and under the body again. This type of restraint keeps the two arms safely and completely restrained and leaves the abdomen exposed (Fig. 6-3).

MUMMY-STYLE SHEET RESTRAINTS

Another method of restraint is the mummy-style sheet restraint. It is made by folding a sheet or a blanket into a triangle and placing it on the radiographic table. The distance from the fold to the lower corner of the sheet should be twice the length of the child. Place the child onto the sheet, with the folds slightly above the shoulders. Loosen or remove the child's clothes. Bring one corner of the sheet over one arm and under the child's body. If both arms are to be restrained, do the same with the other side of the sheet. If the legs are to be restrained, turn the

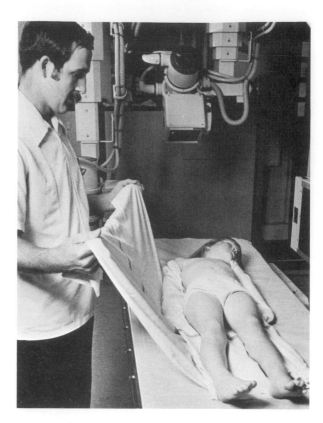

Figure 6-4

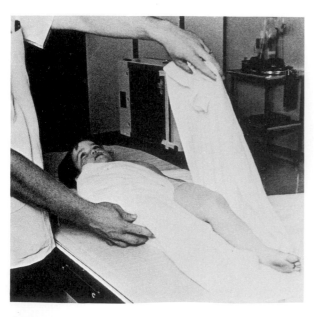

Figure 6-3

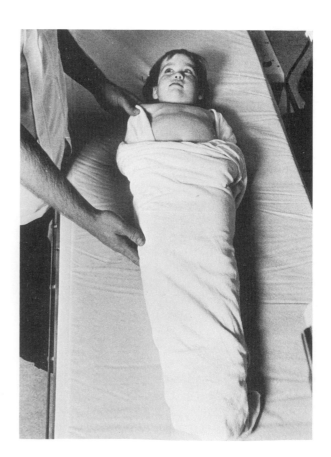

Figure 6-5

sheet and repeat the procedure for the legs (Fig. 6-4). This restraint can be used to restrain one extremity or all extremities (Fig. 6-5).

COMMERCIAL RESTRAINTS

There are commercial restraints that are also recommended. The Pigg-o-stat is a mechanical restraint that is excellent for holding a child safely in an upright position (Fig. 6-6). It is useful for making exposures of the chest or upright abdominal exposures. Another restraint is a plastic mold that has straps to hold the extremities (Fig. 6-7). If it is available, this is the best type of restraint for a procedure such as an intravenous pyelogram.

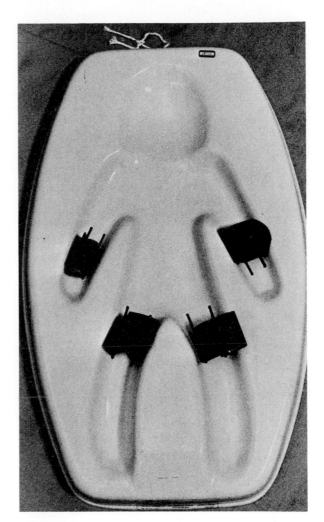

Figure 6-7

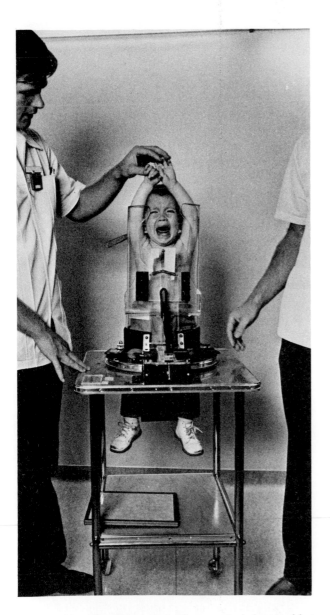

Figure 6-6.   The Pigg-o-stat. The cassette is inserted into slots directly in front of the child.

The geriatric patient

Throughout the life cycle, the body undergoes normal physiologic and anatomic changes. These changes occur at different times from person to person, so one is not able to generalize and say that all persons aged 65 begin to age in a uniform manner. Lifestyle as well as hereditary factors contributes greatly to the aging process.

Generally speaking, as the body ages, the bones become less dense, and fractures occur more easily. This is especially true of the vertebral bodies and the femur. The RT must keep this in mind when moving the elderly patient or directing him to move, because even a slight deviation in the usual pattern of movement may cause a fracture.

As the aging process continues, body tissues lose elasticity. Both the speed and the strength of muscle response diminish. This decrease in tissue elasticity affects the lungs particularly which do not expand and contract as effectively as they did earlier. This in turn increases the likelihood that pulmonary congestion and pneumonia may develop.

The blood vessels also lose their elasticity. This loss may eventually lead to an increase in blood pressure and a decrease in effective circulation to all body parts, which could affect the body's ability to resist infection and to heal.

Because of these factors, the RT must remember that the elderly person tolerates position changes and temperature changes poorly. Allowing the head to be lowered for a long period during an examination may cause the vessels in the head to become engorged and circulation to the extremities to become impaired. If the patient is expected to remain with his feet lowered for long periods, the blood may collect in the lower extremities and cause dizziness or fainting.

Circulatory impairment also causes the nervous system to become less sensitive to pain, heat, and cold. The RT must remember this because the elderly person will become chilled much more quickly than a younger one will. To prevent this problem, offer a blanket or flannel sheet if the patient is to be in one position for any length of time. Skin can easily be traumatized without the patient's awareness until after the injury has occurred, so it is the RT's responsibility to prevent this by using the techniques learned in Chapter 3.

The gag reflex also diminishes with age, and the patient may choke more easily than when he was young. This must be considered when giving contrast agents by mouth to the elderly patient.

The liver, heart, kidneys, and other vital organs continue to function normally as long as the body is not subjected to undue stress. However, even a slight change in normal routine may disturb physiologic homeostasis in the body of the elderly patient. This is important for the RT to remember—if the elderly patient is required to fast prior to a diagnostic examination, the examination should be scheduled for an early morning hour so that the patient can have his breakfast close to the usual time.

The mental processes of the elderly may also diminish. The elderly person who is kept in bed or who is in an unfamiliar environment may become confused. This is likely to happen in an unfamiliar area such as the diagnostic imaging department, especially after a long examination. The RT must be ready to assist the patient back to the dressing room or to the lavatory, because the stress of the examination may cause him to become forgetful. Be certain that the patient is attended before leaving him. The hospitalized patient must be assisted off the diagnostic imaging table and back to his hospital room and back to bed.

Hearing and eyesight are often affected by the aging process; however, the RT must not assume that all aged persons are deaf and blind. He must assess their ability to see and hear. If necessary, he should speak to the patient in an altered manner, but should not automatically raise his voice to all grey-haired people. Often, when a patient has difficulty hearing, it is more effective to speak in a normal voice close to the person's ear.

Increased anxiety may affect the elderly person's ability to interpret directions. To decrease the patient's anxiety level, you should give directions in a quiet area and restate the message as often as necessary. Never give an elderly patient a list of directions to read or a list of verbal instructions and expect that they will be able to understand and follow them. Go over the list with them and have them repeat what the directions state until you are certain that they understand the message.

The patient with a head injury

Injuries to the head are exceedingly common. Each year approximately 10 million head injuries are predicted to occur in the United States. The term *head injury* may refer to any injury of the skull, the brain, or both, which requires medical attention. The RT will be called upon frequently to make diagnostic radiographs of patients brought into the emergency suite with a head injury. These injuries are all potentially serious because they may involve the brain, which is the seat of consciousness and controls every human action.

There are two basic types of head injury, open and closed. With an open injury to the skull or meninges, the brain is vulnerable to damage and infection because its protective casing has been broken. If the injury is closed (also called a *blunt injury*), the brain tissue may swell; the swelling is limited by the confines of the skull, and the resulting pressure may cause extensive brain damage. The brain has little healing power, so any injury to it must be considered potentially permanent and serious.

Fractures at the base of the skull *(basal skull fractures)* often have accompanying fractures of the facial bones. This type of injury may result in a tear in the *dura*, the outer membrane surrounding the brain and spinal cord, and a leakage of cerebral spinal fluid may result.

The RT must consider all patients with head injuries to have accompanying cervical spinal injuries until it is medically disproven. Precautions to alleviate potential extention of these injuries must be taken as a matter of routine.

Signs and symptoms of head injury

Closed injury:
  Varying levels of consciousness ranging from drowsiness, confusion, irritability, and stupor to coma

Lucid periods followed by periods of unconsciousness possible

Loss of reflexes

Changes in vital signs

Headache, visual disturbances, dizziness, and giddiness

Gait abnormalities

Unequal pupil dilatation

Seizures, vomiting, and hemiparesis

Open injury:
Abrasions, contusions, or lacerations apparent on the skull

A break or penetration in the skull or meninges apparent by inspection or on radiographs

Basal fractures may result in leakage of cerebrospinal fluid demonstrated by leakage of blood on the sheet or dressing surrounded by a yellowish stain (the halo sign). Cerebrospinal fluid may leak from the nose, ears, or as a postnasal drip

Varying levels of consciousness

Subconjunctival hemorrhage

Hearing loss

Periorbital ecchymosis (raccoon's eyes)

Facial nerve palsy

RT Action
Keep the head and neck immobilized until injury to the cervical spine is ruled out.

Do not remove sandbags, collars, or dressings; make all radiographs with these in place.

Wear sterile gloves if in contact with open wounds to prevent infection.

Check the patient's vital signs frequently while working with him. Airway obstruction may occur as the result of absence of gag reflex, relaxation of the tongue, or the presence of blood and other products of drainage in the throat.

Apply a sterile pressure dressing if bleeding is profuse, and call for assistance.

Observe the patient for signs and symptoms of hypoxia, changes in level of consciousness, and respiratory arrest.

Notify the nurse or the physician in charge of the patient immediately if any changes occur.

Head-injury patients must not be suctioned through the nasal passages. RTs do not suction but may be called upon to assist with the procedure (Chapter 8).

Be prepared to assist with administration of oxygen and other emergency treatment if the patient's condition requires it.

The patient with a facial injury

Injuries to the facial bones are usually associated with injury to the soft tissues of the face. Often these injuries do not seem serious, but they are all potentially disfiguring. The RT must treat all patients who have serious facial injuries as if they also have basal skull fractures and injuries of the cervical spine until such injuries are ruled out.

Signs and symptoms
Misalignment of the face or teeth

Pain at site of injury

Ecchymosis of the floor of mouth and buccal mucosa

Distortion of facial symmetry

Inability to close the jaw

Edema

Abnormal movement of face or jaw

Flatness of the cheek

Loss of sensation on side of injury

Diplopia (double vision)

Blindness caused by detached retina

Nosebleed

Conjunctival hemorrhage

Paresthesia

Halo sign (indicates basal skull fracture with leaking cerebrospinal fluid)

Changes in level of consciousness; unconscious patient may have respiratory distress or failure caused by obstruction of tongue, loose teeth, bleeding or other body fluids in airway.

RT actions
Observe for airway obstruction. Watch for noisy, labored respirations.

Do not remove sandbags, collars, or other supportive devices or move a patient unless supervised by his physician.

Apply a sterile pressure dressing if bleeding is profuse, and call for assistance.

Patient must not be suctioned through nasal passages.

Wear sterile gloves if in contact with open wounds.

If you find teeth that have fallen out, place them in a container moistened with gauze soaked in sterile water.

Be prepared to assist with oxygen and other emergency treatment if necessary.

Observe for symptoms of shock; notify physician in charge if condition of patient or level of consciousness changes.

The patient with a spinal cord injury

The spinal cord carries messages from the brain to the peripheral nervous system. It is housed in the vertebral canal, which extends down the length of the vertebral column. The spinal column is protected by the fluid in the canal and by the vertebrae—the bony structures encircling the canal. Motor function depends on the transmission of messages from the brain to the spinal nerves on either side of the spinal cord. Injury to or severing of the spinal cord causes message transmission to cease. The result is a cessation of motor function and partial or complete cessation of physical function from the level of damage to the cord to all parts below that level.

Most spinal cord injuries occur in the cervical or lumbar areas because these are the most mobile parts of the spinal column. The spinal cord loses its protection when there is injury to the protective vertebrae, and such an injury may result in compression or complete severing of the cord. Cord tissue, like brain tissue, has little healing power; injuries to it usually cause permanent damage.

Signs and symptoms

Complete transection of spinal cord:
Flaccid paralysis of the skeletal muscles below the level of the injury

Loss of all sensation (touch, pain, temperature, or pressure) below the level of injury; pain at site of injury possible

Absence of somatic and visceral sensations below the site of the injury

Unstable, lowered blood pressure

Loss of ability to perspire below level of injury

Bowel and bladder incontinence

Possible priapism in male

Partial transection of spinal cord:
Asymmetrical, flaccid paralysis below level of injury

Asymmetrical loss of reflexes

Some sensory retention: feeling of pain, temperature, pressure, and touch

Some somatic and visceral sensation

More stable blood pressure

Ability to perspire intact unilaterally

Possible priapism in male

RT actions

Monitor vital signs with special attention to respiration.

Maintain an open airway; call for assistance if respirations become noisy or labored.

Do not allow or request patient to move for radiographs until diagnosis is confirmed and physician supervises moves.

Do not move head or neck even if it is in an awkward position.

Do not remove sand bags, collars, antishock garments, or other supports until diagnosis is confirmed and patient's physician supervises move.

Observe for signs and symptoms of shock, and prepare to assist with emergency CPR. If in respiratory failure, use jaw thrust maneuver to move jaw downward.

If patient is a trauma victim and is unconscious, assume spinal cord injury and treat as such until directed to do otherwise by the patient's physician.

When patient is to be moved, do so with at least four persons assisting and the physician supervising using the log roll method (see Chapter 3).

The patient with a fractured extremity

A fracture may be defined as a disturbance in the continuity of a bone. Fractures can be classified simply as open or closed. The term *open* fracture indicates a visible wound that extends between the fracture and the skin surface. The broken bone itself often breaks through the soft tissue, making the fracture clearly visible.

A *closed* fracture may not be obvious to the untrained eye. Often there is swelling around the injured area, pain, and a deformity of the limb. All or some of these symptoms may be absent and a closed fracture still be present.

Internal injuries caused by fractures of the pelvic bones are a leading cause of death following automobile accidents. The RT caring for trauma patients must always consider the possibility of a fractured pelvis when caring for patients with traumatic injuries. Extreme caution must be used when making initial diagnostic radiographs because the slightest movement may initiate hemorrhage or irreparable damage to a vital organ.

Hip fractures are common accidents in elderly patients as a result of bony changes related to age and disease. This is a common home accident for elderly patients. They too must be treated with the utmost care in diagnostic imaging to prevent any extension of injuries.

Signs and symptoms

Pain and swelling

Functional loss

Deformity of the limb

Grating sound or feel of grating (crepitus) if moved

Discoloration of surrounding tissue caused by hemorrhage within tissue (in closed fracture)

Overt bleeding (open fracture)

Possible signs and symptoms of shock

RT actions

Do not move affected limb or body part.

Patient move must be done under direction of physician in charge of patient's care.

If patient is to be moved, inform him and enlist his support.

Do not remove splints or any type of supports.

If moving a splinted limb, support the joint above and below the fracture, and at the joints.

Move it with one person at the distal end and one at the proximal end. On signal, the limb must be moved with support and as a single unit (Fig. 6-8).

If it is an open fracture, wear sterile gloves if in contact with wound, and use strict infection-control measures.

Observe the patient for signs and symptoms of shock, and be prepared to act if that emergency occurs.

The patient with acute abdominal distress

There are many reasons for acute abdominal pain. Among them are internal injuries that cause hemorrhage, appendicitis, bleeding ulcers, ectopic pregnancy, cholecystitis, pancreatitis, and bowel obstruction. Whatever the cause of the distress, the symptoms are somewhat similar, and for the RT's purposes, may be grouped together. It will be the RT's responsibility to make the diagnostic radiographs as quickly as possible and with the least possible discomfort to the patient. An assistant may be needed to help position and move the patient because he may be too ill to assist. Patients in acute abdominal

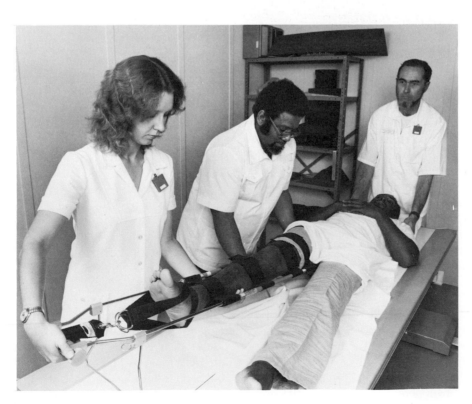

Figure 6-8

distress are frequently sent to the operating room for a surgical procedure following diagnosis.

Signs and symptoms of acute abdominal distress

Severe abdominal pain

A rigid abdomen

Nausea and vomiting

Extreme thirst

Possible symptoms of hypovolemic shock

RT actions

Call for assistance if the patient is too ill to help move himself.

If the patient is unable to stand for upright exposures, use other means of obtaining necessary diagnostic information.

Transport the patient by gurney.

Have an emesis basin and tissues nearby in case vomiting occurs.

Do not give the patient anything to eat or drink.

Observe for signs and symptoms of shock, and be prepared for emergency treatment.

The agitated or confused patient

Patients with emotional problems may come to the emergency suite for treatment that requires diagnostic radiographs, or patients who are hospitalized in mental health units may require diagnostic imaging procedures. These patients are frequently agitated or confused and may become combative. This behavior may be caused by chemical abuse or psychosis of varying etiologies. At times, the confused elderly patient forgets that he is not at home and mistakes the RT for an intruder from whom he must protect himself by attack. Whatever the cause, the RT must take precautions to protect himself and the patient when this type of behavior is threatened.

Patients whom the RT can predict will demonstrate combative behavior are those who have a history of such outbursts or a history of growing confusion and disorientation. Other warning signals are increasing agitation demonstrated by rapid pacing back and forth across the room; a patient in animated and increasingly noisy conversation with a person who is not present; a demonstration of illogical thought processes; refusal to cooperate; distrust of the RT and his explanation of a procedure; examination of the diagnostic imaging room or equipment unnecessarily. Patients who are combative may occasionally display no emotion at all or display irrational fear of a procedure.

Patients who react in a combative or aggressive manner usually do so because they feel that they have no control of what is happening to them. They resort to violent behavior as a means of self-protection.

Before approaching a patient who is not reacting in a rational manner, the RT should discuss the case with the nursing personnel or with the patient's physician. If the patient is behaving in a combative manner or has a history of combativeness, the RT should request assistance with the examination. Trust your instincts about a patient's behavior. Do not isolate yourself with a potentially assaultive patient. Always have a door open, and position yourself so that you are able to leave the room if necessary. If you feel that the patient is apt to become violent, do not begin the procedure without assistance from a person who can protect you and the patient if necessary. The person often chosen to assist in these situations is a security officer.

At times, patients who are agitated or confused react more favorably to persons of one sex or another. If this seems to be the case, have an RT of the preferred sex conduct the procedure.

When approaching a patient who is agitated or confused, do so from the side, not face to face. Never touch a confused or agitated patient without first asking his permission and explaining what you are planning to do. Use simple, concise statements to explain your purpose. If the patient is speaking in a delusional or irrational manner, do not become involved in his conversation. To do so might increase his agitation. If the patient refuses to be radiographed, simply stop what you are doing and return him to his quarters. Explain that you will complete the examination at a later time. To continue to work with an agitated and confused person who is belligerent may cause injury to the RT or to the patient.

If the radiograph is essential to the patient's treatment, he will have to be restrained and supervised by persons in the hospital who are educated to care for such patients.

If the situation escalates beyond control and the patient is actually prepared to strike you, put as much distance as possible between yourself and him. Speak in a calm but firm voice to the patient. Let him know that you are uneasy and ask what can be done to appease him. Ally yourself with the patient by statements such as, "You must be really angry at the people here for putting you through all of these tests." If this does not work, get out of the area and summon help. Do not approach the patient or make any effort to take anything out of his hands.

Summary

The pediatric patient ranges in age from infancy to 14 years of age. The RT must relate to all patients with whom he works in an appropriate and specific manner, regardless of their ages. The infant is usually accompanied by his parents. The RT should attempt to ease their anxiety by giving them an explanation of the procedure to be performed and the approximate amount of time it will take. If it is necessary to restrain the child, the reasons for this procedure should be explained to the child if he is old enough to understand and to his parents. If it is necessary to restrain a child, a restraint made of soft material such as a sheet may be used. If the child is to be restrained by being held, it should be done in a firm, safe manner in order to prevent injury to the child. An RT should never place his body over a child as a restraint. A sheet restraint or a commercial one is less traumatic and more effective. Protective lead aprons should be worn by persons restraining a child.

The RT must assess each elderly patient in order to determine his special needs. The physical limitations brought about by the aging process vary with the individual. The RT would be incorrect if he were to make general assumptions about all persons who are over 65 years of age.

Patients with a spinal cord injury must be moved in a specific manner and only with specific directions from the physician in charge. Supportive devices should not be removed without physician's orders.

Patients with head injuries and facial injuries should be treated as though they also have spinal cord injuries until it is verified that they do not. Basal skull fractures must also be considered if the patient has injuries to the facial bones. Patients with these injuries should not be moved for initial diagnostic radiographs without orders from the physician in charge of their care and with his supervision.

While the RT is working with trauma patients, he should be observing for changes in the level of consciousness, mental status, hemorrhage, shock, and respiratory distress. Patients with fractured extremities should also be moved with great care and under their physician's supervision so that the movement does not increase their pain or extend the injury. If splints or antishock garments are in place, they must not be removed. Strict aseptic practices must be used for patients with open fractures to prevent infection.

Acute abdominal distress is also classified as an emergency. Patients with acute abdominal pain are often very ill and are unable to assist the RT. Radiographs should be made as quickly and gently as possible. An assistant should be on hand to help the RT move the patient in severe pain. The patient may not be able to stand upright while the exposures are being made. If this is so, other methods of obtaining the diagnostic information necessary must be used. Transport these patients by gurney.

The RT may have to work with patients who are agitated, confused, and potentially assaultive. The cause may be chemical abuse, psychosis, or confusion caused by stress, as is occasionally the case in the elderly patient. The RT must be cautious in his approach to patients with this type of problem in order to protect himself and the patient from injury. If the patient refuses treatment, the RT should immediately comply with his refusal and return him to his quarters. If the radiographs are essential to the patient's treatment, the RT should be assisted by personnel who are educated in the care of mentally disturbed patients.

Chapter 6, pre-post test

_____ 1. When caring for a pediatric patient, the best method of transport is always
   a. A gurney
   b. Carrying the child
   c. A crib
   d. Depends on the distance involved and the age of the child

_____ 2. When an RT must schedule an elderly patient for a difficult diagnostic examination, it is best to schedule the examination for
   a. Evening hours, so that the patient has the day to rest
   b. Early morning hours so that the patient can have breakfast as close to the usual time as possible
   c. In the middle of the day so that traffic is less hectic
   d. At a time that is best for you

_____ 3. The RT must consider that all patients with head injuries may also have
   a. Fractures
   b. Seizures
   c. Shock
   d. Cervical spine injuries
   e. Changes in vital signs

_____ 4. What precaution(s) must the RT follow when taking radiographic exposures of a patient who has a head injury?
   a. Keep the head and neck immobilized until

cervical spine injury is ruled out by the physician in charge
b. Wear sterile gloves if there are open wounds
c. Check the patient's vital signs frequently
d. a and b
e. a, b, and c

_____ 5. What precaution(s) must the RT take when caring for a patient with a fractured extremity?
a. Support the joint above and below the fracture and at the joints if moving a splinted limb
b. Do not remove splints without direction of the physician in charge
c. Inform the patient before you move his fractured limb
d. none
e. a, b, and c

_____ 6. When caring for a 6-year-old child, the RT should
a. Explain the procedure to the patient in great detail
b. Tell the patient that there will be no pain or discomfort, regardless of the type of examination
c. Be friendly, honest, and concise in his explanation to the child
d. Routinely restrain the child to be examined

_____ 7. Physiologic changes that come with aging that should be considered by the RT as he works with the elderly patient include
a. A loss of the sensation of pain
b. A loss of sensitivity to heat or cold
c. A diminishing gag reflex
d. A loss of the sense of humor
e. An insensitivity to the manner of the RT's approach

_____ 8. You have been assigned to radiograph Mr. J.J. He has been transported by the local police to the emergency room of the hospital in which you are employed. He is complaining of severe pain in his right leg. As you approach the patient you notice that he is walking rapidly up and down the corridor. His head is bent and he is talking rapidly to persons who are not present. He occasionally stops, looks up at the ceiling, and shouts that he has to "get them." Your best manner of dealing with this situation would be to
a. Walk directly up to the patient, introduce yourself, and explain your purpose in being there
b. Get an assistant, approach the patient from his side, stop slightly away from him and explain your purpose
c. Tell the emergency-room nurse to forget it
d. Have the male orderlies restrain the patient

_____ 9. Assessment of the elderly should include
a. Ability to see and hear
b. Ability to move without assistance
c. Level of understanding
d. a and b
e. a, b, and c

_____ 10. List three factors that the RT must consider when caring for the patient with acute abdominal distress.

_____ 11. If the agitated patient refuses to be radiographed, the RT should
a. Ask the patient to cooperate for just one more minute
b. Explain what he is going to do in short, concise sentences
c. Call for help
d. Stop immediately and return the patient to his quarters

_____ 12. Special care is necessary when caring for a patient whose brain or spinal cord might be injured, because
a. Extreme pain may result from the movement
b. This type of injury heals slowly
c. The incidence of infection is high
d. These tissues have a very little ability to heal

Laboratory reinforcement

1. In the school laboratory, using a mannequin, demonstrate moving a patient who has a fractured femur.

2. Demonstrate in the school laboratory, using a pediatric mannequin, three methods of restraining a child.

Chapter Seven
Patient Care for Barium Studies

Goal of this chapter:

The RT will be able to differentiate between the two types of contrast used in diagnostic imaging, explain and demonstrate the patient preparation necessary for each, and his responsibilities to the patient when they are in progress.

Behavioral objectives:

When the student has completed this chapter, he will be able to do the following:
1. Explain the patient-teaching responsibilities of the RT before, during, and after barium studies, and list content that must be included in each of these teaching presentations
2. Differentiate between positive and negative contrast agents
3. List the medical complications that may result from the administration of barium sulfate
4. List the medical complications that may result from the administration of negative contrast agents
5. List the types of cleansing enemas, demonstrate administration of a cleansing enema in the laboratory, and describe the precautions that must be taken during this procedure
6. List the precautions to be taken when assisting with barium studies
7. Describe the special care considerations when a patient with an ostomy is to receive a barium enema.

Glossary

Anal sphincter circular muscle constricting the outer rectal opening

Aspiration pneumonia inflammation of the lungs caused primarily by foreign matter taken into respiratory tract during inspiration

Barium granuloma a formation of fiberlike growth of intestinal matter mixed with barium usually caused by a perforation

Barium studies radiographic examinations of the digestive system involving administration of barium sulfate

Castile soap a fine, mild soap prepared from olive oil and sodium hydroxide

Catheter a hollow tube passed through the body for removing or injecting fluids into body cavities

Colostomy a surgical procedure that creates an opening between the colon and the abdominal surface of the body

Contrast agent or medium a radiopaque substance used to visualize the soft tissue structures of body systems that blend together and cannot be imaged without the use of a contrast medium

Diverticulitis inflammation of a sac or pouch protruding from walls of the intestines, especially in the colon

Enemas introduction of solutions into rectum and colon to stimulate bowel activity and clean out lower intestine; or as diagnostic aid in x-ray examination of colon with injection of barium sulfate solution

Enterostomal therapist one who is trained to assist patients who have had an ostomy in learning proper methods of caring for their ostomy sites and guide them with emotional adjustment

Fecal impaction a large accumulation of hard, dry feces in the rectum or colon

Flatus expelling of gas from the digestive tract out of a body orifice

Gastric that which originates in the stomach

Gastrointestinal tract the digestive organs from the stomach through intestines forming a continuous pathway

Ileostomy an artificial opening through abdominal wall into small intestine through which feces are expelled

Interstitial space the very small areas between body parts, tissues, or within an organ

Nocturia excessive urination during the night

Perforation of GI tract the puncture or tearing of the bowel that allows contents of the bowel to escape into the abdominal cavity

Peritonitis inflammation of the serous membrane lining the abdominal cavity and surrounding the viscera (abdominal organs). Infectious organisms gain access by way of the perforation

Polyuria excessive secretion and discharge of urine in the amount of several liters above normal

Saline solution a solution consisting of 0.85% sodium (salt) chloride and distilled water considered to be isotonic (same osmolarity) as body fluids

Stoma artificially created opening between two passages and the body surface

Suspension condition of a solid when its particles are mixed with, but not dissolved in, a fluid or another solid

Barium studies and double contrast studies, which include the use of high-density barium and air, are effective methods of detecting pathologic conditions of the upper and lower gastrointestinal tract. These examinations will become routine work for the RT because they are done in great numbers, but they are not routine experiences for the patient receiving the examination. They are stressful and, at best, uncomfortable examinations, which can place the patient in physical and emotional jeopardy. This is particularly true for the very old and the very young patient. It will be the RT's responsibility to keep the patient free of anxiety and as comfortable as possible during these diagnostic procedures. He can do this by careful teaching prior to and following the examination and by thoughtful attention to the patient's needs and potential problems while the study is in progress.

Patient education

The RT as a member of the health-care team has patient-teaching responsibilities that are his professional obligation. He is the specialist in his area of health care; therefore, when the patient comes to his area for treatment, he must be certain that the patient is informed of the care about to be given. This includes the following:

1. A description of the preparation necessary prior to the procedure if correct preparation is essential

2. A description of the purpose of the test, the mechanics of the procedure, and what will be expected of the patient, for instance, frequent position changes or medication to be taken or injected

3. The approximate amount of time that the procedure will take

4. An explanation of any unusual equipment that will be used during the examination

5. The care or activities that will be necessary following the procedure

The possible adverse effects of the procedure should be addressed by the patient's physician. However, the RT must diplomatically explore the patient's knowledge of the procedure to determine if this education has been supplied to the patient. Use the techniques of therapeutic communication described in Chapter 1 to do this effectively. The RT must also be certain that procedures requiring special informed consent forms to be signed by the patient are in order.

The problem-solving process described in Chapter 1 is an effective guideline to be used for patient teaching. First a patient assessment is done to determine the patient's teaching needs; a goal is then set that delineates the expected patient-learning outcomes. A plan must be formulated for the necessary teaching, and the teaching must be evaluated for its effectiveness.

All patients will have different needs that must be met depending on the procedure that is to take place. They also have different learning styles, different levels of education, different socio-cultural backgrounds, and different levels of anxiety that will affect their ability to assimilate the data that you present. The RT must gather and analyze the data that he collects about his patient's ability and style of learning. He must then plan his presentation of the material around the patient's particular needs. Some people respond best to written instruction, some to verbal instruction, and some to an actual demonstration of the items to be used and explanation of how they work.

The RT implements his plan by presenting the information concerning the procedure to the patient in the manner planned. Following implementation, there must be an evaluation of how well the patient has learned the material. This can best be done in diagnostic imaging by the use of immediate feedback from the patient. The RT can have the patient repeat all or some of his instruction or directions and can quickly decide whether the instruction has been effective. If it appears that the patient understands the information, the RT may proceed with his work. However, if the patient seems not to have heard the instruction, it will be necessary to formulate another plan for presenting what the patient needs to know. If the patient has not understood the information or directions given, the RT must not simply proceed with his work with a feeling of frustration. The patient will be feeling the same frustration, and this will increase his anxiety, thus creating an atmosphere of distrust. The end result may be an unsatisfactory procedure.

When a diagnostic examination is completed, the RT must reinforce what he initially taught the patient concerning any follow-up treatment. The anxiety caused by the procedure itself may cause the patient to be somewhat forgetful, and consequently the patient may not remember information or directions given earlier.

Types of contrast media

There are two types of radiographic contrast agents, positive and negative. Positive contrast agents are used to increase organ density and improve radiographic visualization. Negative contrast agents decrease organ density in order to produce contrast. The most commonly used positive contrast agents are barium sulfate and iodinated preparations. The most commonly used negative agents are air, carbon dioxide, oxygen, and nitrous oxide. Iodinated contrast agents will be discussed in Chapter 12.

Negative agents

Carbon dioxide, air, oxygen, and nitrous oxide are the negative contrast agents that are most frequently used. They may be used singly or in combination with a positive contrast medium in examination of the GI tract, cholangiography, arteriography, arthrography, myelography, pneumoencephalography, and cystography. Complications associated with the use of negative contrast media usually result from inadvertent injection of air or oxygen into the bloodstream, producing an air embolus.

When the agent is injected into a joint, the patient may have residual distention of the joint and discomfort caused by gaseous medium.

Barium sulfate

Barium sulfate is the most frequently chosen contrast medium for radiologic examination of the gastrointestinal (GI) tract. It is a white, crystalline powder that is mixed with water to make a suspension. It may be administered by mouth for examination of the upper GI tract, by rectum for examination of the lower GI tract, or by infusion of a thin suspension through a duodenal tube to visualize the jejunum and ileum. The toxic effects of barium are negligible if the suspension remains within the GI tract; however, if there is a break in the gastric mucosa caused by injury or disease, the barium sulfate may pass into the peritoneal cavity or into the bloodstream and result in adverse reactions. When perforation of the GI tract is possible, an absorbable iodinated contrast medium is used in place of barium.

If barium leaks into the peritoneal cavity, peritonitis may result. This possibility increases if the barium is mixed with fecal material. Fibrosis or formation of a barium granuloma may be a further complication. The possibility of leakage of the barium into the venous circulation through a perforation in the gastric mucosa as a result of trauma or disease must also be considered. This would produce an embolus that might be fatal.

Barium sulfate is often constipating. If the patient is not properly instructed following a procedure that involves its use, he may ignore the condition rather than have it treated, and fecal impaction or a bowel obstruction may result.

If the patient reports that a previous administration of oral barium suspension produced a sensation of nausea, the radiologist should be notified before it is administered again because if the patient vomits, aspiration pneumonia might result.

Barium studies of the lower gastrointestinal tract

Proper preparation of the patient for barium studies of the lower GI tract is essential and may seem relatively complex to the patient. This preparation varies somewhat in every institution and with each patient's special needs. It will be the RT's responsibility to learn the specific procedure in his place of employment. If the patient is an outpatient, the RT may be responsible for giving him the appointment for the examination and for instructing him in the preparation. The following directions will generally apply at most institutions, with modifications for particular patients.

If time allows, the patient is instructed to eat foods low in residue for several days prior to the examination. In a low-residue diet, fresh fruits and vegetables, fatty and fried foods, whole-grain cereals and breads are excluded. The patient is encouraged to increase his fluid intake for 2 to 3 days. This regimen will help to clear the lower bowel of waste prior to the examination. Twenty-four hours prior to the examination, a clear liquid diet may be prescribed. A clear liquid diet includes coffee or tea with sugar but no milk, clear gelatin, clear broth, and carbonated beverages.

The afternoon preceding the examination, a laxative is prescribed. The type and quantity will vary depending on the size and physical condition of the patient and on the physician's preference. Laxatives should never be given to a patient without an order from the doctor in charge of the patient because they can be harmful to persons with bowel obstructions and other pathologic conditions of the lower GI tract.

Cleansing enemas are usually prescribed beginning the night before the examination or early the morning of the examination. Since there are several types and variations of cleansing enemas, the RT must become familiar with all of them and must be able to administer one if it is necessary. Occasionally a patient comes to the diagnostic imaging department with his lower bowel poorly prepared for a barium study, and it is necessary for the RT to complete the preparation in the department by giving an additional cleansing enema. By learning the procedure the RT is able to give clear directions to patients who need instruction.

The cleansing enema

The type of cleansing enema to be used is always ordered by the physician. The RT does not decide on the type of enema the patient is to receive, but he may administer a cleansing enema if it is ordered. The most frequently used cleansing enemas include the saline enema, the tap-water enema, the soap suds enema (SS enema), and the oil-retention enema.

Cleansing enemas can influence fluid and electrolyte balance in the body in varying degrees because they all have a different degree of osmolarity, which influences the movement of fluids between the colon and the interstitial spaces beyond the intestinal wall. This means that, in the presence of some cleansing solutions that are instilled into the lower bowel, the bowel extracts fluid from the surrounding interstitial spaces. This happens because the higher osmolarity of the cleansing solution (hyperosmolar) induces the fluid to move across the semipermeable membranes of the intestinal wall. The body fluid that has moved into the large intestine is then excreted from the body along with the enema solution. If an excess of body fluid is excreted from the body, the result is dehydration. This situation can be reversed. An excess of fluid with low osmolarity (hyposmolar) may be instilled into the lower bowel and absorbed into the interstitial spaces surrounding the colon, thus creating a fluid excess in the body. This is called fluid toxicity. These potential hazards must be considered when the physician orders a particular solution for use as a cleansing enema.

The saline enema

There are two types of saline enemas, normal saline and hypertonic saline. Normal saline is the safest solution to use for a cleansing enema because it has the same osmolarity as that in the interstitial spaces that surround the colon; therefore, it will not change the fluid balance in the body. It is the only safe fluid to use for cleansing enemas for children because they can tolerate very little change in fluid and electrolyte balance. This solution is also considered for the elderly patient for this reason.

In hospitals, commercially prepared normal saline is available in containers of varying sizes. For an adult patient, 750 to 1000 ml is the average amount used. The amount of fluid used for infants and children varies with their age and weight. If children are to be given a cleansing enema, it should be given by a nurse educated in caring for pediatric patients. If commercial preparations of normal saline are not available or are too expensive for the patient to purchase, a normal saline solution can be made by adding 1 teaspoon of table salt per 500 milliters of water.

Hypertonic solution pulls fluid from the interstitial spaces around the sigmoid colon and fills it with fluid, thereby initiating peristalsis. Only a small amount is required to do this (120 to 180 ml). Hypertonic saline enemas are often available under the name Fleet enema (Fig. 7-1).

The Fleet enema

The Fleet enema is a commercial enema containing water and Fleet Phospho-Soda. It is packaged in a small plastic container with a prelubricated tip. The tip is inserted into the rectum, and the liquid is squeezed into the rectum from the plastic bottle. The patient is asked to retain the fluid for several minutes and then to evacuate it. The Fleet enema is quick, easy to use, and effective for relief of constipation or fecal impaction, or for eliminating barium sulfate residue after a radiographic examination.

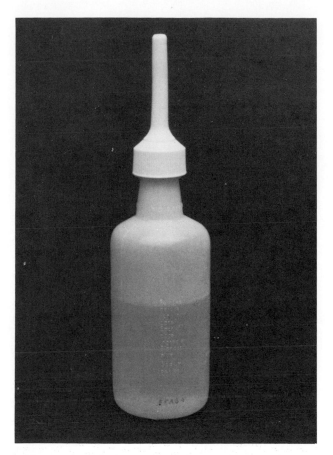

Figure 7-1. Hypertonic saline enema set (Fleet enema).

The oil-retention enema

The oil-retention enema is given for relief of chronic constipation, fecal impaction, or for eliminating barium sulfate residue after a radiographic examination. A small amount of mineral oil or olive oil (120 to 140 ml) is instilled into the rectum, and the patient is requested to retain the oil for as long a time as possible, preferably up to 1 hour, and then expel it. The oil lubricates the rectum and colon and softens the fecal material, thereby making it easier to expel.

Although the RT will probably not be administering this type of enema, he must be knowledgeable about it so that he can discuss it as part of his patient-teaching plan. Oil-retention enemas are usually commercially prepared and can be purchased in a container ready for use with a prelubricated tip. The tip is inserted into the anus, and the oil is slowly instilled into the rectum.

The tap-water enema

Tap water may be used to cleanse the bowel prior to diagnostic imaging procedures; however, the RT must remember that there is the potential for fluid toxicity if this is used. The procedure for administration is the same as for the soap suds enema, which will be described in the next paragraphs.

The soap suds enema (SS enema)

Soap may be added to tap water or to normal saline to increase the irritation of the intestine, thereby promoting peristalsis and defecation. The only soap safe to use for this purpose is a pure castile soap. Detergents and strong soaps may result in intestinal inflammation. For each 1000 ml of liquid, 5 ml of soap is recommended. The SS enema is the cleansing enema most frequently used prior to barium studies of the lower GI tract. The procedure for administering a cleansing enema to an adult patient is as follows:

1. The RT must ascertain that the treatment is ordered by the patient's physician or the radiologist in charge of performing the procedure. Giving an enema to persons with some gastrointestinal diseases is contraindicated.

2. Go to the patient and explain that a cleansing enema has been ordered, why it has been ordered, and explain the procedure to him.

3. Wash your hands; then assemble the equipment that is needed for the procedure. This will include
   a. A plastic container that holds 1000 ml of fluid. This may be a bucket or a plastic bag with an attached plastic tubing.
   b. A plastic tubing with a 22 to 26 French lumen (French measurement is discussed in Chapter 10) about 4 feet long with a smooth, perforated tip and a clamping device (Fig. 7-2)
   c. The liquid to be instilled
   d. Liquid castile soap (5 ml)
   e. Water-soluble lubricant
   f. A paper or cloth pad to place under the patient's hips, paper towels to receive the soiled enema tip, and a towel to protect the table where the equipment is placed
   g. A bedpan
   h. The patient's shoes or slippers and a robe
   i. Clean, disposable gloves
   j. A drape sheet to cover the patient

4. Attach the tubing to the container if this has not been done and clamp the clamp closed.

5. Go to a utility area that has a sink and hot and cold running water. Prepare the enema solution. The water used should be warmed to 105° F (41°

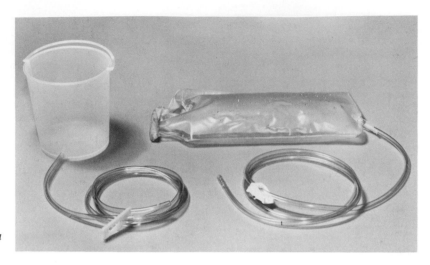

Figure 7-2. Two types of cleansing-enema sets.

C). Fill the container with 1000 ml of water and place the soap in the container and mix it.

6. Open the clamp and allow some of the fluid to run through the tubing into the sink to displace the air and to ensure that the enema set is working correctly (Fig. 7-3).

7. Take the equipment assembled on a tray if one is available. Place it on a table or stand near the patient. Close the door or otherwise arrange for privacy.

8. Drape the patient with the drape sheet and position him in a left Sims' position. Arrange the drape sheet so that only the area of the buttocks that must be exposed for insertion of the enema tip is exposed. Place the towel under the patient's hips to avoid soiling the table or sheet on which the patient is lying (Fig. 7-4).

9. Explain to the patient that you are about to begin the instillation of the fluid. Tell him that he may feel some cramping as the fluid runs in; if this

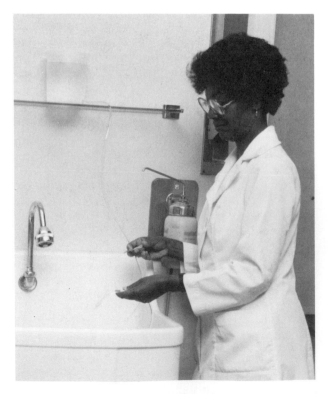

Figure 7-3. Allow the air in the tubing to be displaced by the enema solution.

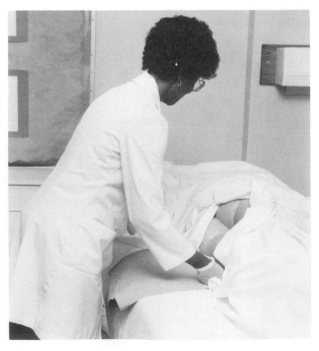

Figure 7-4. Place a towel under the patient's hips.

is the case, tell him to inform you and that you will stop the instillation until the cramping stops. Also inform the patient that he should try to retain the fluid for as long as he is able. Explain that there is a bedpan at hand if he is unable to get to the bathroom. If the patient is on a radiographic table, have a stepping stool ready to assist the patient off the table.

10. Tell the patient when you are about to insert the tube and ask him to exhale as you do this.

11. Don your gloves. Lubricate the tip of the tube if it does not come in a kit in which it is prelubricated.

12. Lift the patient's right buttocks with the heel of your hand to expose the anus.

13. Ask the patient to slowly exhale and gently insert the enema tip into the rectum toward the umbilicus 3 to 4 inches (Fig. 7-5). Make certain that you are visualizing the anus as you insert the tip to prevent injuring the patient. Do not insert the tube forcefully as the mucous membranes may be damaged (Fig. 7-6).

14. When the tip is inserted, hold it in place with your nondominant hand and release the tube clamp with the other hand. Then raise the container of fluid 18 inches (Fig. 7-7).

15. Allow the fluid to run in slowly. It should take about 10 minutes for all the fluid to be instilled. If the physician orders the transverse and ascending colon to be cleansed, the patient may be asked to turn onto his back and then onto

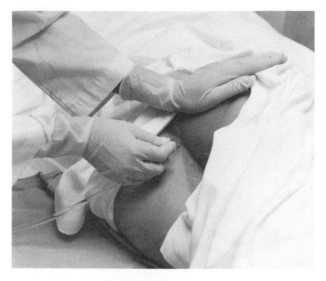

*Figure 7-6.   **Insert the tube gently to prevent injury.***

his right side as the fluid is being instilled. The quantity of fluid that a patient can retain will vary, but if possible, at least 500 ml of fluid should be instilled. Instruct the patient to tell you when he is unable to take more fluid.

16. Clamp the tube before the fluid has reached the bottom of the container so that air will not enter the rectum.

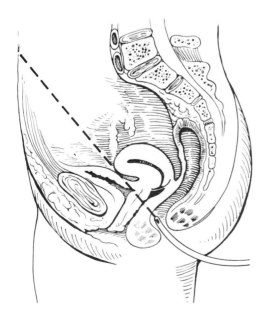

Figure 7-5

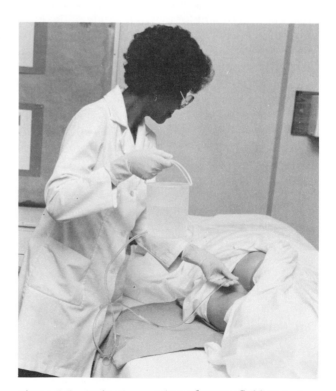

*Figure 7-7.   **Raise the container of enema fluid 18 inches.***

17. Gently remove the enema tip, wrap it in a paper towel, and place it in the enema container. Dispose of the set in the appropriate receptable, and remove your gloves according to the rules of medical asepsis.

18. If the patient is able, have him rest quietly on the table for as long as he can before going to the lavatory to expel the enema. Stay close by to assist him to the bathroom. If the patient cannot go to the lavatory, place him on a bedpan; don gloves to remove the bedpan as discussed in Chapter 3.

The RT can clean the area and wash his hands as for heavy contamination while the patient is expelling the enema. Instruct the patient not to flush the commode until the expelled material has been assessed. The RT must note the color, quantity, and consistency of the fecal material. Preparation for some barium studies requires that a second or even a third enema be administered so that the bowel is thoroughly cleansed. This process is referred to as giving enemas ''till clear'' and means that the enema fluid returns with no fecal matter present. This procedure must not be repeated more than three times because the patient's fluid balance may be jeopardized.

The self-administered cleansing enema

If a patient is coming from his home to the diagnostic imaging department for a barium study of the lower bowel, he must be taught to administer his own enemas effectively. The RT must be able to assume this teaching responsibility. The patient should be instructed to purchase an enema kit when he goes to the pharmacy for his laxative medication. The enema prescribed is usually a cleansing enema; the adult patient will be required to add 1000 ml water and 20 ml liquid soap. Carefully explain to the patient the type of enema set needed, because there will be many to choose from. Even if the laxative has the desired effect, explain to the patient that he will not be adequately prepared if he does not take his enemas as instructed.

Next, explain the preparation of the enema to the patient as described earlier in this chapter. The enema should be taken on the morning of the examination. If the patient has no one at home to assist him, explain that he should place a terry towel or newspaper on the floor near the toilet in his bathroom at home. Instruct him to place the enema set with the prelubricated tubing on a low stool or chair near him so that when he is lying down, the solution will be about 18 to 24 inches above the hip level. Since the enema solution must cleanse the entire colon, the procedure must not be performed with the patient in a sitting position. He may insert the enema tip while lying on his left side. Explain that if he changes position from his left side to his back and then to his right side while the enema is being instilled, he will be more certain that the solution is reaching his entire colon. The RT should also instruct the patient to try to relax by taking deep breaths during the procedure so that he will be able to hold the solution more easily. If the procedure is unsuccessful the first time, or if the patient has been directed to take enemas ''until clear'' he will be required to repeat this procedure.

The barium enema

Barium studies and double-contrast studies using high-density barium and air are used to diagnose pathologic conditions of the lower GI tract. A much larger catheter is required than is used for cleansing enemas to allow the viscous fluid to be instilled into the lower bowel. The catheter may have a plain tip or an inflatable cuff attached (Figs. 7-8 and 7-9). The cuff is inflated after the tip is inserted in order to hold the catheter in place and prevent involuntary expulsion of barium. Barium solution is usually available in a prepared, prepackaged form. When mixing the solution, the RT should remember that its consistency should be dense. After the solution is mixed, it should remain dense for some time before resettling. Foam is undesirable in the mixture because if it is present, the barium suspension will not coat the mucosal walls evenly.

The RT should have ready for use a plastic container of barium that has been well mixed (Fig. 7-10). The quantity needed for examination of an adult is generally 1500 ml, though it may vary. The barium solution is passed through the tubing in the same manner as the solution for a cleansing enema in order to displace the air in the tubing before inserting the tip. Premixed preparations of barium should be remixed so that the suspension is uniform, and they should be administered at room temperature.

The bag containing the barium is hung from a metal standard. A clamp on the tubing opens and closes the tubing easily. The bag should be placed about 30 inches above the table. The RT must not begin instillation of barium until the radiologist is present in the room to direct the procedure. The RT may insert the rectal catheter. The procedure is much the same as for the cleansing enema. The RT washes his hands, places the patient in the Sims' position, and drapes him so that only the anal area is exposed. The tip of the catheter is heavily lubricated. The RT then dons clean, disposable gloves. The patient is then

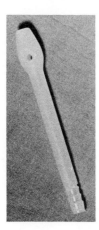

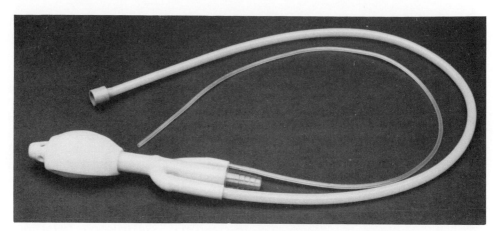

Figure 7-8.   Plain tip.   *Figure 7-9.   Tip with inflatable cuff and second lumen for air insufflation.*

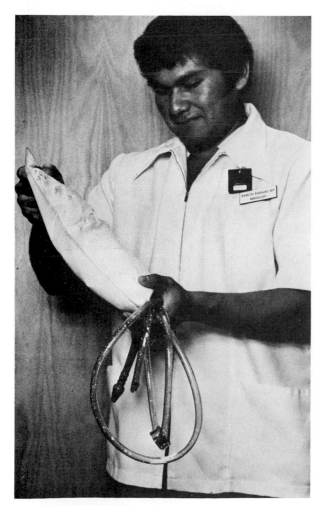

Figure 7-10

instructed to exhale slowly as the tip of the catheter is inserted 3 to 4 inches or until it passes the anal sphincter. Do not use force to insert the catheter because to do so might cause laceration of the mucous membranes. If the tip cannot be easily inserted, stop the procedure and ask the radiologist to complete the task. The patient may be returned to a supine position after the catheter is in place.

When a retention-type catheter with an inflatable cuff is used to administer barium, the cuff may be inflated with a hand inflation pump or with a syringe. The RT must be certain that the cuff is inserted beyond the rectal sphincter before it is inflated. Inflate the cuff initially with no more than 30 ml of air for an adult patient. If more air is desired, the radiologist may add more (Fig. 7-11). An inflatable cuff is not used for an infant or a child.

Every effort must be made by the RT to keep the patient as comfortable as possible during this examination. If the patient cannot hold the barium and cannot tolerate the inflatable cuff, an inflatable bedpan may be placed under him during the procedure (Fig. 7-12). Inform the patient that he will be moved into several positions to afford maximum visualization while the examination is in progress. Explain that the radiologist will be giving instructions to the RT that the patient may mistakenly think are being addressed to him. Tell him that these commands will consist of single words—"open," "close," "off," "on"—that the patient can ignore. Inform the patient of the approximate amount of barium that he will be given. Also explain that he will have an urge to defecate and will be taken to the lavatory immediately following the procedure.

Air is often placed into the bowel during this examination. If this is the case, it must be done by the physician. If barium has been instilled first, the patient is usually allowed to evacuate some of the barium

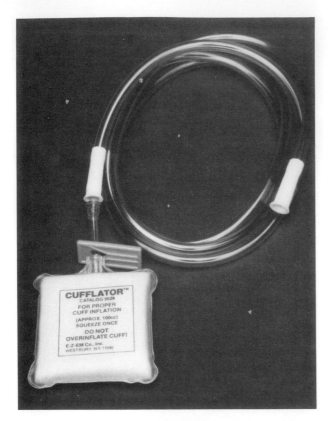

Figure 7-11.   Hand inflation pump.

before the air instillation. A rectal catheter with an air-insufflating mechanism attached is then inserted, and air is injected as a second contrast medium. The patient will be extremely uncomfortable during this study, and the RT should remain close to him in order to help reassure him and help him move about.

When removing a rectal catheter that has an inflatable cuff attached, the RT must be certain that the cuff is deflated before removing the catheter. The barium is sometimes removed by gravity flow before

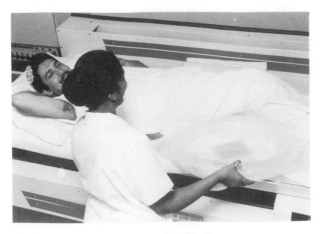

Figure 7-12.   Placing an inflatable bed pan.

the catheter tip is removed, and the air is then permitted to escape from the cuff. Following this, the RT gently removes the catheter. If there is any resistance, the radiologist should be summoned to remove it.

The RT must assist the patient to the lavatory following barium enemas. It may be necessary to allow the patient to evacuate some of the barium into a bedpan before attempting the trip. Stay with the patient until the problem is resolved because he will need assistance and direction.

Instructions following barium studies of the lower GI tract

A patient must never be dismissed from the diagnostic imaging department following a procedure without instruction in postexamination care. This is particularly true for the patient who has received barium because, without adequate care, the patient may retain barium, which can cause fecal impaction or intestinal obstruction. He may also suffer from extreme dehydration as a result of preparation for the test.

The RT must explain to the patient that his stools will be white or very light-colored until all of the barium is expelled. Some physicians regularly prescribe a laxative medication or an enema following barium studies. If he does not, tell the patient that if he has not had a bowel movement within 24 hours following the test, that he should contact his physician. Stress the importance of eliminating the barium.

It is also of extreme importance that the patient increase his fluid intake and the fiber in his diet for several days if this is not medically contraindicated. The patient should be instructed to rest following the examination. If he feels weak or faint; has abdominal pain, constipation, or rectal bleeding; is not passing flatus; has polyuria, nocturia, or abdominal distention, he must contact his physician immediately.

The patient with an intestinal stoma

There are pathologic conditions of the lower GI tract that require creation of a stoma through which the contents of the bowel can be eliminated. A stoma is created by bringing a loop of bowel to the skin surface of the abdomen. Some diseases that might be treated in this manner are cancer, diverticulitis, and ulcerative colitis. Traumatic injuries of the bowel may also require this type of treatment. The surgical procedure done to repair the bowel and create the ostomy is named by the area of bowel on which the operation

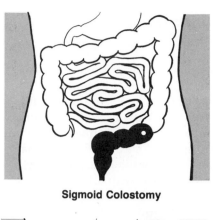

Sigmoid Colostomy

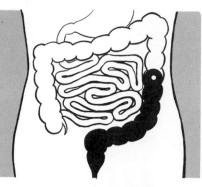

Descending Colostomy

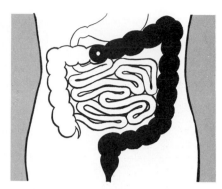

Transverse (Single B) Colostomy

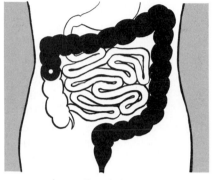

Ascending Colostomy

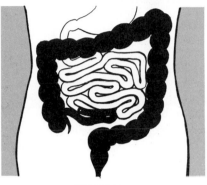

Ileostomy

Figure 7-13. Location of various colostomies and the location of an ileostomy. (Wolff LV, Weitzel MH, Zornow RA: Fundamentals of Nursing, 7th ed. Philadelphia, JB Lippincott, 1987) (Redrawn after Types of Ostomies. Copyright © 1979, Hollister Incorporated. All rights reserved)

is done. For instance, if the opening is from the colon, it is called a colostomy, from the ileum, an ileostomy (Fig. 7-13). The stoma may be temporary, done in order to rest and heal a diseased portion of the bowel, or permanent, done in order to remove a diseased or traumatized portion of the bowel.

The stoma may have either one or two openings depending on the type of surgery that was performed. In the latter, one opening will be toward the rectum and the other toward the small bowel. One opening, called the proximal stoma, will emit fecal material. The other opening, the distal stoma, will be relatively nonfunctioning and will emit only mucus. Some stoma patients (also called ostomy patients) have had their rectum and lower bowel removed. Others do not. A patient who has an ostomy may require barium studies for further diagnosis or study of the progression of their disease.

The RT must recognize that an ostomy produces a major change in a patient's body image and that many persons with a new colostomy or ileostomy stoma will be going through the grieving process. This is particularly true of younger patients. They may be angry, depressed, in a stage of denial, or just beginning to accept the fact that they must learn to live with this handicap.

Caring for the patient with a new ostomy requires sensitivity and a matter-of-fact attitude. It is suggested that the RT student who has never seen an ostomy

should observe the diagnostic studies being performed for these patients until he can care for them easily.

The ostomy patient will have a dressing or drainage pouch in place over the area of his stoma (Fig. 7-14). The dressing must be removed by an RT wearing clean gloves, then placed in a plastic bag and disposed of in a receptacle intended for contaminated waste. The gloves are then removed, and hands are washed. Procedure for dressing change will

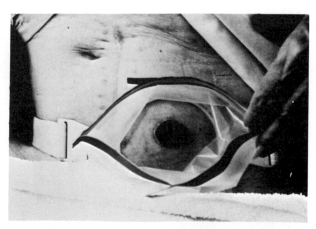

Figure 7-14. A colostomy stoma with an irrigation bag in place.

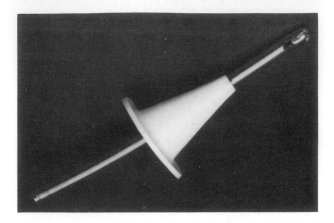

Figure 7-15.   Cone tip for colostomy patients.

be discussed in Chapter 9. A drainage pouch should be removed and put aside in a safe place to be reused. Gloves are worn by the RT to do this. The patient may want to do this himself or direct the RT in his care. The pouch must be kept clean and dry.

A patient who has a colostomy or ileostomy and is going to have a barium studies of the lower GI tract needs special instruction to be adequately prepared. If the hospital in which you are employed has an enterostomal therapist, the patient should be referred to this person for instruction. If not, the radiologist and the patient's physician should give the instructions before and after the procedure. All ostomy patients should be instructed to bring an extra pouch with them if they are coming from outside the hospital. Dietary, laxative, and cleansing preparations will vary depending on the type and location of the ostomy.

Administering a barium enema to a patient with an ostomy

Ostomy patients will have barium studies for diagnostic purposes, and the procedure is somewhat different than it is for a person with normally functioning bowels. The RT assisting with a barium examination for an ostomy patient must plan the procedure with the physician in charge and the patient before beginning to ensure the patient's comfort and safety. A cone-shaped tip with a long drainage bag that attaches to it following the procedure is frequently the instillation instrument of choice (Fig. 7-15). Occasionally a small catheter with an inflatable cuff is used. If the patient has had the ostomy for some time, he may prefer to insert the tip himself.

The RT will lubricate the tip of the cone and hand it to the patient for insertion (Fig. 7-17). He then puts on clean, disposable gloves so that he may assist the patient. A smaller amount of barium solution is needed for some ostomy patients.

Once the cone or catheter has been inserted, the procedure is the same as for other patients. Barium must not be instilled until the physician who is conducting the examination is present to supervise the procedure. If the patient's rectum and lower bowel are present, barium may be instilled into the ostomy and also into the lower bowel through the rectum.

When the procedure is completed, the drainage bag can be attached to the cone and the barium drained into it. When the drainage is complete, the patient whose physical condition permits it may be taken to the lavatory with the drainage bag still in place to be cleansed and to replace his ostomy pouch.

The RT should give the patient as much assistance as is needed. The patient should be offered a towel

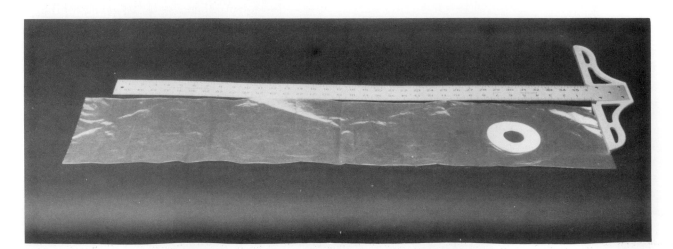

Figure 7-16.   Drainage bag used with cone tip.

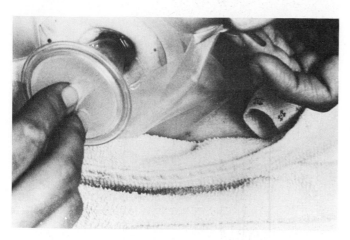

Figure 7-17. The lubricated cone is gently placed over the stoma and is held in place with the hand. (Wolff LV, Weitzel MH, Zornow RA: Fundamentals of Nursing, 7th ed. Philadelphia, JB Lippincott, 1987) (Printed with permission of Hollister Inc.)

and wash cloth, and any articles he needs should be made available to him.

Barium studies of the upper GI tract

Barium studies of the upper GI tract may be called *barium swallows* or *upper GI series.* They are performed to diagnose pathologic conditions of the pharynx, esophagus, stomach, duodenum, and jejunum.

Preparation for this examination varies depending upon the reason for the test and institutional preferences. The RT will be responsible for learning the requirements of the institution in which he is employed. The preparation usually includes instruction that the patient have nothing to eat or drink for 8 hours prior to the examination. Smoking and chew-ing gum should be discouraged because of the resulting increase in gastric secretion which may cause dilution of the contrast agent. Medications are also restricted for the 8 hours prior to the examination in most instances. Enemas are usually not required unless a barium enema will follow.

The RT should inform the patient that he will be given 12 to 14 ounces of flavored barium to drink. A thick solution is often given and is later followed by a thin solution. This solution does not have an unpleasant taste, but the chalkiness may be difficult to tolerate. It may be less distasteful for the patient if he drinks the substance through a straw. Double contrast with air is often used. If this is the case, the patient should be informed of this and the fact that he will have a feeling of fullness. He should also be told that during the examination he will be positioned in upright, supine, and side-lying positions while the passage of barium is viewed fluoroscopically. Spot films are also taken. The usual length of the study is 30 to 40 minutes.

Instructions following barium studies of the upper GI tract

The RT must inform patients that they should increase their fluid intake and increase the amount of fiber in their diet for several days following the test if it is not medically contraindicated. They may resume eating immediately unless another examination is to follow. The patient should expect that his stools will be light in color and that, if he does not have a bowel movement in 24 hours, he should have his physician prescribe a laxative. The patient must not allow himself to become constipated, because fecal impaction or bowel obstruction may result. If rectal bleeding occurs, he must notify his physican immediately.

Summary

There are two types of contrast agents, positive and negative. The most commonly used positive agents are barium sulfate and iodinated preparations. The most commonly used negative agents are air, carbon dioxide, oxygen, and nitrous oxide. Double-contrast studies combining barium sulfate and air are common.

Barium studies are frequently conducted in the diagnostic imaging department to diagnose pathologic conditions of the upper and lower GI tracts. Correct preparation for these examinations is essential for a successful outcome. It is the RT's professional responsibility to teach the patient the correct methods of preparing for barium studies and for the care and precautions he must take following these or any diagnostic imaging procedures.

The problem-solving process should be used as an outline for the RT's teaching presentations. Evaluation of the teaching plan can be in the form of patient repetition of directions given by the RT to make certain that he has assimilated the instructions and is able to carry them out.

Preparation for barium studies of the lower GI tract usually requires cleansing enemas. The types of cleansing enemas with which the RT must be familiar are saline enemas, the oil-retention enema, the tap-water enema, and the SS enema. The RT must be able to perform the cleansing enema correctly and be able to instruct a patient to administer these to himself if this is necessary. The hazards of the enema procedure must be kept in mind, and care must be taken to prevent injuries.

The patient with a colostomy or ileostomy may also require a barium enema. The procedure varies for these patients. The catheter used has an inflatable balloon to prevent expulsion of the barium and is smaller than the catheter used for rectal barium enemas. The RT must be sensitive in his care of the ostomy patients because they are often in the process of grieving over a recently acquired handicap. An RT who is not accustomed to seeing this type of stoma should work with a specially trained technologist or simply observe the procedure until he feels comfortable enough to relate to the ostomy patient in a therapeutic manner.

Barium studies of the upper GI tract are frequently done to diagnose pathology of the pharynx, esophagus, stomach, duodenum, and jejunum. The preparation before and after these studies varies somewhat from that of the lower GI series. The RT must familiarize himself with this information so that he can correctly instruct the patient and keep him as comfortable and anxiety-free as is possible during the procedure.

Chapter 7, pre-post test

1. List and differentiate between the two types of contrast agents.

____ 2. Under which circumstance is barium not the contrast agent of choice?
   a. There is a possible perforation of the GI mucosa.
   b. The patient is a diabetic.
   c. There is an emotional problem.
   d. There is a potential diagosis of paralytic ileus.

____ 3. As a specialist in his area of health care, the RT has patient-teaching responsibilities. These responsibilities include
   a. A description of the preparation, purpose, time involved, and equipment used for examinations
   b. A description of the adverse reactions possible and the diagnosis made during the examination
   c. The toxic effects of the barium and the amount of work involved for the RT
   d. The risk to the patient, the family, and the health-care team

____ 4. Barium is a relatively nontoxic contrast agent; therefore, no special precautions need be taken.
   a. True
   b. False

____ 5. The amount of solution prescribed for a cleansing enema prior to barium studies of the lower GI tract is usually
   a. 10 ml
   b. 1000 ml
   c. 500 ml
   d. 900 ml

____ 6. The only safe soap to use for a cleansing enema is
   a. Liquid detergent
   b. Oatmeal soap
   c. Nonperfumed soap
   d. Castile soap
   e. Hypoallergenic soap

____ 7. Following a barium study, the RT must instruct the patient in follow-up care. These instructions will include
   a. Description of the appearance of his stools
   b. Instructions to call the patient's physician if he does not have a bowel movement within 24 hours
   c. Need for increased fluid intake and fiber in the diet if not contraindicated
   d. a and b
   e. a, b, and c

____ 8. The RT must recognize that the patient with an ostomy has suffered a change in his body image and may be going through
   a. The grieving process
   b. The process of self-examination
   c. The aging process
   d. The self-actualization process

9. List the equipment needed for a cleansing enema.

____ 10. The type of cleansing enema prescribed for a pediatric patient would probably be
   a. An SS enema
   b. A tap-water enema
   c. An oil-retention enema
   d. A saline enema

Laboratory reinforcement

1. Demonstrate the administration of a cleansing enema in the school laboratory using a mannequin as the patient.

2. Using a classmate as a patient, explain how he should prepare prior to receiving a barium enema for diagnostic purposes.

Chapter Eight

Care of Patients with Drainage Tubes or in Need of Suctioning

---

Goal of this chapter:

The RT student will learn to care for or assist with patients who have nasogastric (NG) tubes, nasointestinal (NI) tubes, chest tubes, tracheostomy tubes, tissue drains, or those in need of suctioning.

Behavioral objectives:

When the student has completed this chapter, he will be able to do the following:
1. List the reasons for passage of an NG tube or NI tube and the equipment necessary if one of these must be inserted while a patient is in the diagnostic imaging department
2. Give a written explanation of the care needed for a patient in the diagnostic imaging department who is receiving continuous gastric suctioning
3. Demonstrate and explain the method of transfer from a hospital ward to the diagnostic imaging department for a patient who is receiving gastric suctioning
4. Explain the RT's responsibilities in assessing the need for and preparing for oropharyngeal or nasopharyngeal suctioning
5. List the precautions that the RT must take when working with a patient who has a tracheostomy tube in place
6. List the precautions that the RT must take when working with the patient who has a chest tube with water-seal drainage in place
7. List the precautions the RT must take if a patient has a tissue drain in place

Glossary

Aspiration drawing in; inhaling or drawing out as by suction—foreign objects can be aspirated into the lungs

Cannula a tube used to allow fluids or oxygen into the body

Decompression removal or slow reduction of pressure produced by air or gas within the body

Drain free flow or withdrawal of fluids from a wound or surgery by means of gauze or tubing

Drainage pus, serum, blood, or other fluids from a body wound or abcess

Fluoroscopy used in medicine to visualize the motion of internal body structures and fluids by use of an x-ray tube and TV monitor screen

French scale or measurement a system used to indicate diameter of tubes, catheters, or instruments; each unit on scale in approximately ⅓ mm (0.33)

Gomco suction electrically operated, portable machine attached to a gastric tube to provide continuous drainage from stomach

Hemostat a clamplike instrument used to control flow of fluids, barium, or blood into or out of the body

115

Impermeable bag impenetrable; not allowing fluids to seep through

Intubation a tube passed into larynx to administer oxygen for breathing or to dialate a stricture

Levin tube named for New Orleans physician of 1900s; a catheter, usually introduced through the nose and extends through the stomach into the duodenum

Lumen the hollow space within an artery, vein, intestine, tube, or instrument such as a syringe needle

Pathology condition produced by a disease; involves changes in structure and function

Pleural space or cavity area between the parietal (lining of chest wall or of wall of thorax and diaphragm) and visceral membrane layers (lungs)

Radiopaque a material or substance not allowing x-rays to pass through or penetrate, *e.g.*, lead or barium sulfate

Tension pneumothorax air entering pleural space as a result of perforation, which cannot leave by route of entry; the resulting pressure increase can lead to a collapsed lung

Vomitus material ejected from the stomach by vomiting; gastric contents ejected through the mouth

Nasogastric (NG) tubes and nasointestinal (NI) tubes are inserted for therapeutic and diagnostic purposes. These tubes have a hollow lumen through which secretions and air may be evacuated, or medications, nourishment, or diagnostic contrast agents may be instilled. The RT must be able to care for and transport patients with these tubes in place. He must also understand the purposes of gastric suction and be able to attach or discontinue it when the physician's orders require this treatment.

Studies are done in diagnostic imaging that require the passage of NG or NI tubes prior to the examination. The RT will not insert these tubes, but he may be asked to prepare the patient if the tube is to be placed in the department. He must know what type of equipment to assemble for the procedure.

Occasionally it will be necessary for the patient who has vomited or who has an accumulation of blood or secretions in his mouth or throat to be suctioned while the RT is caring for him. The RT does not perform the suctioning procedure, but he must be able to assess a patient's need for suctioning and be able to prepare the equipment so that the procedure may be done quickly in order to prevent aspiration of fluid into the lungs or to prevent respiratory failure.

Patients with tracheostomy tubes in place may also need diagnostic imaging examinations. They will require proper care by the RT in order to prevent injury and to keep them comfortable while the examination is in progress.

Chest tubes are inserted following surgical procedures, injury, or diseases of the lungs in order to permit drainage of fluid or air out of the pleural space. If air and fluid become trapped in the pleural space, pressure will build and create what is called a *tension pneumothorax*. If this condition is not relieved, the resulting respiratory distress may produce a life-threatening situation. The RT must learn the precautions he must take when caring for patients with chest tubes in place.

Following surgical procedures, a variety of tissue drains are placed in the areas of the body that tolerate an accumulation of fluid poorly. The RT must be able to recognize these drains and direct patient care in a manner that prevents dislodging these if they are present.

Nasogastric and nasointestinal tubes

NG tubes are plastic or rubber tubes inserted through the nasopharynx into the stomach. If a patient has an anatomical or physiologic reason why the nose cannot be used, the tube may be inserted through the mouth over the tongue. They are used to keep the stomach free of gastric contents and air (this assists with healing before and after operative procedures); they may also be used for diagnostic examinations or for the administration of medications directly into the stomach.

NI tubes are inserted in much the same way as NG tubes are, but they are allowed to pass on into the intestines by means of peristalsis. They are also used for decompression, diagnosis, and treatment purposes.

The two most common NG tubes used for gastric decompression are the Levin and Salem-Sump tubes. The Levin tube is a single-lumen tube with holes near its tip (Fig. 8-1). The Salem-Sump tube is a double-lumen tube, which is radiopaque. The opening of the second lumen is a blue extension off of the proximal end of the tube (the end that remains outside) called a "pig tail" (Fig. 8-2). This end is always left open to room air for the purpose of maintaining a continuous flow of atmospheric air into the stomach, thereby controlling the amount of suction pressure that may be placed on the gastric mucosa. This is a means of preventing injury and ulceration of these tissues.

There are several kinds of NI tubes that may be used, depending on the patient's diagnosis and physician's preference. These tubes are longer than NG tubes and have an inflatable bag at the distal end, the end that goes into the gastrointestinal (GI) tract, which is weighted with mercury. They are threaded through the nose into the stomach and then allowed to pass into the intestine. This passage is assisted by the weighted bag.

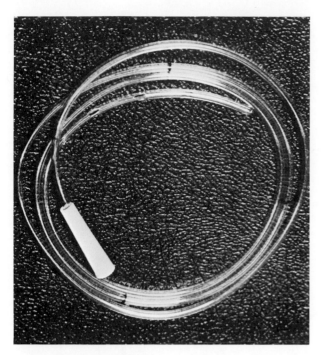

Figure 8-1.   A Levin tube.

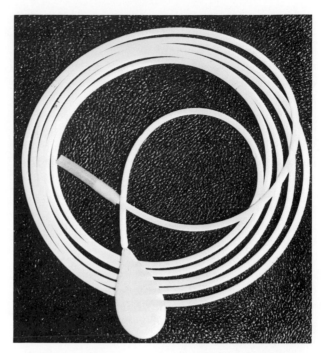

Figure 8-3.   The Cantor tube—a nasointestinal tube.

Three of the most commonly used NI tubes are the Cantor, the Harris, and the Miller-Abbott. The Cantor and Harris tubes have a single lumen; the Miller-Abbott tube is a double-lumen tube (Fig. 8-3). One lumen of the Miller-Abbott tube is used for intestinal decompression; the other is for insertion of mercury following insertion. Some single-lumen tubes are weighted with a metal tip. The progress of the tube may be followed in the diagnostic imaging department fluoroscopically.

Passage of nasogastric and nasointestinal tubes

RTs are not responsible for inserting NG or NI tubes. A registered nurse usually inserts an NG tube; a phy-

sician, the NI tube. However, the RT may be requested to assist with the passage of a gastric tube and will frequently care for patients who have them in place.

Patients with NG or NI tubes in place are often uncomfortable and may be very ill. While in the diagnostic imaging department, they should be informed of the treatment plan that will be followed and not be left unattended. Care must be taken to prevent accidental withdrawal of the tube after it has been inserted.

The materials needed for passage of an NG or NI tube are the following: a tube of the correct type and size (usually a 14 to 16 French lumen is used for an adult patient); rubber tubes (placed in a basin of ice prior to insertion to make the rubber more rigid and to facilitate passage); clean, disposable gloves; an emesis basin, a towel, a glass of water, and a drinking straw; a 20- to 50-ml aspirating or bulb syringe; water-soluble lubricant; wide hypoallergenic tape; a stethoscope; a tongue blade; a safety pin and rubber band; normal saline solution; and a suction machine if suction is to be used.

This procedure is uncomfortable and frightening for the patient. If this procedure is to take place in the diagnostic imaging department, the RT must explain to the patient what is to be done and for what reason. The patient should be assured that if he concentrates on swallowing and breathing as the tube is inserted, the procedure will go smoothly and quickly.

Place the patient in a Fowler's position with pillows supporting his head and shoulders. Have tissues

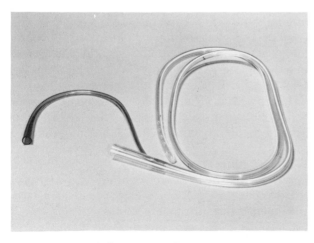

Figure 8-2.   A Salem sump tube.

and an emesis basin close by for patient use. The procedure is begun by the nurse or physician measuring the distance from the nose to the stomach externally (Fig. 8-4). Levin tubes have black markings on them that indicate how far the tube has been inserted.

When the physician or nurse is ready to insert the tube, the RT may lubricate the distal end of the tube with water-soluble lubricant and hand it to him. The patient is instructed to swallow water through a straw as the procedure begins. If the patient is unable to take fluids, he may simply swallow air through the straw. The tube should go down easily with little force. The RT should stand beside the patient and encourage him to swallow.

When the tube is believed to be in the stomach, its position is verified by placing the diaphragm of the stethoscope over the gastric region and injecting 10 ml to 20 ml of air into the stomach. If a whooshing sound is heard as the air enters the stomach, the tube is in the correct position (Fig. 8-5). If not, the tube is immediately removed, because it may be in the trachea instead of the stomach.

Another method of determining the position of the NG tube that may be used is to attach the syringe to the portal of the NG tube and draw back the plunger. If gastric fluid returns, the tube is in the stomach.

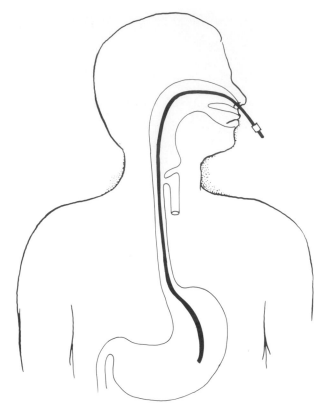

Figure 8-5. Position of the Levin tube in the stomach.

The external end of the tube may also be placed into a glass of water. If the water bubbles, the tube is believed to be in the trachea and is removed.

When it is certain that the tube has reached the stomach, reassure the patient and make him comfortable. NG tubes are taped in place, but NI tubes are not taped, because their position is achieved through peristaltic action.

A safe and secure method of taping is the butterfly method. A piece of tape approximately 2 inches long is cut or torn lengthwise, and the remaining 2-inch piece is left intact. Wrap the intact piece of tape around the tubing. At the front of the tubing, crisscross the two pieces of tape and place them over the bridge of the nose (Fig. 8-6). A second piece of tape may be placed over the first two so that they will remain in place (Fig. 8-7).

Patients with gastric tubes in place are very uncomfortable and may be very ill. They should be reassured frequently and not left alone until they feel secure.

The RT must take care to tape the Levin tube securely so that it is not accidentally withdrawn. It should never be necessary to repeat passage of a gastric tube because of careless handling. There should be no pulling pressure on the tube. Patients with gastric tubes in place are not to eat or drink anything unless it is specifically ordered by the physician.

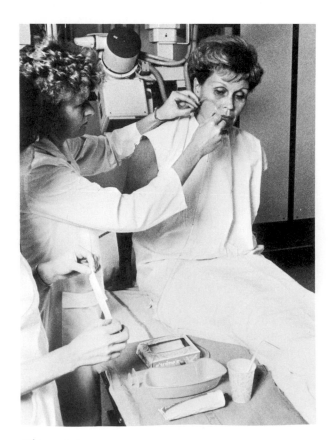

Figure 8-4

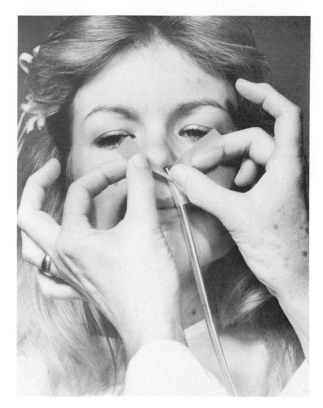

Figure 8-6

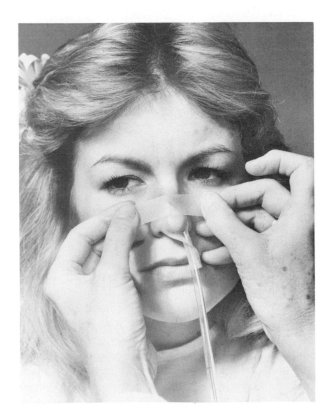

Figure 8-7

Removing gastric tubes

The Levin tube is removed easily; however, the RT must never assume that simply because a diagnostic imaging examination that involved its use is complete, that the tube may be removed. The physician must order its removal or it should be left in place. If its removal is ordered by the physician in charge of the patient, the RT may remove it.

Items needed to remove an NG tube are as follows: an emesis basin, tissues, several thicknesses of paper toweling, an impermeable bag for disposal, and clean, disposable gloves. The RT will identify the patient and explain the procedure to him. Wash your hands, then turn off and disconnect the suction apparatus, if there is one in place. Gently remove the tape from the patient's nose and make certain that the tubing is free from the patient's facial skin. Don clean gloves, ask the patient to take in a deep breath as you gently withdraw the tube, wrap it in the paper toweling, and place it in the disposal bag. If there is any resistance, stop the procedure and ask the radiologist to assist in the tube withdrawal.

NI tubes are not removed by the RT. The physician or registered nurse may remove the tube, or it is sometimes allowed to be passed through the intestinal tract and removed rectally.

Transferring patients with nasogastric suction

NG and NI suction tubes are used before or after surgical procedures that involve the digestive system to keep the stomach and bowel free of gastric contents and for gastric decompression. An NG or NI tube is attached to a suction apparatus, which is either portable or piped into the room from a central hospital unit (Figs. 8-8 and 8-9). The suction is maintained either continuously or intermittently as the patient's needs demand.

When the RT is responsible for transferring a patient who is having either continuous or intermittent gastric suctioning, he must verify the physician's orders before making the transfer. If it is permissible to discontinue the suction, he must know the length of time that it can be interrupted safely. If it is for only a short time, he must be certain that suction can be reestablished in the diagnostic imaging department. This can be accomplished by taking the patient's portable suction machine with him or by using the suction available in the department. The RT must also know the amount of suction pressure that is required so that he can adjust the pressure accurately. The amount of pressure ordered varies, and the RT can determine the correct level by reading the physician's orders or by asking the nurse in charge of the patient

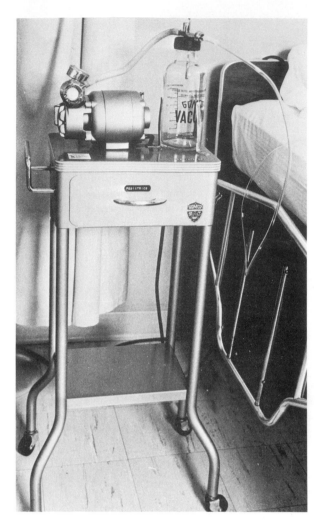

Figure 8-8. A portable, electrically operated suction machine. The pressure control valve and the pressure indicator are located above the motor. The drainage runs into the vacuum bottle on the right. The tubing at right is connected to the gastric tube.

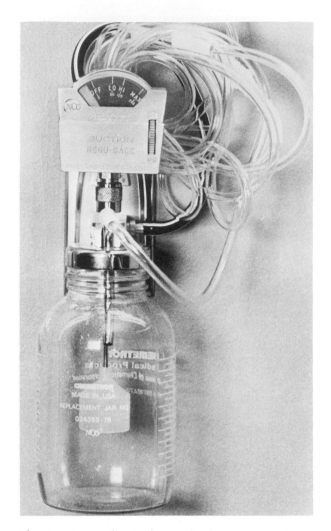

Figure 8-9. Suction equipment is often used in radiology departments, and suction may be piped to the department from a central area in the hospital. This particular model is activated by turning the valve at the top (right), just below the pressure gauge. The suction pressure is regulated by adjusting the valve (center) above the vacuum collecting bottle.

to do this. The maximum amount of suction that can be used is a pressure equal to 25 mm Hg for an adult patient. More than this can damage the gastric mucosa.

If the suction must be discontinued for a period of time, the RT may do this. If the tube is a single-lumen tube, the RT will need the following materials: a pair of clean, disposable gloves, a clamping device, a package of sterile gauze sponges, and two rubber bands.

Explain the procedure to the patient, then wash your hands, open the package of sponges, and don the gloves. Turn off the suction; clamp or plug the gastric tube with the clamp or stopper (Fig. 8-10), and place one gauze pad over the end of the tube and secure it with a rubber band. Then cover the connecting end of the suction tubing or the adapter with the other sponge, and secure it with a rubber

band. This gauze covering will keep both ends of the tubing clean while not in use (Fig. 8-11). Secure the suction tubing on the machine so that it will not fall onto the floor, and make certain that the NG or NI tube will not be dislodged during the transfer. Then proceed with the transfer by wheelchair or gurney as required. If the suction is to be restarted in the diagnostic imaging department on arrival, set the suction pressure gauge, turn on the suction, and reattach it to the tubing. This procedure is repeated when transferring the patient back to his room.

If the NG tube is a double-lumen tube, it must never be clamped closed with a hemostat or regular clamping device, because this may cause the lumens to adhere to each other and destroy the double-lumen effect. To prevent leakage from this type of tube, the barrel of a pistonlike syringe may be inserted into

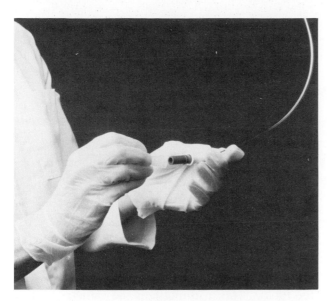

Figure 8-10.   Clamping gastric tube with plug.

the suction–drainage lumen, and it is then pinned to the patient's gown with the barrel upward (Fig. 8-12).

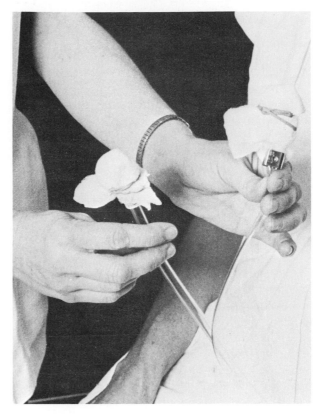

Figure 8-11

The patient requiring emergency suctioning

Occasionally an infant, a child, an unconscious person, a patient with head or facial injuries, or a very weak and debilitated patient will be unable to clear vomitus, sputum, or other drainage from the nose, mouth, nasopharynx, or oropharynx by coughing or swallowing while being cared for by the RT. Signs that indictate that a patient may need to receive nasopharyngeal or oropharyngeal suctioning are audible rattling or gurgling sounds coming from the patient's throat, gagging, or breathing with difficulty. Patients with these symptoms may require mechanical suctioning to remove the secretions in order to prevent aspiration or respiratory arrest. If this is necessary, it is usually an emergency procedure. Although it is not within the scope of the RT's practice to perform suctioning procedures, he must be able to assess the patient's need for suctioning, call for the physician or the registered nurse to do this, and assist with the procedure.

It is the RT's responsibility to examine the emergency suctioning equipment in his department each day in order to be certain that it is in good working order and that all necessary items are available. The items that must be on hand for suctioning the oropharynx or nasopharynx are as follows:

1. A wall outlet or a working portable suction machine

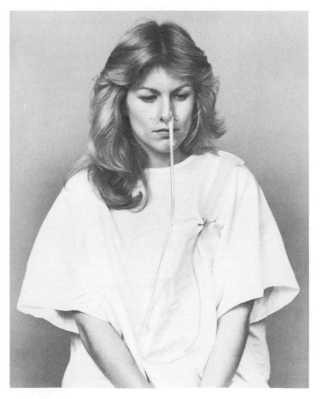

Figure 8-12

2. Adapters for all wall outlets

3. Sterile gloves of various sizes

4. Tubing

5. Sterile disposable suctioning sets that contain suction catheters of various sizes and either a y or thumb-control connector

6. Sterile containers for sterile solution

7. Sterile normal saline solution

8. Tongue depressors padded with gauze

9. An oxygen source

10. Packets of sterile, water-soluble lubricant

Catheters for emergency suctioning may vary in size from a 10- to an 18-French lumen for adults (22 inches long) and 5- to 8-French lumen (15 inches long) for children (Fig. 8-13). Pressure settings will vary depending on the patient's age and will usually be higher than those used for NG or NI suctioning. Sterile technique is recommended for nasopharyngeal suctioning because the respiratory tract is easily infected. Introducing new microorganisms into the respiratory tract must be avoided. Maintenance of sterile technique is discussed in Chapter 9.

Before suctioning begins, the RT should wash his hands and assemble the necessary equipment for the physician or nurse. Place the patient in a semi-Fowler's position with his head turned toward the side if he is alert and has a functioning gag reflex. An unconscious patient or a child should be placed in a lateral (side-lying) position with no pillow. Have adequate lighting available. (A portable gooseneck lamp may be used.) Place a towel over the patient's chest. After the patient is prepared, the person who will do the suctioning will open the sterile packet containing the catheter and the connector and put

on sterile gloves, pick up the catheter, and connect it to the suction adapter. He must keep the hand that will touch the suction catheter sterile; the other hand becomes contaminated. The RT may pour a small amount of normal saline into a sterile container and turn on the suction machine and adjust the pressure as directed by the physician or nurse. The suction pressure for adults is approximately 110 mm Hg to 150 mm Hg on a wall-mounted outlet. Wall outlets are usually more powerful than portable machines. For infants the requirements vary from 50 mm Hg to 95 mm Hg for wall-mounted outlets. For older children the setting for wall outlet suction varies from 100 mm Hg to 120 mm Hg.

The person doing the suctioning may test the suction by placing the catheter tip into the sterile normal saline solution and drawing a small amount through the tubing. This also moistens the catheter tip and thereby lubricates it. The catheter tip is then placed into the patient's oropharynx or nasopharynx. Suctioning must not begin until the catheter is in place. The suction is activated by placing the thumb over the opening on the connector (Fig. 8-14). The actual suctioning procedure should not take more than 15 seconds. Suctioning for longer periods compromises the patient's oxygen supply. The catheter is withdrawn by a gentle rotating motion. The catheter tip is placed into the normal saline, and the solution is passed through the catheter in order to cleanse it. A padded tongue blade may be used to keep the tongue depressed during oropharyngeal suctioning.

If further suctioning is needed, a period of 20 to 30 seconds is allowed for the patient to rest between catheter insertions. If the patient is able, he should be asked to cough and deep breathe between suctionings. For infants and children, the actual suctioning should not last longer than 10 seconds with 1- to 3-minute rest periods. If both oropharyngeal and nasopharyngeal passages are to be suctioned, a

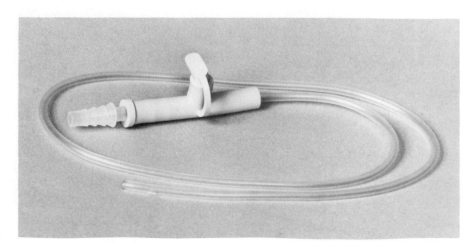

Figure 8-13. A suction catheter.

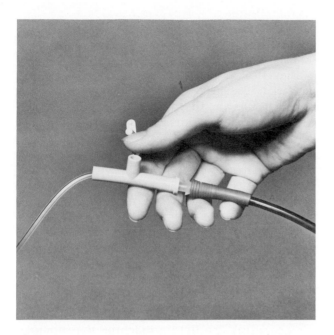

Figure 8-14

patient's condition permits, the diagnostic imaging procedure may continue.

The patient with a tracheostomy

A tracheostomy is an opening into the trachea created surgically either to relieve respiratory distress caused by obstruction of the upper airway or to improve respiratory function by permitting better access of air to the lower respiratory tract. This may be done as either a temporary or a permanent measure. Patients requiring this procedure may have suffered traumatic injury or may have a tumor or an infectious disease that interferes with respiration. Once the surgical incision is made and the opening exists, a tracheostomy tube is inserted into the opening. Tracheostomy tubes are equipped with an obturator in order to ensure safe insertion; the obturator is removed as soon as the tube is in place (Fig. 8-15).

There are several types of tracheostomy tubes. They are usually made of plastic but may be metal. They have a cuff that helps to seal the tracheostomy to prevent air leaks and aspiration of gastric contents (Fig. 8-16). Most tracheostomy tubes have an inner cannula that is locked into place (Fig. 8-17). The tracheostomy tube is held in place at the back of the neck with ties or tapes. Tracheostomy tubes used for infants and small children do not usually have the cuff, because they fit tightly enough without one.

Patients with newly inserted tracheostomy tubes are very fearful. They are unable to speak because the opening in the windpipe prevents air from being forced from the lungs past the vocal cords and into the larynx. They are afraid of choking because they are unable to remove secretions that accumulate in

fresh catheter is used for each. Sterile, water-soluble lubricant is applied to the tip of a catheter to be inserted into the nasal passages. During this procedure, the RT should reassure the patient. If he fights the procedure, it may have to be discontinued.

After suctioning has been completed, place the used disposable equipment into a plastic bag, seal the bag, and dispose of it in the proper waste receptacle. The drainage tubing and collecting bottle from a portable suction machine should be cleaned and replaced. Clean, disposable gloves must be worn by the RT while he is cleaning and disposing of this equipment because he may come into direct contact with the patient's secretions during the process. Sterile supplies should be replenished immediately. If the

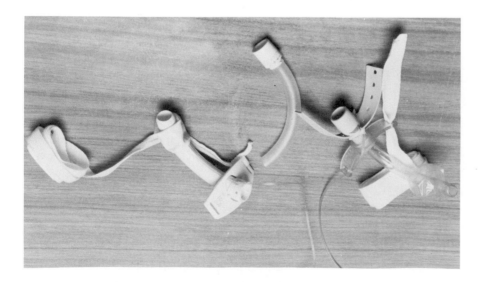

Figure 8-15. Two types of tracheostomy tubes. Tube on left with obturator removed. Obturator is beside tube.

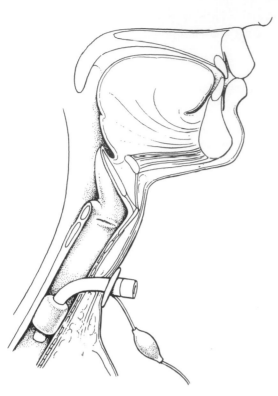

Figure 8-16.   Tracheostomy tube placement. (Brunner L, Suddarth DM: Lippincott Manual of Nursing Practice. Philadelphia, JB Lippincott, 1986)

the tracheostomy tube. These secretions must be suctioned out by a registered nurse (Fig. 8-18). If a patient with a new tracheostomy is brought to the diagnostic imaging department, he should be accompanied by a nurse qualified to care for him. Sterile suction catheters and suctioning equipment as listed above and oxygen administration equipment must be prepared before the patient arrives in the department. The semi-Fowler's position is usually most

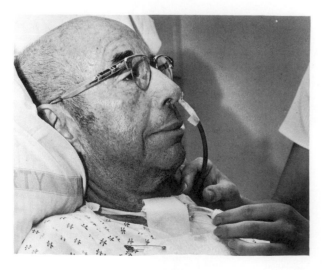

Figure 8-17.   Removing the inner cannula from a tracheostomy tube.

comfortable for these patients, and the RT should provide bolsters or pillows in order that the best position for the patient may be maintained.

The RT caring for the patient with a tracheostomy must plan his care with the patient's nurse and the patient before any diagnostic imaging procedure is begun. The tracheostomy tube must not be removed nor the tapes holding it in place untied for any reason because the tracheostomy tube may be dislodged and not be able to be replaced immediately. The RT must explain all procedures that the patient will receive to him in order to alleviate his anxiety. A pencil and a writing pad should be provided for the patient on which he may write any comments or responses that he wants to make. If the patient appears to be breathing noisily or with difficulty, the RT must immediately stop working and allow the nurse to suction the patient or otherwise relieve his discomfort.

The patient who is critically ill may be assisted by a mechanical ventilating machine that operates through the tracheostomy. Patients in this condition frequently require portable bedside radiographs. The RT must never turn off or interfere with mechanical ventilating equipment. Any alterations in this equipment must be made by the nurse in charge of the patient's care. The patient's nurse should remain close by while the RT is working with the patient.

The patient with a chest tube and water-sealed drainage

The pressure in the pleural cavity is normally lower than atmospheric pressure, but disease or injury can interfere with this. The result of increased pressure in the pleural cavity is collapse of the lungs (pneumothorax). A chest tube is inserted into the pleural cavity and attached to water-sealed drainage to remove air and fluid from the intrapleural space in order to reestablish normal intrapleural pressure and allow the lungs to expand normally.

A water-sealed drainage system is established by connecting the chest tube, which originates in the area of pathology in the pleural cavity, to a glass-connecting tube, which ends in a bottle containing sterile water. The glass tube leading from the chest tube remains below water level at all times to maintain the seal. When the patient inspires, air and fluid from the interpleural spaces go into the drainage tube and are eliminated. Since the water in the drainage system is heavier than air, it cannot be drawn into the tube on inspiration, nor can air from the atmosphere enter because of the water seal.

There are several variations of the water-sealed system. There may be one, two, or three bottles present. Additional bottles, also with water seals, are added for drainage from the patient's pleural cavity

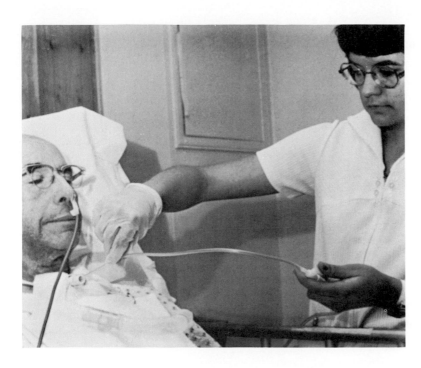

Figure 8-18. Nurse suctioning a tracheostomy tube.

and for suction regulation if suction is also attached to the chest tube. There are a number of commercial water-sealed drainage systems on the market. Some of these are disposable, and some have traditional glass bottles (Figs. 8-19 and 8-20).

When the RT is caring for a patient with a chest tube and water-sealed drainage he must remember to follow these procedures:

1. Keep the tubing as straight as possible. If it is long, loosely coil it on the patient's bed and do not allow it to fall below the level of the patient's chest.

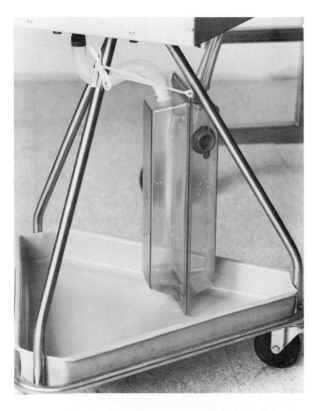

Figure 8-19. A disposable water-sealed pleural drainage set.

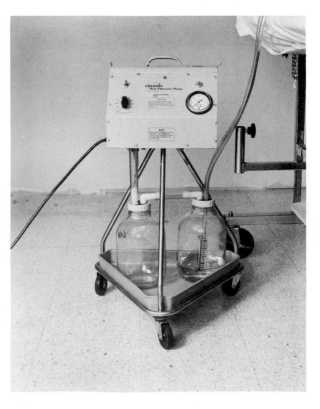

Figure 8-20. A nondisposable water-sealed pleural drainage set connected to an Emerson suction pump.

2. All connections must be kept tight, *i.e.*, chest tube connected tightly to drainage tube; stoppers fitted tightly into receptacles.

3. Water seals must be maintained at all times. If a water-sealed bottle tips, it must be righted immediately.

4. Continuous bubbling in a water-sealed system is not normal; intermittent bubbling is. If the RT notices continuous bubbling in a water-sealed system, he must bring it to the attention of the patient's nurse or the radiologist immediately.

5. Do not empty water-sealed bottles or raise them. The water seal must remain below the patient's chest.

6. Do not clamp chest tubes.

7. If a water seal is below the level of the tube, notify the nurse in charge of the patient immediately.

8. The drainage tube from the chest should be long enough to allow free patient movement. If the patient must be moved for radiographic exposures, do not allow tension to be placed on the chest tube or the patient to be positioned in a way that causes the tubing to kink or be sealed off.

Tissue drains

Tissue drains are placed at or near wound sites or operative sites when large amounts of drainage are expected. This drainage interferes with the healing

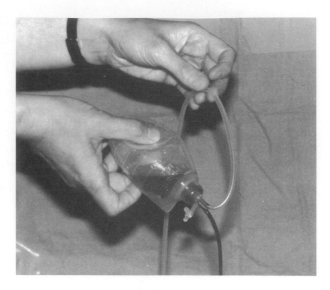

Figure 8-22.   Jackson-Pratt drain. (Patrick ML, Woods SL, Craven RF et al: Medical-Surgical Nursing. Philadelphia, JB Lippincott, 1986)

process because it is reabsorbed by the body too slowly. In some circumstances it may produce infection or result in formation of fistulas.

The Hemovac, the Jackson-Pratt, and the Penrose drains are three of the most common postoperative tissue drains. They are often placed in areas where the surgical procedure calls for large amounts of tissue dissection or in areas with an increased blood supply such as the breast, the neck, or the kidney. They will also be found in the abdominal area. One end of the

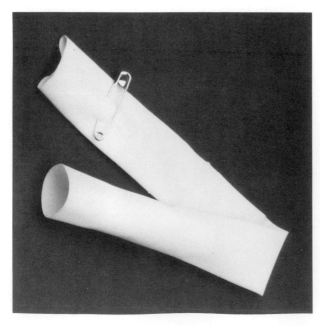

Figure 8-21.   Penrose drain.

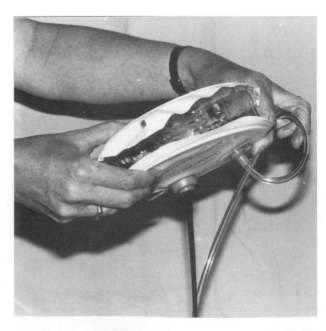

Figure 8-23.   Hemovac drain. (Patrick ML, Woods SL, Craven RF et al: Medical-Surgical Nursing. Philadelphia, JB Lippincott, 1986)

tube or drain is placed in or near the operative site, and the other end exits through the body wall. They are removed by the surgeon when the drainage diminishes.

The Penrose drain is a soft rubber tube, which is kept from slipping into the surgical wound or beneath the body wall by a sterile safety pin (Fig. 8-21). It is allowed to drain into the surgical dressing.

The Jackson-Pratt and Hemovac drains are plastic drainage tubes that maintain constant, low, negative pressure by means of a small bulb, which is squeezed together and slowly expands to create low-pressure suction (Figs. 8-22 and 8-23). The drainage goes from the tubing into the bulb.

Other types of drains are placed into the hollow organs of the body and may be sutured in place and attached to collecting bags. Some of these are the T tube, which is often placed into the common bile duct; the gastrostomy tube, which is placed in the stomach; the cecostomy tube, placed in the cecum; and the cystostomy tube, which is placed in the kidney.

All these drains must be identified during the RT's assessment of his patient; he must plan care to prevent any tension on these drains, which might dislodge them partially or completely. Infection control must also be considered. The presence of a tissue drain indicates that the patient has an opening directly into the body where infection may be easily introduced. If the care that the RT must give to his patient includes touching an area where a drain is inserted, he must use surgical aseptic technique to prevent introduction of new microorganisms into the wound. This will require hand-washing and donning sterile gloves (Chapter 9). If the RT may come into contact with drainage from these areas, he must wear gloves and wash his hands correctly after their removal.

Summary

NG and NI tubes are inserted to maintain gastric or intestinal decompression, to diagnose diseases of the GI tract, to treat diseases of the GI tract, and to feed patients who are unable to swallow food in the normal manner. Mechanical suction often accompanies NG and NI intubation. The RT must be prepared to assist with passage of an NG tube and to transfer patients who have NG and NI tubes in place and are receiving gastric suction.

Before transferring a patient who has a gastric tube in place and is receiving continuous gastric suction, the RT must learn whether it is permissible to discontinue the suction and, if so, for how long. The patient should be moved carefully. If the suction is continuous, it must be restarted as soon as the patient reaches the diagnostic imaging department at the same pressure as was used in his room.

The Salem-Sump gastric tube is a double-lumen tube designed to maintain a continuous flow of atmospheric air into the stomach. This tube must never be clamped with a regular clamp or hemostat, since such clamping may destroy the double-lumen effect of the tube.

The gastric tubes most often used in the radiology department are the Levin tube and the Cantor tube. The Levin tube enters the stomach, and the Cantor, the small intestine. The RT must learn to assist with their passage and care.

Levin tubes may be removed by the RT if he receives a physician's order to do so. They should be gently withdrawn and wrapped in several thicknesses of paper toweling, placed in an impermeable bag, and disposed of in the contaminated waste. If the tube is not easily removed, the radiologist should be called to remove it. NI tubes are not removed by the RT. Either a registered nurse or the physician removes it, or it is allowed to pass through the intestinal tract and is removed rectally.

The RT will not perform nasopharyngeal or oropharyngeal suctioning procedures, but he must be able to assess the patient's need for suctioning. He is responsible for having the equipment prepared and for assisting with the procedure. When it is required, it is usually an emergency procedure done to prevent aspiration of secretions into the lungs or respiratory arrest.

The patient with a tracheostomy may require diagnostic imaging examination. The RT must understand that these patients may be extremely apprehensive. They are unable to speak and unable to clear their tracheostomy tube of secretions that accumulate. A nurse who is able to suction a tracheostomy should accompany the patient who has a new tracheostomy to the diagnostic imaging department. It is the RT's responsibility to stop whatever he is doing for the patient at any time the patient needs to be suctioned.

The RT must be able to care for patients who have chest tubes that are connected to water-sealed drainage. He must remember to keep the tubing coiled at the patient's chest level, to keep all connections tightly sealed, to maintain the water seal at all times, to notify the nurse or physician if there is continuous bubbling in the water-sealed bottle, not to lift the water-sealed bottle above the patient's chest level, not to clamp or kink the drainage tube, and to notify the patient's nurse immediately if the water is below the level of the drainage tube.

There are various tissue drains used for the purpose of removing excessive fluid from an operative site to hasten the healing process and prevent infection. The RT must be aware of the presence of a tissue drain in any patient for whom he is caring. If a tissue drain is present, the RT must not allow tension to be placed on the drain that might dislodge it. He must also take appropriate infection-control precautions when caring for the patient who has a drain in place.

Chapter 8, pre-post test

_____ 1. When the RT is caring for a patient who has an NG tube in place in his department, he needs to
   a. Find out if the tube is to be reconnected to suction; if so, the amount of pressure needed
   b. Take care not to dislodge the tube
   c. Remove the tube before the patient leaves the department
   d. a and b
   e. a, b, and c

_____ 2. The items that must be on hand for patients who may need suctioning in the diagnostic imaging department are
   1. A portable wall outlet or portable suction machine
   2. A rectal tube
   3. Sterile gloves of all sizes
   4. An oily base lubricant
   5. A hemostat
   6. Sterile, disposable suction sets (or sterile basins and suction catheters)
   7. Sterile normal saline solution
   8. an oxygen source

   a. Items 1,2,3,4, and 8
   b. Items 2,3,5,7, and 8
   c. Items 2,4,5,6, and 8
   d. Items 1,3,6,7, and 8

_____ 3. If a patient has been suctioned in the room assigned to a particular RT, it is his responsibility to remove the used items and clean the suction receptacle. What materials will he need to perform this task safely?
   a. Clean, disposable gloves and a paper bag for waste
   b. An impermeable waste bag for waste materials
   c. Disinfectant, sterile gloves, and a paper bag
   d. Clean, disposable gloves and an impermeable bag for waste

_____ 4. The following are two points to remember when caring for a patient with a new tracheostomy in place:
   a. He may need to be suctioned, and he will be talkative.

   b. He will be anxious, and he will be unable to speak.
   c. He will be in the stage of denial, and he will express his anger.
   d. He will be unconscious, and he will be accompanied by a nurse.

_____ 5. When caring for a patient who has a chest tube with water-seal drainage, what must the RT remember?
   a. The water seal must be maintained at all times, and if the water-seal bottle tips, it must be righted immediately.
   b. Continuous bubbling into the water-sealed system is an indication that all is well, and the tube may be clamped if necessary.
   c. a is correct.
   d. b is correct.

_____ 6. Signs and symptoms that indicate a patient's need for oropharyngeal suctioning are
   a. Audible rattling and gurgling sounds from the patient's throat
   b. Gagging
   c. Breathing with difficulty
   d. a and b
   e. a, b, and c

_____ 7. If an RT is caring for a patient who has a tissue drain in place, he must
   a. Disregard these drains, because they are not his concern
   b. Prevent tension on the drain and use surgical aseptic technique if in direct contact with the drain
   c. Measure intake and output from the drain
   d. Remove the drain because it will impede the success of the radiograph

8. List three reasons why a patient might have NG or NI intubation, and explain the RT's responsibilities if such a tube is in place in a patient to whom he is assigned.

_____ 9. When disconnecting a Salem-Sump gastric tube (a tube with a double lumen), the RT must
   a. Clamp the tube with a regular clamp and then place sterile gauze over each end
   b. Clamp the tube closed with a hemostat
   c. Increase the amount of suction pressure
   d. Place a piston syringe in the open end of the gastric tube or place the "pig tail" over it
   e. Decrease the amount of suction pressure

____ 10. When working with a patient who has a chest tube in place, the RT must take which of the following precautions:
   a. Clamping the tube before beginning work
   b. Placing the drainage bottle on the patient's bed

   c. Calling the porter to wipe up the floor if the drainage bottle breaks
   d. a, b, and c
   e. none of the above

Laboratory reinforcement

1. Using a mannequin, demonstrate in the school laboratory how to disconnect a Levin tube and then a Salem-Sump tube.

2. Simulate in the school laboratory the preparation the RT would make for nasopharyngeal suctioning, including preparing the required equipment.

Chapter Nine

Surgical Aseptic Technique for Radiologic Technologists

Goal of this chapter:

The RT student will be able to list the principles of surgical asepsis and be able to create and maintain a sterile field when it is called for in his department or in the operating room.

Behavioral objectives:

When the student has completed this chapter, he will be able to do the following:
1. Define surgical asepsis and differentiate between medical asepsis and surgical asepsis
2. List the most common means of transmitting microorganisms in the operating room (OR) and in the special procedures area
3. Differentiate between disinfection and sterilization
4. List the methods of sterilization and disinfection
5. List the rules of surgical asepsis
6. Demonstrate the correct method of opening a sterile pack in order to prevent contamination
7. Demonstrate the correct method of placing a sterile object on a sterile field
8. Demonstrate the correct method of putting on a sterile gown and sterile gloves
9. Demonstrate skin preparation for a sterile procedure
10. Demonstrate the correct method of removing and reapplying a dressing

Glossary

Ampule a small glass container that can be sealed and its contents sterilized

Fenestrated having one or more openings; used in sterile procedures

Laminar air flow filtered air moving along separate parallel flow planes to various hospital areas; helps prevent contamination in sterile areas

Ratchet the section of the forceps that allows the instrument to remain closed and firmly locked until released

Sterile field an area protected from microorganisms, usually by a sterile sheet or covering onto which only sterile objects may be placed

Sterile pack usually contains all necessary items for a particular medical or surgical procedure and needs only be opened using sterile precautions

Parenteral medications medicines given any other route than the alimentary canal

Surgical asepsis must be differentiated from medical asepsis. In Chapter 2 *medical asepsis* was defined as any practice that helps reduce the number and spread of microorganisms. The term *surgical asepsis* was defined as the complete removal of all microorganisms and their spores from the surface of any object on which they might exist. One may then say an object is *sterile*. The practice of surgical asepsis begins with cleaning the object in a medically aseptic way. It is followed by a sterilization procedure, utilizing either heat or chemical action to accomplish the total removal of microorganisms and spores. Any medical procedure that involves penetration of body tissues (an invasive procedure) requires the use of surgical aseptic technique. This includes major and minor surgical procedures and administration of parenteral medications. It is also used for catheterization of the urinary bladder, tracheostomy care, and dressing changes.

Many diagnostic imaging examinations involve penetration of body tissues, so they must be done by means of surgical aseptic technique. Frequently, the RT is called to the OR for radiographic examinations while a major surgical procedure is in progress. He must be able to do his work in the OR without contaminating the surgical field.

All invasive procedures require special skin preparation before they are begun. The purpose of skin preparation (skin prep) is to remove any skin oils, dirt, and as many microorganisms as is possible to prevent their entry into the operative site and reduce the chances of an infection. Since the RT is often responsible for the skin prep in his department, he must learn to do it correctly.

Occasionally the radiologist will request that a dressing be removed or reapplied. Microorganisms must not be introduced into the wound during this process. Draining wounds are a potential source of contamination for the RT and for others in the department. The RT must be able to remove or reapply a dressing by using aseptic technique in order to protect the patient, himself, and others from infection.

The RT frequently participates in procedures that call for the use of surgical asepsis. If he is not skilled in its use, he may be responsible for contaminating a surgical field. This causes loss of time while the field is resterilized. If the contamination is not recognized, microorganisms may be introduced into the surgical wound, ultimately resulting in infection. It is the duty of all health workers who participate in sterile procedures to maintain strict surgical aseptic technique at all times because the patient's well-being is at stake.

The environment and surgical asepsis

The means of transmission of microorganisms was discussed in Chapter 2. To review, the methods of transmission are contact, both direct and indirect; droplet; vehicle; and airborne. Every possible effort

is made in the OR and special procedures areas to protect the patient from spread of microorganisms, because the patient who comes to these areas is easy prey to infection. This is done by creating an environment that establishes barriers to the spread of microbes. All persons who enter these areas are expected to follow the rules established to maintain these barriers.

OR departments have strict dress and behavior protocols that are strictly enforced. The RT who is assigned to work in this area is expected to follow these protocols.

Comfortable, supportive shoes must be worn. Clogs, sandals, and tennis shoes are prohibited for safety reasons. Meticulous personal hygiene is required. Jewelry and nail polish are prohibited, because they harbor microorganisms. Any health worker who has an acute infection or skin lesion must not work in the OR or special procedures area. All persons working in the OR change their outer clothing and don special OR garments called *scrub suits* and protective shoe covers before entering the OR suite. If the RT must leave the operating suite to develop films and return, he must change his clothes before reentering. Hair must be completely covered with a surgical cap or hood at all times when in the operating suite. Hands and arms are scrubbed as described for surgical asepsis before the RT begins his work in the OR or special procedures room.

A clean surgical mask is worn over the mouth and nose when an operation or other sterile procedure is in progress. The RT who must use radiographic equipment in the OR must clean it with a disinfectant solution before bringing it into the area. Many hospitals have radiographic equipment that is never removed from the operating suite, and it is cleaned routinely before and after every use by the housecleaning department.

Hands and forearms are scrubbed in a specified manner by persons participating in invasive surgical procedures. When this is completed, they dry their hands with sterile towels, dress in a sterile gown, and put on sterile gloves. Medical personnel dressed in sterile attire and ready to participate in a sterile procedure are called *sterile* or *scrubbed*. After a person is scrubbed, he must not touch anything that is not sterile. If he does, he is considered contaminated and must change whatever has been contaminated so that he is sterile once again.

The person who assists the sterile medical personnel is called the circulating nurse. The circulating nurse wears a scrub suit, a cap to cover the hair, and a mask, but does not don a sterile gown and sterile gloves. Her duty is to obtain the necessary equipment for the procedure and to place it on the sterile field in a manner that maintains its sterility.

A sterile field is an area that has been prepared to receive sterile equipment. It is touched only by the sterile personnel. The circulating nurse monitors the sterile field and counts the sponges, needles, and instruments before and after each surgical procedure, because all of these must be accounted for.

Sterile linens and other equipment and supplies used for sterile procedures must be packaged in a particular manner to be considered safe for use. They must also be stored in a manner that protects them from infection.

Any break in sterile technique increases the patient's susceptibility to infection. Those involved in carrying out a sterile procedure must constantly be aware of which areas and articles are sterile. If a sterile article is touched by an unsterile one, it must be replaced by an article that is sterile. A contaminated area must be made sterile again. Correct sterilization techniques must be learned and followed. Correct methods of opening sterile packs and donning sterile gown and gloves must also be learned and used without fail.

The use of contaminated instruments or gloves, a wet or damp sterile field, and microorganisms blown onto a surgical site are the most common causes of contamination. Ventilating ducts must have special filters in order to prevent dust particles from entering the room. Laminar air flow may be used to prevent drafts that transport dirt particles and microbes into the OR. Doors must always be kept closed during surgical procedures.

The RT whose work involves sterile procedures must develop a sense of responsibility and maintain the highest standards possible when practicing surgical asepsis. The patient's welfare depends on this.

Methods of sterilization

Removal of microorganisms and their spores must be complete, or the article is not sterile. The method used to attain sterilization depends on the nature of the item to be sterilized. All effective methods of sterilization have advantages and disadvantages. The methods currently used include (1) steam under pressure, (2) gas, (3) chemicals, (4) dry heat, and (5) ionizing radiation.

Steam under pressure

Using steam under pressure is an effective and convenient means of sterilization for items that can withstand high temperatures and moisture. It is fast, convenient, and economical. Steam that is not pres-

surized cannot reach temperatures high enough to kill all microorganisms and their spores. Pressure is attained in a chamber called an *autoclave.*

There are several types of autoclaves designed to sterilize with steam under pressure. Whatever type is chosen must allow the steam to penetrate every fiber of the article in order to accomplish its purpose. Some bacterial spores continue to live for longer than 3 hours in temperatures as high as 240° F (115° C), but none can live if the temperature is raised to 250° F (121° C) for longer than 15 minutes, so the temperature within the autoclave must reach this range for this period of time on every fiber to be sterilized. The time required to do this depends upon the contents of the pack and the temperature in the autoclave.

Indicators are placed in the center and outside of each pack to be sterilized. When the indicator changes color, it is proof that the contents of the pack have been exposed sufficiently to steam to change the color of the indicator, but it does not guarantee the sterility of the pack. There are variations among indicators used, and the RT must familiarize himself with the types used in his place of employment.

Gas

Sterilization by gas is the method of choice for sterilizing items that cannot withstand moisture and high temperatures. A mixture of ethylene oxide and carbon dioxide or fluorinated hydrocarbon is used because ethylene oxide gas alone is inflammable and explosive.

Gas sterilizers are heated from 120° F to 140° F (49° C to 60° C) with a humidity of 40% to 80%. This humidity is lower than is achieved with steam under pressure. The items to be sterilized, size, gas concentration, and temperature dictate time needed for sterilization to be achieved.

Gas sterilization should not be used for items that can be sterilized with steam. Glass ampules of medication with rubber stoppers should not be gas-sterilized, because the gas may penetrate through the rubber stopper and change the chemical composition of the solution.

Chemicals

Chemical sterilization is used when an item cannot withstand heat, when gas sterilization is not available, or when the aeration time is lengthy. The only chemicals that may be used for sterilization purposes are those registered as sterilants by the United States Environmental Protection Agency and used as directed by the manufacturer. The chemical solution of choice at present is 2% activated, buffered alkaline glutaraldehyde, which will kill spores on items immersed in solution for at least 10 hours.

Dry heat

Dry heat is used to sterilize anhydrous oils (oils containing no water), petroleum products, and bulk powders. It may also be used to sterilize some delicate cutting instruments that may be corroded or discolored by other methods of sterilization. It is a slow, uneven method rarely used in hospitals. The time it takes to sterilize with dry heat varies from 1 to 6 hours.

Ionizing radiation

Ionizing radiation is not used in institutions, but it is used in commercial sterilization. Cobalt-60 is the most common source of radiation sterilization. Ionic energy is converted to thermal energy during this process and causes the death of microorganisms and their spores.

Disinfection

All items that penetrate the skin or mucous membranes must be sterile. Articles or surfaces that cannot be sterilized in the OR or special procedures area must be disinfected. Tables, floors, walls, and equipment used in areas where the patient is to have an invasive procedure are included in this category. Skin around the area to be penetrated is also disinfected. When skin is disinfected, the solutions used are called *antiseptics*. The term *disinfection* means that as many microorganisms as possible are eliminated from the surfaces by physical or chemical means. Spores are often not destroyed by disinfection.

Chemical disinfectants are numerous and vary in their effectiveness for destroying microorganisms. In order for a chemical disinfectant to be accepted for hospital use, it must be effective against *Staphylococcus aureus, Salmonella choleraesulis,* and *Pseudomonas aeruginosa.* If an agent is not pseudomonacidal it may be used, but the label must state that it does not destroy *Pseudomonas aeruginosa.* The nature of the contamination and the area or object to be disinfected are also taken into consideration when a disinfectant is selected for use. The manufacturer's directions must be followed carefully when using any chemical.

Physical methods of disinfecting are boiling in water and ultraviolet irradiation. Boiling may be used as a means of disinfection if no other method is available; however, many spores are able to resist the heat of boiling (212° F or 100° C) for many hours.

In order to increase the effectiveness of boiling, sodium carbonate may be added to the water in quantity to make a 2% solution. It should not be added if the material being boiled is made of rubber, because sodium carbonate will destroy the rubber. If an object is to be disinfected by boiling and sodium carbonate is added to the water, it should be boiled for 15 minutes. If sodium carbonate has not been added, boiling time should be 30 minutes.

Ultraviolet rays kill microorganisms when they come into direct contact with them. This is not a practical means of disinfecting for hospital use because there is no assurance that the ultraviolet has actually come into contact with microbes, which are in a constantly mobile state because of air currents.

Packaging and storing sterile supplies

There are several acceptable materials that can be used for packaging items that are to be sterilized. They are cloth, nonwoven fabrics, paper, and plastic. Whichever material is chosen for use, the following restrictions must be considered:

1. The sterilizing agent must be able to penetrate the material.

2. The sterilizing agent must be able to escape at the end of the sterilizing process.

3. Items packaged must be covered completely by the wrapper and securely fastened with tape or a heat seal that does not lend itself to reuse.

4. Pins, staples, or other sharp, penetrating objects must not be used to fasten packages, because they allow a port for contaminants to enter the pack when removed.

5. Contents must be identifiable, and evidence of exposure to the sterilizing agent must be present. Indicator tape with stripes that change color when exposed to the sterilizing agent is the most frequently used.

6. Packaging must be impermeable to dust, microbes, and moisture and must be able to maintain the sterility of the contents until opened.

7. The wrapper must be strong enough to remain damage-free.

8. Items must be wrapped to allow opening and removing them without contamination.

9. The wrapping material must be free of toxic ingredients and dyes and be economical.

A special area is designated in hospitals for the preparation of sterile supplies by a method that is followed at all times. Cloth wrappers are made of muslin of a specified weight. If this material is used for wrapping, it must be used in quadruple thickness, usually accomplished by using two double-thickness wrappers together. Nonwoven fabrics are available in three thicknesses: light, medium, and heavy. Lightweight nonwoven fabrics must be used in four thicknesses and mediumweight in double thickness. Heavyweight nonwoven material is usually used for surgical drapes in single thickness.

All sterile items are stored in the same place, separate from nonsterile items. A sterile package must have an expiration date printed on it. The RT must check the sterilization date carefully to be certain that the shelf life (the time that the package may be considered sterile while being stored) has not been exceeded. If there is no date on the package, it must be considered unsterile.

All storage areas for sterile materials must be clean, dust-free, vermin-free, and draft-free. Generally speaking, items that have been sterilized in the hospital and wrapped in cloth or paper wrappers are considered sterile for 30 days if they are in a closed cupboard. If they are on an open shelf, they are considered sterile for 21 days. Extremes of temperature and humidity must be avoided, and traffic in the storage area should be light. Items sealed in plastic bags immediately after sterilization are considered sterile for 6 to 12 months, provided the seal is not broken.

Commercially packaged sterilized items are considered sterile until the seal is broken or the package has been damaged or until the expiration date on the package has been passed.

Rules for surgical asepsis

The basic rules for surgical aseptic technique apply whenever and wherever the sterile procedure is done. The RT must commit these rules to memory and use them whether he is in his own department or in the OR. They are as follows:

1. Know which areas and objects are sterile and which are not.

2. If the sterility of an object is questionable, it is not to be considered sterile.

3. Sterile objects and persons must be kept separate from those that are unsterile.

4. When any item that must be sterile becomes contaminated, the contamination must be remedied immediately.

5. When tabletops are to be used as areas for creating a sterile field, they must be clean, and a sterile drape must be placed over them.

6. Personnel must be clothed in a sterile gown and gloves if they are to be considered sterile.

7. Any sterile instrument or sterile area that is touched by an unsterile object or person is contaminated by microorganisms.

8. A contaminated area on a sterile field must be covered by a folded sterile towel or a drape of double thickness.

9. If a sterile person's gown or gloves become contaminated, they must be changed.

10. A sterile field must be created just prior to its use.

11. Once a sterile field has been prepared, it must not be left unattended, because it may become contaminated accidently and not be observed.

12. An unsterile person does not reach across a sterile field.

13. A sterile person does not lean over an unsterile area.

14. A sterile field ends at the level of the tabletop or at the waist of the sterile person's gown.

15. Anything that drops below the tabletop or a sterile person's waistline is no longer sterile. The only parts of a sterile gown considered sterile are the areas from the waist to the shoulders in front and the sleeves.

16. The edges of a sterile wrapper are not considered sterile and must not touch a sterile object.

17. Any part of a sterile drape that falls below the tabletop is considered unsterile and is not brought up to table level.

18. Sterile drapes are placed by the sterile person who drapes the area closest to him first to protect his sterile gown.

19. A sterile person must remain within the sterile area. He does not lean on tables or against the wall.

20. If one sterile person must pass another, they must pass each other back-to-back.

21. The sterile person faces the sterile field and keeps his sterile gloved hands above his waist and in front of his chest. He avoids touching any area of his body.

22. Any sterile material or pack that becomes dampened or wet is considered unsterile.

23. Any objects that are wet with sporicidal solution and are placed on the sterile field must be placed on a folded sterile towel in order for the moisture to be absorbed.

24. A wet area on a sterile field must be covered with several thicknesses of sterile toweling or an impervious drape.

25. All areas that are used for sterile procedures, including floors, should be well cleaned with disinfectant solution after each procedure. Mops used should be disposable and used only one time.

26. Air conditioning units must be kept clean, and filters should be changed frequently to prevent their blowing bacteria on sterile fields.

27. Ventilation ducts must have special filters in order to prevent particles from entering the OR or special procedures room.

28. When pouring a sterile solution, place the lid face upward and do not touch the inside of the lid or the lip of the flask. Pour off a small amount of solution before the remainder is poured into the sterile container.

29. When a sterile solution is to be poured into a container on a sterile field, the container is placed at the edge of the sterile filed by the sterile person.

Commercial packs

Commercial packs are usually wrapped in paper or plastic wrappers. They are frequently sealed in plastic to ensure prolonged sterility. Directions for opening the containers in such a way that there is no contamination are printed on the pack and should be read before opening. The most common type of pack is sealed at the edges. The seal can be separated at the top and peeled back until the sterile article is exposed. The pack can either be opened completely and the contents made available for the sterile person to pick up, or the contents can be dropped onto the sterile field. Packs must never be cut open or pierced with a knife or sharp object. Do not tear packs open, and do not allow the contents to slide over the edges of the pack. They should be flipped or lifted out.

Opening sterile packs

The RT must be prepared to open sterile packs and either place their contents on the sterile field or hand them to the sterile person without contaminating them. There is a standard method for this procedure, which can be done without difficulty after it is practiced.

Cloth-wrapped packs

The RT should already have washed his hands. When a request for a sterile item is received, the RT obtains the correct pack and returns it to the procedure room. A cloth-wrapped pack will be sealed with indicator tape. The lines in the tape will be dark gray if the pack has been correctly sterilized.

The pack is placed on a clean tabletop with the sealed end toward the RT (Fig. 9-1). Remove the tape and discard it. Open corner 1 back and away from the pack (Fig. 9-2). Next, open corners 2 and 3 (Figs. 9-3 and 9-4). Then open corner 4 and drop it toward your body (Fig. 9-5). Do not touch the sterile contents of the pack. This can now become a sterile field, and more sterile items may be placed in the center of the drape. Or the sterile contents of the pack can now be placed on another sterile field.

To move the contents to another sterile field, grasp the underside of the wrapper and let the edges fall over your hand. Hold the contents forward for the sterile person to grasp (Fig. 9-6). If it is preferable that the RT place the contents on the sterile field, he must grasp the corners of the wrapper with the other hand so that they do not brush the field. The RT reaches slightly over the sterile field and several inches above it and drops the contents of the pack onto the field (Fig. 9-7).

Sterile forceps

A sterile forceps—usually a large serrated ring forceps with ratchet closures—may be used to transfer objects

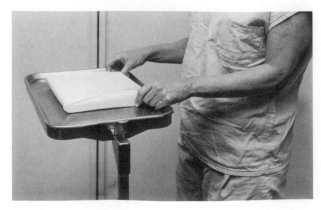

Figure 9.1

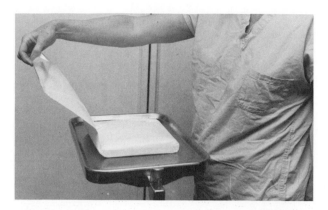

Figure 9.2

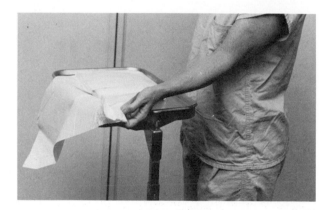

Figure 9.3.   Open the second corner.

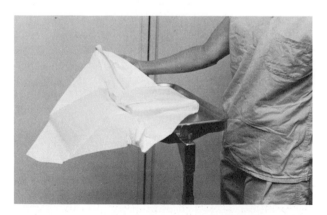

Figure 9.4

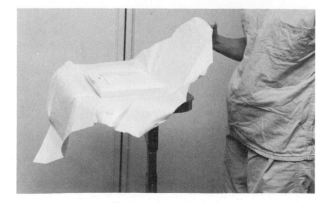

Figure 9.5

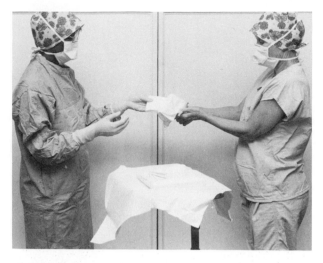

Figure 9.6

from one sterile area to another. It is packaged in a sterile wrapper. The package should be opened so that there is a sterile surface on which to place the forceps when it is not in use. Only the tips of the forceps are sterile.

When an object is to be transferred with a sterile forceps, the procedure is as follows: Open the sterile pack. Grasp the forceps by the handle, open the ratchet, and grasp the object to be transferred. Close the ratchet around the object. Transfer the object to the new location. Open the ratchet and drop the sterile object onto the sterile field. Replace the forceps on its sterile wrapper with the handles away from the center of the wrapper (Fig. 9-8). The forceps must not be used for more than one procedure. If it is not kept in constant sight of the person using it, it should not be considered sterile and another must be obtained for use.

The surgical scrub

Although the RT is not often the ''sterile person'' in the OR or special procedures area, he must be able

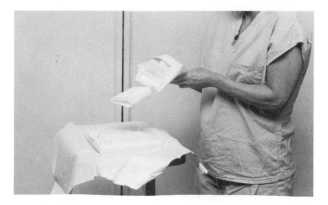

Figure 9.7

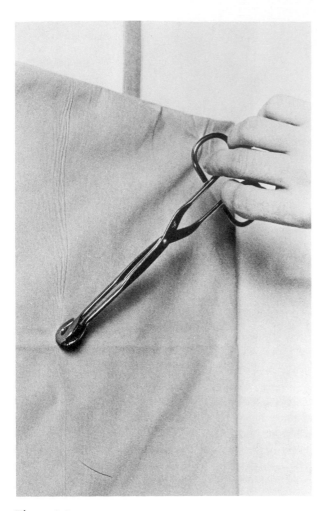

Figure 9.8

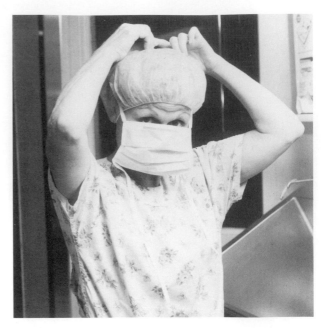

Figure 9.9

to perform this function if the situation calls for it. To begin, regular exterior clothing is changed for a scrub suit, and shoe covers are placed over your shoes. The shoe covers are made of a heavy paper and have a built-in conductive strip that prevents the production of static electricity. A surgical cap or hood is then put on to cover all hair. Hoods are used if the person has a beard. All jewelry is removed. If pierced-ear studs are worn, they must be covered by the cap.

If the procedure to be performed in the OR or special procedures room involves fluoroscopy or the team is unable to protect themselves while radiographic exposures are being taken, protective lead garments must be worn over the scrub suit and under the sterile gown. These protective garments, which should include a lead apron, a thyroid shield, and special glasses, should be put on before the surgical scrub is begun.

A face mask is removed from the container. Handle the mask only by the ties. Place the mask on your face so that it covers the nose and mouth (Fig. 9-9). Tie it at the back of the head and neck. Make certain that it is comfortable and secure. The mask must

never be touched after it is in place, because it quickly becomes contaminated. Masks must be changed between each procedure and are never to be worn around the neck to be pulled up again over the face.

At this point the procedure will vary with the OR assignment. If the RT is to take radiographic exposures, he should scrub for 3 minutes with an antiseptic soap, dry his hands with paper towels, and proceed to his position in the OR. If he is to put on a sterile gown and gloves, he must do a surgical scrub.

The procedure for the surgical scrub varies from hospital to hospital, but either the timed method or the brush count method is used. Some institutions require an initial 10-minute scrub and subsequent 5-minute or reduced brush stroke scrubs for each case following the initial scrub during a 24-hour period. The antimicrobial agents most commonly used for surgical scrub at this time are an iodine complex and detergent (Iodophors), chlorhexidine gluconate in 4% solution, and in cases of allergy to other agents, hexachlorophene or triclosan.

The surgical scrub is performed to remove as many microorganisms as possible from the skin of the hands and lower arms by mechanical and chemical means prior to a sterile procedure. The arms should be bare to at least 4 inches above the elbows. The procedure for the timed or stroke method surgical scrub is as follows:

1. Approach the sink. Adjust the water temperature and pressure. Most surgical scrub areas have knee or foot regulators for water faucets. If they do not, the faucet handles should be turned on, adjusted, and not touched again.

2. Obtain a scrub brush. Brushes must be single-use and disposable. Combination sponge-brushes with the antimicrobial agent permeated through them are most commonly used. Wet the hands and forearms to approximately 2 inches above the elbow. Hold the hands up and allow the water to flow downward toward the elbows from the cleanest area to least clean and apply the antimicrobial agent (Fig. 9-10).

3. Scrub hands and arms using a firm rotary motion. Fingers, hands, and arms should be considered to have four sides, all of which must be thoroughly cleaned. An anatomical pattern should be followed, beginning with the thumb and proceeding to each finger. Next do the dorsal surface of the hand, the palm, and up the wrist ending 2 inches above the elbow. Wash all four sides of the arm. Scrubbing for the OR always begins with the hands because they are in direct contact with the sterile field (Fig. 9-11).

4. A nail cleaner is included with the scrub brush. After the first hand and arm scrub, clean under each fingernail with this nail cleaner and dispose

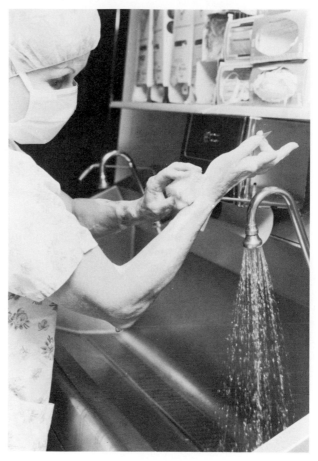

Figure 9.11

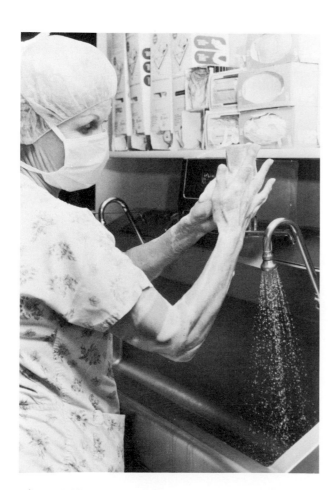

Figure 9.10

of it (Fig. 9-12). Rinse hands and arms, and re-scrub in the same pattern until all brush strokes are complete or until the time is up (Fig. 9-13).

5. When the scrub is complete, drop the brush into the sink or a receptacle prepared to receive the used brushes. Do not touch the sink or the receptacle. Remember to hold the hands up above the waist and higher than the elbows during and after the surgical scrub.

6. Proceed to the area where a sterile towel, sterile gown, and sterile gloves have been prepared for you.

7. Pick up the sterile towel, which is folded on top of the sterile gown, by one corner and let it unfold in front of you at waist level. Do not let the towel touch your scrub suit (Fig. 9-14).

8. Dry one hand and one arm with each end of the towel.

9. When hands and arms are thoroughly dry, drop the towel to the floor or into a receptacle for this purpose, being careful to keep hands held up above the waist (Fig. 9-15).

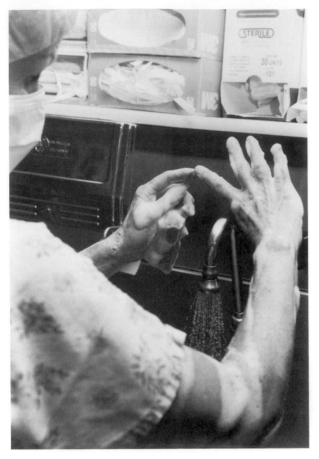

Figure 9.12

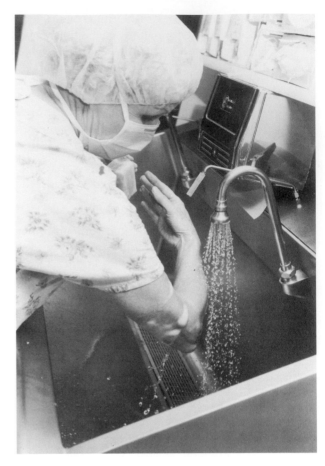

Figure 9.13

Sterile gowning and gloving

If the RT must open his own sterile gown and glove packs, he must do so before the surgical scrub. Usually an assistant is on hand to do this for the person who is scrubbing.

Gowning

The sterile gown is made of either a synthetic non-woven material or of cloth. Grasp the gown and remove it from the table. Step away from the table. The gown will be folded inside out. Hold the gown away from your body and allow it to unfold length-wise without touching the floor (Fig. 9-16). Open the gown and hold it by the shoulder seams. Place both arms into the arm holes of the gown and wait for assistance (Fig. 9-17). Your assistant or the circulating nurse will place her hands into the inside of the gown at the shoulders and pull the gown over the shoulders and arms until the hands are exposed if open-gloving technique is to be used. If closed-

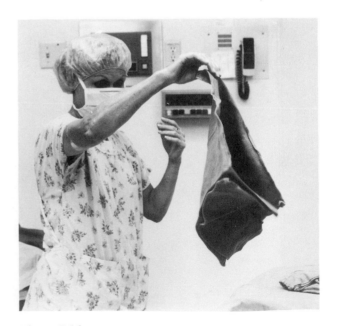

Figure 9.14

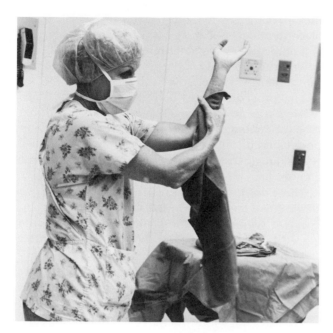

Figure 9.15

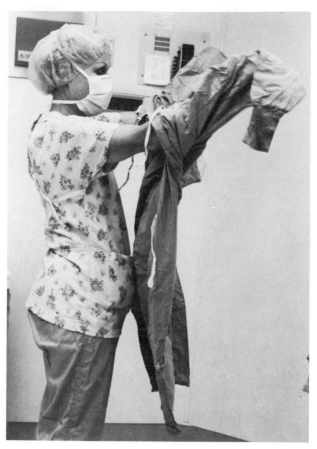

Figure 9.17

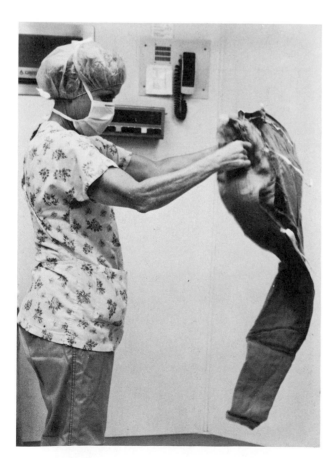

Figure 9.16

gloving technique is to be used, the cuffs of the gown sleeves will be left to cover the hands (Fig. 9-18).

Gloving

There are two methods of gloving for sterile procedures: open and closed. For the RT's purposes, the open method is more practical. Setting up for a sterile procedure, as well as performing certain minor sterile procedures, requires the use of sterile gloves, but not a sterile gown. If this is the case, the RT should wash his hands according to the rules of medical asepsis described in Chapter 2 and proceed with gloving by the open method.

The glove wrapper is opened, and the gloves are exposed. Sterile gloves are always packaged folded down at the cuff and powdered so that they may be put on more easily.

Pick up the right glove with the left hand at the folded cuff. Slide the right hand into the glove, leaving the cuff of the glove folded down. When it is over the hand, leave it and pick up the left glove with the gloved right hand under the fold (Fig. 9-19), *A* through *E*). Pull the glove over the hand and over

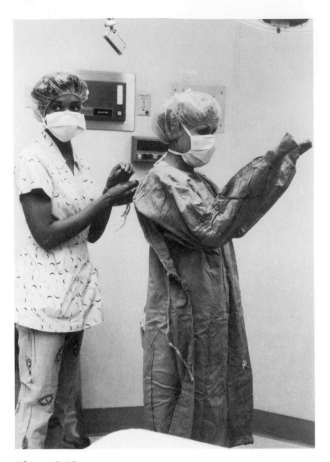

Figure 9.18

the cuff of the gown in one motion (Fig. 9-20). Then place the fingers of the gloved left hand under the cuff of the right glove and pull it over the cuff of the gown. After the cuffs of the gloves cover the cuffs of the sterile gown, the gloves can be adjusted.

This procedure must be practiced several times before it is perfected. The RT must not be discouraged if he contaminates his gloves the first few times that he puts them on. The important thing is to notice when the gloves become contaminated and ask for another pair.

The closed method is restricted to use when a sterile gown has been donned and the hands remain enclosed within the cuffs of the gown. The sterile glove pack is opened before the procedure begins.

With the left hand (or nondominant hand) covered by the gown sleeve cuff, pick up the right glove and place it palm-side down on the palm of the right hand, which is also covered by the cuff of the second sleeve. The fingers of the glove should be pointing toward the elbow (Figs. 9-21, 9-22). Grasp the cuff of the glove through the gown with the right hand. The covered left hand pulls the glove over the right hand, gently inserting the fingers into the finger spaces of the glove. Be certain that the cuff of the glove covers the cuff of the gown (Figs. 9-23, 9-24).

With the gloved right (or dominant) hand, pick up the next glove and place it on the palm of the left

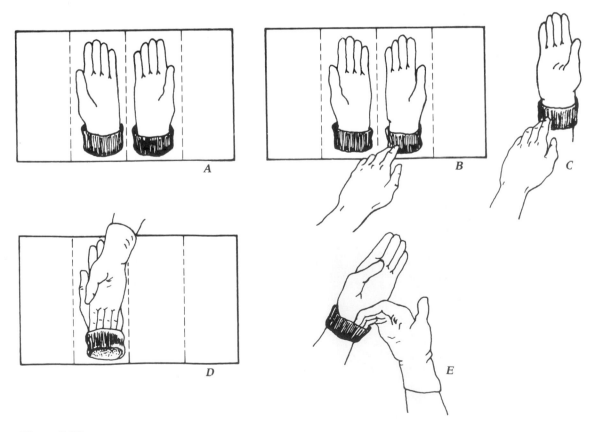

Figure 9.19

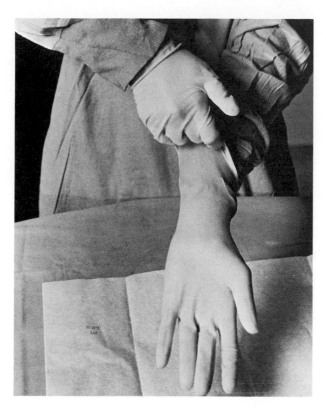

Figure 9.20

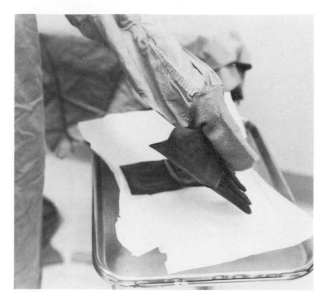

Figure 9.21

hand with the fingers pointing to the elbow. Grasp the cuff of the glove through the sleeve cuff and with the gloved right hand, pull the second glove into place (Fig. 9-25).

Taking radiographs in the operating room

When the RT is called to the OR, he must know what equipment the institution has available for this purpose. In many hospitals, radiographic equipment remains in the operating suite at all times. In smaller institutions, the RT will have to transfer a portable radiographic machine from his own department.

The RT is also responsible for protecting himself and the persons in the OR from radiation. He must know if the institution in which he is employed has protective lead garments available at all times in the OR suite or if he must transport them along with his portable machine for his own use and the use of the OR team.

The RT must clean his portable radiographic machine and the cassettes that will be used with a disinfectant solution before he transfers them into the operating room where he will be working. All necessary equipment must be prepared and cleaned before the RT changes into a scrub suit and scrubs.

Frequently the need for a radiograph is anticipated, and cassettes may be placed before the surgical procedure begins. At other times, the need is not anticipated, and the RT will have to place his machine and cassettes after the sterile field has been created and the surgery begun. If this is the case, the cassette may be passed to the scrub nurse by the RT. The scrub nurse receives it in a sterile plastic bag and places it at the RT's direction. The RT places the cassette in the bag carefully to avoid contaminating the outside of the bag and the scrub nurse's gloves (Fig. 9-26).

If the RT must place the cassette himself, the OR team will make room for him. He can direct the team

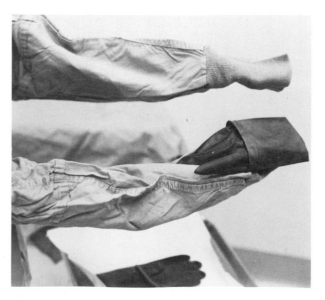

Figure 9.22

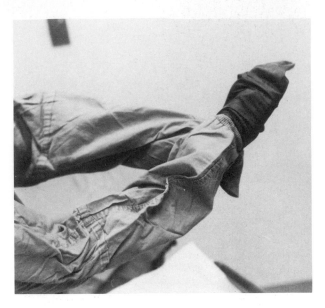

Figure 9.23

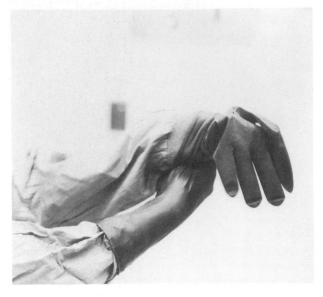

Figure 9.25

to stand behind plastic screens placed to protect them from radiation while he makes the necessary exposures. Care must be taken to prevent contamination of the surgical field. Approach the operating table and place the cassette by lifting the surgical drapes from the bottom underside only (Fig. 9-27).

Skin preparation for sterile procedures

All invasive procedures are apt to introduce microorganisms into the open wound. To make the operative site or the procedure site as free of micro-

organisms as possible and to decrease the possibility of infection, the skin is disinfected before beginning the procedure. This is done by mechanical and chemical methods that are called *skin prep* or *prepping the skin*. Skin prep solutions are called antiseptics rather than disinfectants. The RT is often expected to do the skin prep in the special procedures area.

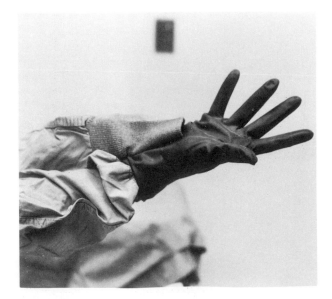

Figure 9.24

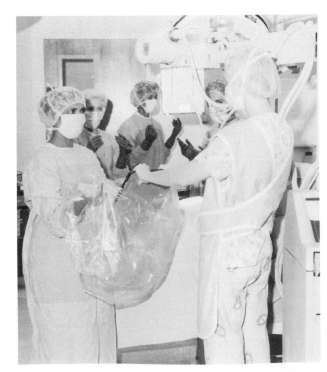

Figure 9.26

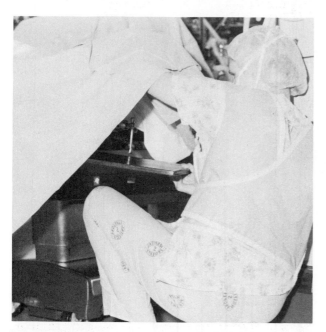

Figure 9.27

Mechanical methods of skin preparation

The mechanical method of skin preparation includes the removal of hair as necessary and a friction scrub with an antiseptic soap and water. Hair removal can break or injure the skin and should be done only when it is essential to prevent infection. It must be done only with an order from the physician in charge of the patient and as close to the time of the procedure as possible.

If hair removal is ordered, the RT should wash his hands and obtain a prep set that includes a small basin, a sponge permeated with antiseptic soap, one or two disposable razors, a sponge for rinsing, and a towel. Clean gloves are worn by the RT for this procedure. Explain the procedure to the patient and place him in a comfortable position.

Fill the basin with warm water, don the clean gloves, wet the soap sponge, and soak and soap the area to be shaved thoroughly. Shave the skin using short, firm strokes. Hold the skin taut and shave in the direction of hair growth. Remove only as much hair as necessary. After all unwanted hair has been removed, rinse the area with sterile water and dry it with the towel.

After all unwanted hair has been removed, the area is draped with towels in order to designate the upper and lower limits of the area to be prepped. The radiologist will explain how large an area he desires to have prepared. Usually it will be an area of approximately 6 to 10 inches in diameter around the puncture area.

Often, prepackaged prep trays are available that contain two small basins (one for sterile water and one for antiseptic), a set of large sponges, sterile towels, sterile gloves, and the antiseptic detergent solution. A flask of sterile water must also be on hand. The water should be no colder than room temperature. If the umbilicus is in the area to be prepared, four sterile applicators should be included. If the area to be prepared includes the vagina, a long sponge holder and eight to ten gauze sponges should be added. The physician will do the vaginal prep. The antiseptic detergent solutions most commonly used for skin preparation are iodophors, chlorhexidine gluconate, and, in special circumstances, hexachlorophene or triclosan.

After all of the necessary equipment has been assembled and the patient has been prepared, open the sterile pack. Pour sterile water into one of the basins. If the antiseptic agent is not in the sterile set, pour it into the other sterile basin. Then put on the sterile gloves using the open-gloving technique. Wet a sponge with water and then with soap solution and begin scrubbing in the center of the area to be prepared, working slowly outward in a circular motion. Use a firm stroke—friction is as important in the removal of microorganisms as is the antiseptic. Do not rewash the skin that has already been scrubbed with this sponge. When you reach the edges of the area being scrubbed, remove the sponge from the sterile field, discard it, and obtain another one. Repeat the procedure using the other sponge (Fig. 9-28). If the umbilicus is to be prepared, clean it with cotton applicators soaked in the antiseptic detergent.

This scrubbing procedure should last from 3 to 10 minutes. The skin must then be rinsed well with sterile water, or the lather may be wiped away without rinsing. The routine varies depending upon the procedure, the antiseptic used, and the policy of the institution. Before any skin preparation with antiseptics, the RT must ask the patient if he is allergic to iodine or any other antiseptic solutions. If the answer is positive, he must inform the physician, who will choose a substitute. The RT must carefully inspect the patient's skin during the skin prep. If it shows any sign of irritation or rash, the procedure should be stopped, and the antiseptic thoroughly rinsed off with sterile water. The radiologist should then be notified of the patient's sensitivity so that another chemical may be chosen that is not harmful to him. Do not allow solution to drain off the area being prepped and pool under the patient during the procedure, because this may burn the skin.

Chemical methods of skin preparation

After the scrub, which is a combination of mechanical and chemical preparation of the skin, the skin around

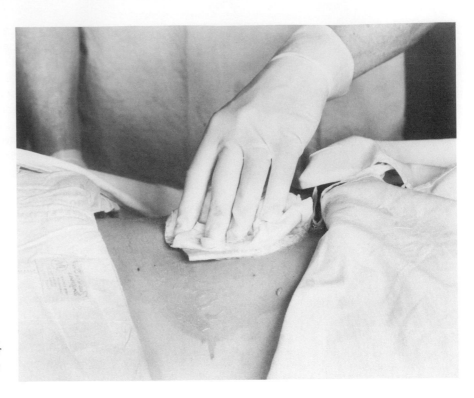

Figure 9.28. Repeat the scrub, beginning again in the center of the area to be prepared for the sterile procedure.

the area to be incised is often painted with an antiseptic solution. Application of an antiseptic to the skin destroys some bacteria and acts as a deterrent to bacterial growth (is bacteriostatic) for a short period of time. Isopropyl alcohol or povidone-iodine are often used. Alcohol must never be used on mucous membranes or on an open wound, because it coagulates protein and therefore may cause harm.

If the skin is to be painted with antiseptic after the scrub, it should be done with a circular motion, beginning at the center of the area to be prepped and working outward (Fig. 9-29). Many special procedure sets have long-handled sponges and a receptacle for this purpose. Use the antiseptic of your institution's choice and follow the directions listed in the previous paragraph. If there are no special skin-prep sponges, gauze sponges folded and grasped in a sterile ring forcep and dipped into a small sterile container of disinfectant may be used.

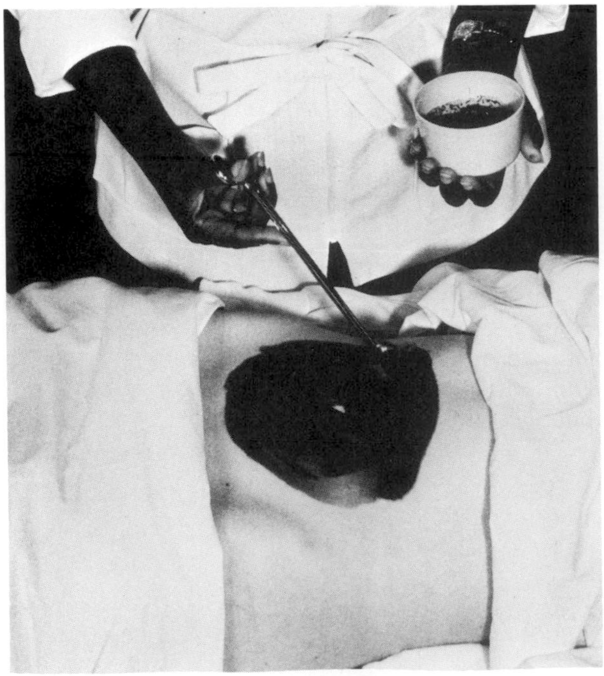

Figure 9.29. Begin at the center of the area being prepared and work outward in a circular motion.

Draping

After the skin has been mechanically and chemically prepared and allowed to dry, sterile drapes may be applied. They are placed around the area of skin that has been prepared. The type of sterile drape used differs with each procedure. In the diagnostic imaging department, the drapes are usually a single-thickness, impermeable material that is disposable. A fenestrated drape is often used. If this is the case, the drape should be applied in such a way that the opening leaves only the operative site exposed.

If sterile towels are used, they should be placed so that they are well within the limits of the area prepared, and they should be folded and placed so

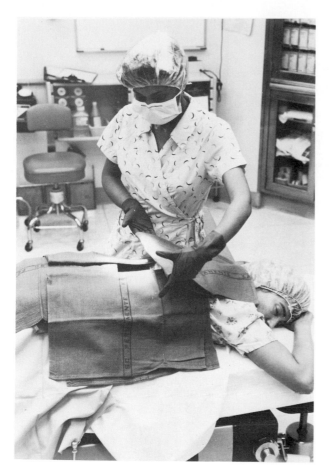

Figure 9.30

that they overlap and the folds face the operative site (Fig. 9-30).

Usually the physician places the sterile drapes after he has donned sterile gloves for the procedure. The RT must have the sterile pack that contains the drapes open and ready. Many prepackaged procedure sets contain sterile drapes. If the RT is to place the sterile drapes, he must first open a set of sterile gloves for himself. Then the pack containing the drapes is opened. The sterile gloves are then donned, and the drapes are placed. The part of the drape closest to the RT is placed first so that the sterility of the RT's gloves is maintained, or he holds the drape to protect his gloves (Fig. 9-31). Once the drape is in place, it may not be moved, because the underside of the drape would then be contaminated by touching the patient's skin.

Changing dressings

The RT must not remove dressings or reapply them unless such action is ordered by the physician. When the physician requests that a dressing be removed for

a procedure in the diagnostic imaging department, the RT must be able to remove it without contaminating the wound or himself in the process.

All dressings must be treated as if they are contaminated, because wound drainage may harbor pathogenic microorganisms. Before you remove a dressing, obtain clean gloves and a waterproof bag into which the soiled dressing will be placed. Open the bag and fold a large cuff over the opening. Dressings should not be touched with bare hands. Have everything in readiness before beginning to remove the dressing. Wash your hands, place the patient in a comfortable position, an explain to him what you are going to do. Provide privacy for the patient by closing the door and keeping his entire body covered except the affected area. Loosen the adhesive tape that holds the dressing in place. This must be done with care to prevent pain and skin damage. If the tape is difficult to remove, use a commercial tape remover to loosen it. Pull the tape toward the wound while supporting the skin with the other hand. Remove the dressing carefully with a gloved hand, and place it in the bag (Figs. 9-32, 9-33). Be cautious when removing the dressing and watch for any drain that may have been placed in or near the wound. It may be easily dislodged. After placing the soiled dressing into the bag, remove your gloves correctly and drop them into the bag. Place your hands under the cuff in the bag and unfold it upward; close the bag and place it into a contaminated waste receptacle. Wash your hands. If the dressing does not come off easily, stop the procedure and notify the physician. Never use force to remove a dressing; to do so may cause further damage to a wound.

When a dressing is reapplied, sterile technique must be used. Wash your hands and obtain the necessary equipment: a sterile towel, gauze pads, tape, a bag for refuse, and sterile gloves. Occasionally, if the wound is draining, it will be necessary to apply a larger dressing over the small gauze pads to absorb the drainage.

When the materials are assembled, approach the patient and explain the procedure to him. If the dressing has not been removed, remove it in the manner just described. Open the sterile towel to double thickness, and use it as a sterile field on which to place the sterile dressings. Open the dressings and place them on the sterile towel (Fig. 9-34). Prepare the tape by having it cut into the lengths needed for use.

If the skin around the wound is soiled or damp, add a small container and several small gauze sponges to the sterile set. Pour sterile water or sterile normal saline solution into the container. Put on sterile gloves and pick up and fold the small sponges. Moisten them in the sterile solution and cleanse the skin around the wound from the site outward. Do not wash the

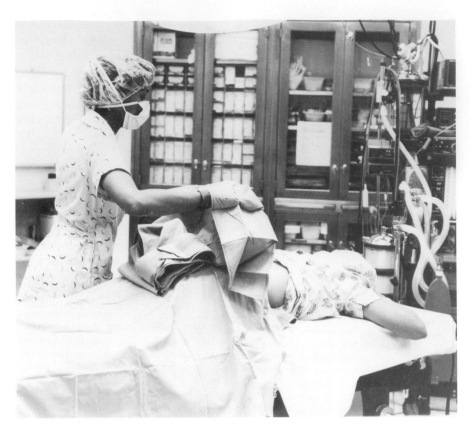

Figure 9.31

wound itself and do not apply any medications or antiseptics to the wound.

After the skin is dry, apply the dry sterile dressing (Fig. 9-35). If the wound is draining, add extra gauze dressings in order to absorb the drainage. Remove your gloves and drop them into the refuse bag. Tape the dressing in place, cover the patient, and make him comfortable. Wash your hands and dispose of the waste material correctly.

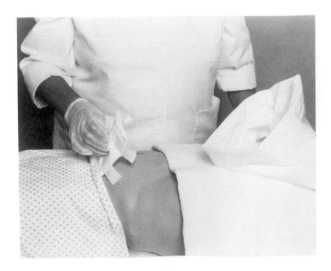

Figure 9.32

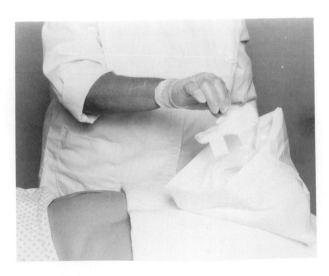

Figure 9.33

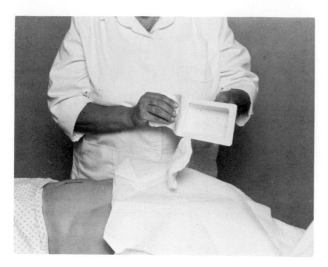

Figure 9.34

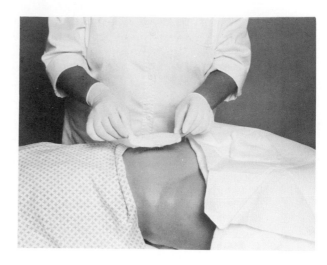

Figure 9.35

Summary

The RT must participate in examinations that require sterile technique both in the OR and in the diagnostic imaging department. Any health worker who participates in sterile procedures must practice meticulous surgical asepsis in order to prevent contamination and resultant patient infection.

The most common means of spreading microorganisms in the OR and special procedures area are the use of contaminated instruments and gloves, the wetting of a sterile field, and failure to control air currents across sterile fields. All of these situations can be prevented by use of flawless surgical aseptic technique.

There are several methods of rendering an article sterile, that is, completely removing microorganisms and their spores. They are steam under pressure, ethylene oxide gas, dry heat, chemicals, and ionizing radiation.

Sterilization indicators are used inside and outside packs before they are exposed to the sterilization process. They are an indication that the article has been exposed to a particular sterilization process. The RT must be able to read and understand the indicators used in the institution in which he works.

Mechanical and chemical methods are used to disinfect objects and surfaces that cannot be sterilized. Chemical disinfectants that are acceptable for hospital use must be able to destroy *Staphylococcus aureus, Salmonella choleraesulis,* and *Pseudomonas aeruginosa.* In order to ensure their effectiveness, the manufacturer's directions must be followed exactly.

Mechanical disinfecting methods are boiling and ultraviolet irradiation. Boiling is used as a means of disinfection only if no other method is available, because many microorganisms and their spores can withstand the boiling temperature for many hours. Ultraviolet rays kill microorganisms when they come into direct contact with them; however, it is an inefficient method of disinfection and is seldom used in hospitals.

The RT must learn the rules of surgical asepsis, because all invasive medical procedures require its use. He must learn to differentiate sterile objects from unsterile objects. He must learn to open sterile packs correctly to prevent contamination. When there is a question about the sterility of an item, it is always considered to be unsterile.

A surgical scrub is performed in the OR before a sterile gown and gloves are donned for a surgical procedure. The RT will not usually be the sterile person, because he will be in the OR to make radiographic exposures. He must become familiar with all OR practices, however, so that he can do his work without contaminating the sterile field.

Preparation of the skin for surgical penetration involves removing as many microorganisms as possible from the operative site. This reduces the possibility of infection from the procedure. Mechanical and chemical methods are used to prepare the skin, followed by application of sterile drapes around the operative area.

The RT may be required to remove or reapply a dressing. These procedures should be performed using aseptic technique. Any dressing that is removed must be assumed to harbor pathogenic microorganisms. Soiled dressings must not be touched with bare hands. Gloves must be used. The soiled dressings must be wrapped in a waterproof bag and disposed of properly in order to prevent contamination.

When dressings are removed or reapplied, the patient must be protected from infection. The RT must also protect himself and others in his department. Use of aseptic technique and proper methods of waste disposal will accomplish these goals.

Chapter 9, pre-post test

_____ 1. Which of the following is the best definition of surgical asepsis?
   a. Removing as many microorganisms as possible by mechanical and chemical methods
   b. Removing as many microorganisms and spores as possible by autoclaving
   c. Complete removal of microorganisms and spores
   d. Scrubbing, gowning, and gloving to prevent contamination

_____ 2. Which of the following procedures does not require the use of surgical aseptic technique?
   a. An intramuscular injection
   b. An intravenous injection
   c. An intrathecal procedure
   d. An arteriogram
   e. A gastrointestinal series

_____ 3. All items that penetrate the skin or mucous membrane must be
   a. Disinfected
   b. Sterile

_____ 4. Methods of disinfection are
   a. Steam under pressure and ionizing radiation
   b. Boiling and ultraviolet light
   c. Dry heat
   d. Ethylene oxide gas

_____ 5. You are the new RT in charge of maintaining a special procedures suite at the local community hospital. Since most procedures done in this suite demand sterile technique, you must consider
   a. The type of disinfectant solutions that the housekeepers will use to clean the area before and after each procedure
   b. How often the air filters are changed
   c. How sterile packs and instruments are packaged and stored
   d. a and b
   e. a, b, and c

_____ 6. Any dressing removed in the diagnostic imaging department should be considered
   a. Sterile
   b. Surgically aseptic
   c. Contaminated
   d. Medically aseptic

_____ 7. Sterile drapes are placed by the sterile person. They drape
   a. The area farthest away from them first
   b. The area nearest the invasive site first
   c. The area closest to them first

_____ 8. The skin is disinfected before beginning all invasive procedures to
   a. Protect the sterile drapes from contamination
   b. Decrease the possibility of introducing microorganisms into the open wound
   c. To protect the health worker from infection
   d. To ensure the success of the procedure

_____ 9. Removal of hair is done in preparation for an invasive procedure
   a. As close to the time of the invasive procedure as possible
   b. The night before the procedure
   c. Any time at all

_____ 10. When preparing the skin for a sterile procedure, the RT should scrub
   a. From the outside inward
   b. In a back and forth motion
   c. In a circular motion from inside to outside

_____ 11. Before the RT uses a sterile pack, he must check
   a. Its shelf life
   b. Its expiration date
   c. Its list of contents
   d. Its method of sterilization

_____ 12. Boiling is an acceptable means of sterilization.
   a. True
   b. False

_____ 13. Common means of transmitting microorganisms in the OR or special procedures room include
   a. Use of contaminated gloves or instruments
   b. Allowing a sterile field to become wet or damp
   c. Allowing microorganisms to be blown onto a surgical site
   d. None of the above
   e. All are correct

_____ 14. In order to maintain a sterile field, the person who has created it must never leave it unattended.
   a. True
   b. False

_____ 15. If an object on a sterile field drops below the "sterile person's" waistline, it may still be considered sterile.
   a. True
   b. False

_____ 16. The edges of a sterile wrapper may be considered sterile.
   a. True
   b. False

Laboratory reinforcement

1. Demonstrate in the school laboratory the proper techniques for scrubbing, gowning, and gloving for the OR.

2. Demonstrate in the school laboratory how to open a large sterile pack in such a way as to create a sterile field.

3. The radiologist is scrubbed, and he asks the RT to get him a #16 French catheter. Demonstrate in the school laboratory the placement of this catheter on the sterile field without causing contamination.

4. Mrs. Brown is in the radiology department to have radiographs of her ankle prepared. There is an open wound on the ankle covered by a large dressing. The dressing must be removed for the procedure and reapplied after the exposures are completed. The radiologist asks the RT to do this. Demonstrate in the laboratory how you will remove and reapply the dressing.

5. Demonstrate in the school laboratory how to prepare the skin for an examination that involves a puncture of the lumbar spine.

6. Demonstrate in the school laboratory how you would drape the skin for a sterile procedure.

Chapter Ten
Catheterization of the Urinary Bladder

Goal of this chapter:

The radiologic technology student must be able to insert a catheter into the urinary bladder using correct methodology and care for patients who have retention catheters in place.

Behavioral objectives:

When the student has completed this chapter, he will be able to do the following:
1. Demonstrate the correct method of inserting a straight and a retention catheter into the urinary bladder
2. Explain the proper method of transporting a patient who has an indwelling catheter in place
3. Explain the most important considerations in caring for the patient who has an indwelling catheter in place
4. Demonstrate the correct method of removing an indwelling catheter
5. Describe alternate methods of catheterization of the urinary bladder and the RT's responsibility for patient care when these methods are used

Glossary

Glans a gland found on head of clitoris *or* cone-shaped head of penis containing urethral orifice

Meatus external opening into body
Reflux backward flow, usually unnatural, *i.e.,* urine up ureter during micturation

Sphincter circular band of muscle constricting an orifice; contracts to close opening as urethral sphincter

Catheterization of the urinary bladder refers to the insertion of a plastic, silicone, or rubber tube through the urethral meatus into the bladder. Catheters are inserted into the urinary bladder to keep it empty while the surrounding tissues heal following surgical procedures; to drain, irrigate, or instill medication into the bladder; to assist the incontinent patient to control urinary flow; to begin bladder retraining; or to diagnose diseases or injury to the bladder.

The RT may be required to care for patients who have indwelling catheters in place; in addition, he

may be expected to insert a catheter into the urinary bladder. Therefore, it is necessary for him to learn the correct methods of insertion and of catheter care.

Preparation for catheterization

The urinary bladder is easily infected, so any object or solution that is inserted into it must be sterile. Poor technique when performing catheterization of the urinary bladder or when caring for a patient who has an indwelling catheter in place may result in infection or injury.

Catheterization is not performed without a specific order from the physician in charge of the patient, and the RT must not perform the procedure by himself until he has been adequately supervised and is certain that he understands the technique required. It is less stressful for some patients if male nurses or technologists catheterize male patients, and female nurses or technologists catheterize female patients.

When the RT has been requested to catheterize a patient by a physician, he must establish whether an indwelling or straight catheter is to be used. An indwelling catheter is inserted and left in place to allow for continuous drainage of urine. A straight catheter is used to empty the bladder and is then removed. Most hospitals provide prepared sterile trays for catheterization with the desired type and size of catheter and the necessary equipment included. A set is chosen depending on the type of catheter to be inserted.

The equipment needed to perform a catheterization is as follows:

1. A straight or indwelling catheter (#14 or #16 for an adult female; #16 to #20 for an adult male)

2. Antiseptic solution

3. Cotton balls for cleansing

4. Water-soluble lubricant

5. A specimen bottle

6. A receptacle for draining urine for a straight catheterization

7. A closed system drainage set for an indwelling catheterization

8. Sterile gloves

9. Sterile drapes

10. Sterile forceps

A drape sheet and an extra means of casting light on the perineal area are also needed. Do not attempt to catheterize a female patient unless adequate lighting is provided. Catheter sizes and tips vary and are graded according to lumen size, usually on the French scale. The size of the catheter is listed on the prepared catheterization set (Fig. 10-1).

A straight catheter is a single-lumen tube. Retention catheters have a double lumen with an inflatable balloon at one end. One lumen allows for continuous urinary drainage, and the other is a passageway for instilling sterile water into the balloon. The balloon holds the catheter in place after it is inserted into the bladder. The indwelling catheter also has a valve at one end that serves as a portal for the instillation of sterile water (Fig. 10-2). The RT may occasionally see a third type of catheter that has three lumens. The third lumen provides a passage for irrigation solution and is used for patients in need of continuous bladder irrigation.

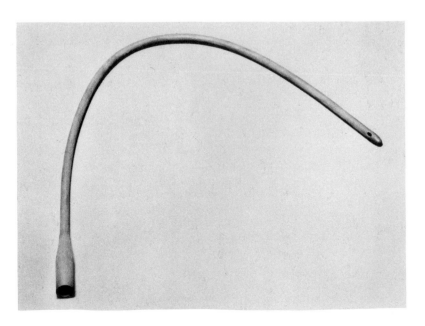

Figure 10.1. A plain French-tipped, or straight, catheter.

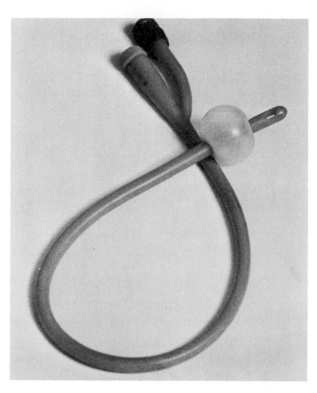

Figure 10.2. A Foley catheter with the balloon inflated.

2. Drape the patient with a sheet so that only the perineum is exposed. If she is disabled and cannot maintain this position, the RT may need assistance in order to maintain adequate exposure.

3. Adjust the light so that it shines directly on the perineal area (Fig. 10-3). It is difficult to locate the urinary meatus in many women unless adequate lighting is available.

4. Open the sterile pack, which may be conveniently placed between the patient's legs if she is cooperative and will not contaminate the sterile field. If this is not the case, the tray must be opened on a Mayo stand at the side of the table. You may use the outer plastic covering of the pack as a waste receptacle or provide an impermeable waste bag. Place it in a convenient spot away from the sterile field and in a place where your hand will not cross the sterile field as you place soiled items into the bag.

5. Put on the sterile gloves. The gloves are usually the uppermost item in the sterile pack and will

Female catheterization

When the RT receives an order from the patient's physician to perform a catheterization, he must determine the type of catheter to be inserted. He then assembles the equipment necessary, washes his hands as described for 2 minutes and approaches the patient, identifies her, and explains what is to be done. Patients are often embarrassed and apprehensive about this procedure, so a good explanation and reassurance that there will be little, if any, pain are vital to the success of the procedure. Inform the patient that there will be a slight sensation of pressure when the catheter is inserted. Provide privacy for her by using a screen or by closing the door to the procedure room. Assess the patient's ability to maintain a position that allows for adequate exposure of the perineum. Assess the perineal area for soiling at this time. If the perineum is soiled, obtain wash cloths, soap, warm water, and clean, disposable gloves and cleanse the area before beginning the procedure. Then proceed with the steps for catheterization.

1. Position the patient on her back; have her flex her knees and relax her thighs so as to externally rotate them. This is called the *dorsal recumbent* position.

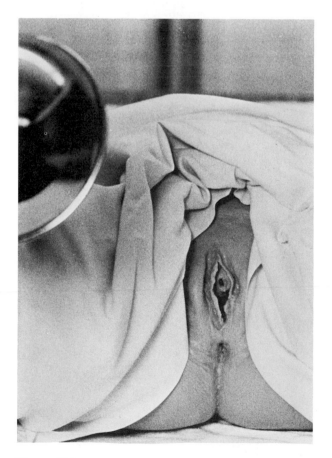

Figure 10.3

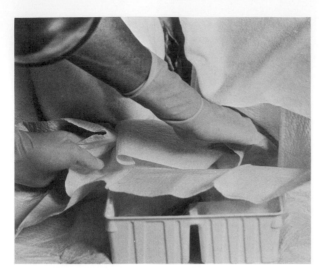

Figure 10.4

be cuffed for donning by use of the open-gloving technique for sterile gloving.

6. Pick up the first sterile drape. Cover your hands with the drape to protect your gloves from con-

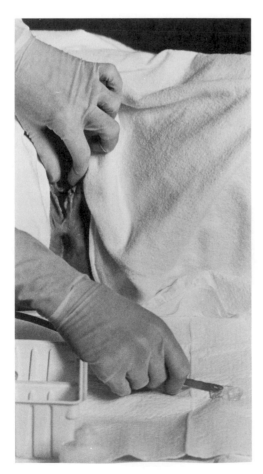

Figure 10.5

tamination. Place the drape slightly under the patient's hips extending to the front of the buttocks to cover the table (Fig. 10-4).

7. Place the second drape, which is a fenestrated drape allowing for only perineal exposure. This drape is frequently omitted.

8. Open the container of sterile, water-soluble lubricant and lubricate the catheter tip (about ½ inch [1.2 cm] for the female patient) (Fig. 10-5).

9. Open the antiseptic solution and pour it over all except two of the cotton balls. An iodophor solution is usually included in the sterile catheterization sets. Keep one or two cotton balls dry to wipe away the excess antiseptic.

10. If the catheterization being done is an indwelling type, the syringe containing sterile water will be attached to the inflation valve at this time. The balloon may be tested by pushing the plunger down and instilling 2 or 3 ml of solution into the balloon to be certain that it will not leak. After this has been determined, withdraw the water, and leave the syringe tip connected to the valve to be used later.

11. With the nondominant hand, separate the labia minora until the urethral meatus is clearly visible. This glove is now contaminated and will be maintained in this position to maintain exposure until the procedure is complete.

12. Pick up the forceps and then pick up one cotton ball that is saturated with antiseptic solution with the forceps.

13. Cleanse the distal side of the meatus with a single downward stroke and then drop the contaminated cotton ball into the waste receptacle prepared earlier (Fig. 10-6).

14. Pick up another cotton ball saturated with antiseptic solution and wipe down the proximal side and discard. Then take a third cotton ball and wipe down the center directly over the meatus and discard.

15. Keep the contaminated, nondominant hand in place, and with the dominant hand, which is sterile, pick up the lubricated catheter and insert it into the urethra (Fig. 10-7). The catheter will usually pass unobstructed into the bladder. If there is any resistance, do not continue the procedure. The female urethra is 1½ to 2 inches (3.7 cm to 5 cm) in length. When urine begins to flow from the catheter, the catheter has passed through the sphincter and into the bladder. When this occurs, insert the catheter about 1 inch more, then remove your hand from the

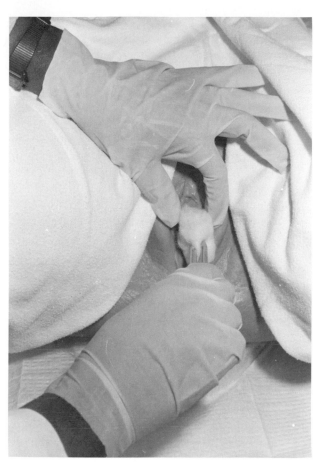

Figure 10.6

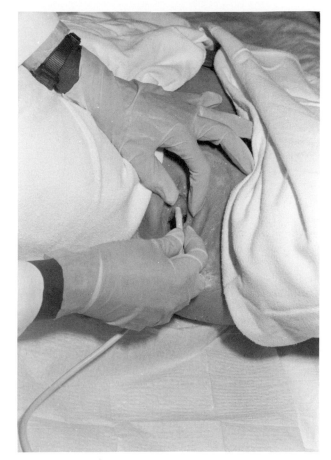

Figure 10.7

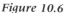

perineum, continuing to hold the catheter in place until the bladder is emptied.

16. If a straight catheter is being used, have the drainage basin in place so that it will catch the urine. Allow it to drain without interference unless a urine specimen is to be obtained. If this is the case, after the initial flow of urine, place the end of the catheter into the opening of the specimen bottle and collect a specimen of about 30 ml of urine. Then close the lid of the container and allow the remaining urine to drain into the collecting basin.

17. If an indwelling catheter is being used, a drainage tube may be attached at the distal end of the catheter, and the urine will flow into the tubing and on into the drainage bag that is attached. Insert the catheter 1 inch more (2.5 cm), and then you may remove your hand from the perineum.

18. If the catheter is to be indwelling, pick up the syringe, which you have already attached to the

valve, and push in the plunger until all of the water in the syringe has been injected into the balloon. It is most often filled with 5 ml to 10 ml of sterile water (Fig. 10-8). Then immediately remove the syringe from the valve. Most indwelling catheter valves are self-sealing, so when the syringe is removed, the procedure is complete.

19. Gently tug on the catheter to be certain that it will be retained. If there is resistance, the balloon is properly inflated.

20. Remove the soiled equipment and make the patient comfortable. Remove your gloves and wash your hands.

21. If the catheter is to remain in place for some time, it should be taped to the inner thigh in order to prevent it from becoming dislodged. Make certain that there is no tension placed on the catheter as it is taped. Arrangements for urinary drainage must be made, depending on the procedure that is to follow.

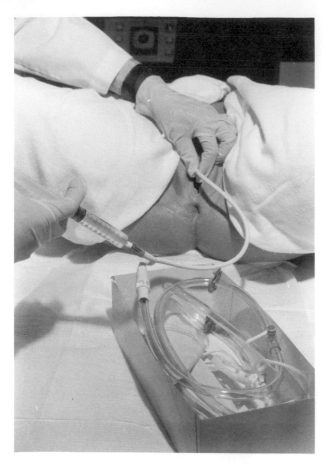

Figure 10.8

Male catheterization

The equipment needed for catheterizing males is the same as for catheterizing females, though a slightly larger catheter is usually required (#16 to #20). The patient is placed in a supine position with his legs slightly abducted. His torso is covered to the pubis, and his legs are covered to the pubis so that exposure is minimal. Make certain that the patient's pubic area is clean. If he is not circumcised, withdraw the foreskin of the penis and clean the urethral meatus. Wear clean, disposable gloves to do this, and remove them upon completion. Have good lighting available. Then begin the procedure by washing your hands as for surgical asepsis.

1. Open the sterile pack on a Mayo stand beside the patient or on the patient's thighs if he can be depended upon not to contaminate the sterile field. Pick up the catheter and lubricate it heavily from the tip down about 5 to 7 inches (12.5 cm to 17.5 cm), as more lubricant is required to facilitate passage of the catheter for males than for females.

2. Prepare the pack as in steps 4 through 10 for female catheterization. Place the first sterile drape over the thigh up to the scrotum and the fenestrated drape over the pubic area leaving the penis exposed.

3. Grasp the penis firmly at the shaft with the non-dominant hand, retract the foreskin and keep it retracted until the procedure is complete. Slightly spread the urinary meatus between the thumb and forefinger. If the penis is not firmly held, an erection may be stimulated. This hand is now contaminated and continues to hold the penis in position until the procedure is complete.

4. Pick up the forceps, and with it, a cotton ball saturated with antiseptic solution. Cleanse from the urethral meatus to the glans using a circular motion. Then drop the cotton ball into the waste receptacle.

5. Repeat this procedure two more times.

6. Pick up the lubricated catheter with the remaining sterile hand. Ask the patient to bear down as if he were trying to urinate, because this action will relax the sphincter.

7. Using gentle, constant pressure, insert the catheter (Fig. 10-9). Too much force may cause a spasm of the sphincter and delay insertion. Do not try to proceed if there is an obstruction; withdraw the catheter and notify the physician.

8. When the urine begins to flow you will know that the catheter is in the bladder; insert the

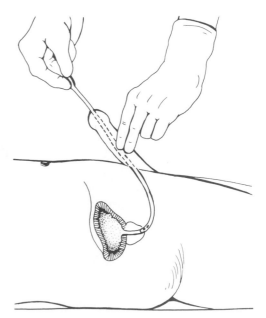

Figure 10.9

catheter slightly further (another ½ inch or 1.2 cm). The adult male urethra is 5½ inches to 7 inches in length (13.75 to 17.5 cm).

9. Depending on the type of catheter used for the procedure, follow steps 16 through 20 for female catheterization listed previously. Replace the foreskin over the glans.

10. If the indwelling catheter is to be in place for some time, it should be taped to the lower abdomen using nonallergenic tape, with the penis directed toward the patient's chest. Allow slack so that there is no tension on the catheter. This position minimizes trauma to the urethra by straightening the angle of the penoscrotal junction.

Removing an indwelling catheter

A physician's order is needed before an indwelling catheter may be removed. Equipment needed will be a 10-ml syringe or a calibrated medicine glass, several thicknesses of paper toweling, a nonpermeable disposable bag, and clean, disposable gloves.

When you receive an order from the physician in charge of the patient to remove an indwelling catheter, collect the equipment necessary and wash your hands. Identify the patient and explain the procedure to him. There is usually little, if any, discomfort with this procedure.

1. Uncover the patient just enough to see the insertion point of the catheter. Ask the female patient to separate her legs slightly and remove the tape that holds the catheter in place. Put on the clean gloves, and place the paper toweling under the catheter.

2. Insert the tip of the syringe into the valve port and pull back on the plunger until all of the sterile water from the retention balloon is removed; then disconnect the plunger from the valve (Fig. 10-10). Another method is to place the calibrated medicine glass under the valve and cut off the tip of the valve. Then allow the sterile water from the retention balloon to drain into the glass (Fig. 10-11).

3. When the water is completely removed from the balloon, wrap the paper toweling around the catheter and gently withdraw it from the bladder. If there is any resistance, stop the procedure and notify the physician. The catheter should come out easily.

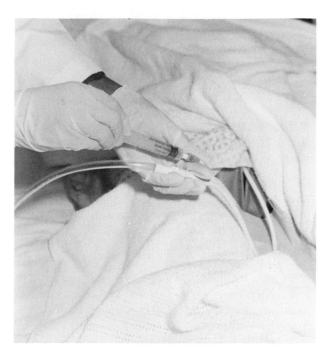

Figure 10.10

4. Wrap the catheter in the toweling and place it and the drainage set into the nonpermeable bag. Before placing the catheter in the bag, measure the urine in the collecting bag and empty it. Place the soiled equipment into the container for con-

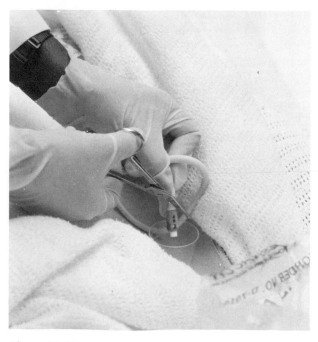

Figure 10.11

taminated waste, remove your gloves, and wash your hands.

5. Return to the patient to make certain that he is comfortable.

Catheter care in the diagnostic imaging department

Often patients must be transported to the diagnostic imaging department with indwelling catheters in place. If this is the case, the RT must keep the drainage bag below the level of the urinary bladder so that the gravity flow is maintained (Fig. 10-12). The drainage tubing must be placed over the patient's leg and coiled on the gurney or table top, not below the level of the patient's hips. If urine is allowed to flow back into the bladder, or if drainage is obstructed, a urinary tract infection may result. If the drainage bag is to be lifted above the patient during a move, the drainage tubing should be clamped and the drainage bag emptied before the move is begun in order to prevent a backflow of urine.

If the bag is to be emptied, equipment needed will be six alcohol sponges; clean, disposable gloves; and a measuring receptacle. Withdraw the emptying spout from its housing, and wipe it several times with alcohol sponges from top to bottom. Release the clamp that keeps the spout closed, and allow the urine to drain into the graduated receptacle (Fig. 10-13). When the drainage bag is empty, reclamp the spout, wipe it again with alcohol wipes, and replace it in the housing.

When you are moving a patient with a catheter in place, care must be taken to avoid undue tension on the catheter. Pulling on the catheter can cause the patient great discomfort or injury if it becomes dislodged.

If the patient is transported by wheelchair and the patient has an indwelling catheter, the drainage bag should be attached to the underpart of the wheelchair. The tubing must be coiled at the level of the patient's hips. Care must be taken not to allow the tubing or drainage bag to touch the floor. Never place a drainage bag on the patient's lap or abdomen during transport, because this may cause a reflux of urine into the bladder.

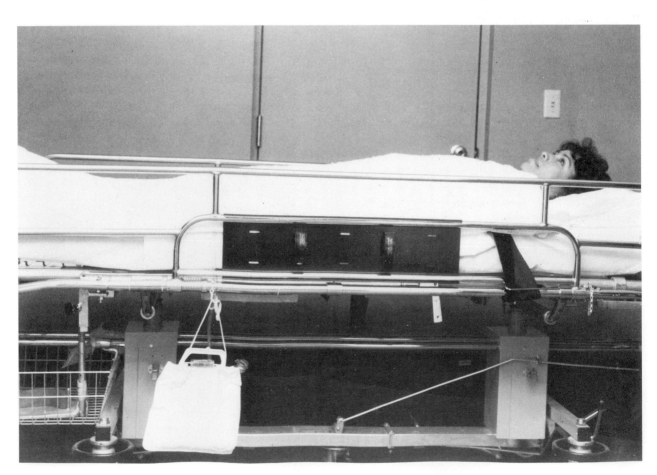

Figure 10.12

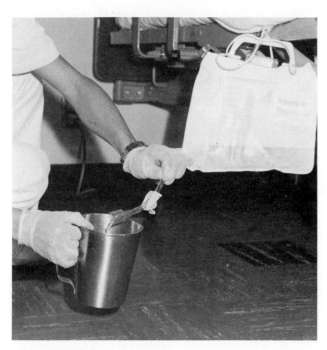

Figure 10.13

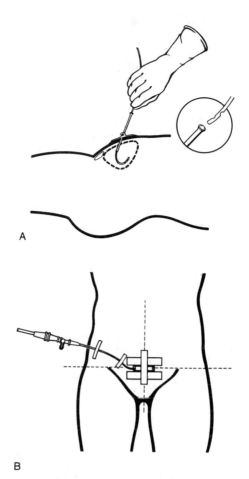

Disconnecting the catheter from its closed drainage system should be avoided. Maintenance of a closed urinary drainage system is essential if infection is to be prevented. Once the closed drainage system has been invaded, it should not be reconnected. The patient must have a new catheter with new closed system drainage reinserted if catheter drainage of the bladder is to be continued.

Figure 10.14. (A) Introduction of suprapubic catheter. (B) The body seal and catheter are taped to the abdomen. (Brunner L, Suddarth DM: Lippincott Manual of Nursing Practice. Philadelphia, JB Lippincott, 1986. Courtesy of Dow Corning Corp.)

Alternative methods of urinary drainage

There are two common methods of dealing with urinary drainage on a temporary or permanent basis, which the RT must recognize. These are the suprapubic catheter (also called a cystocatheter) and the condom catheter.

The *suprapubic catheter* is placed directly into the bladder by means of an abdominal incision. This method is sometimes chosen to divert the flow of urine from the urethral route following gynecologic surgery, urethral injuries, prostatic obstructions, or for chronic incontinence or loss of bladder control. This method of urinary drainage is believed to reduce risk of infection as a long-term method of bladder drainage and to facilitate normal urination following surgical procedures. The catheter is attached to a closed urinary drainage system, and the catheter is secured with sutures, tape, or a body seal system (Fig. 10-14).

The RT caring for a patient with a suprapubic catheter must guard against placing tension on the catheter. He must also follow the same rules of asepsis as for patients with other closed-system urinary drainage. That is, the drainage bag must be kept below the patient's bladder level at all times and not lifted over the patient. The bag must be emptied before moving the patient with direction of the nurse in charge of the patient.

The *condom catheter* is an externally applied drainage device used for male patients who are incontinent or comatose whose bladder continues to empty spontaneously. The condom catheter is a soft rubber sheath that is placed over the penis and secured with a special type of adhesive material. The distal end of the condom has an opening that fits onto a drainage tube and terminates in a drainage bag that attaches to the patient's thigh. The drainage bag can be emptied easily when necessary.

The condom catheter is changed every 24 to 48

hours and has the advantage of reducing urinary tract infections in men who are unable to urinate normally. The RT caring for patients who have condom catheters in place must guard against dislodging the catheter from the drainage tube or twisting the condom and causing pain or skin irritation.

Summary

Catheterization of the urinary bladder is the process of inserting a plastic, rubber, or silicone tube through the urethral meatus into the urinary bladder. There are two types of catheters that the RT may have to insert: the straight and the indwelling catheter. Catheter insertion or removal requires a physician's order. Surgical aseptic technique is required for catheter insertion to prevent urinary tract infection.

The same type of equipment is required for catheterization of both males and females, although the procedure varies slightly because of anatomic differences. A larger catheter is required for the adult male. Prior to a catheterization procedure, the patient must be given adequate explanation, reassurance, and privacy to reduce embarrassment and anxiety.

Correct care of the indwelling catheter while the patient is being transported to the diagnostic imaging department or cared for there is necessary for the prevention of urinary tract infection or injury. The RT must be certain that the drainage bag remains below the level of the urinary bladder in order to ensure gravity flow of urine. Closed-system drainage of the urinary bladder should not be broken, and tension on the catheter must be avoided.

Alternative methods of urinary drainage are by suprapubic catheter and external condom catheter. Patients who have these types of urinary drainage require precautionary care to prevent urinary tract infections and injury.

Chapter 10, pre-post test

_____ 1. When performing a urethral catheterization, how will the RT know that the catheter is in the bladder?
   a. The patient will relax
   b. There will be a mucoid discharge
   c. Urine will start to flow
   d. There is no way of knowing

_____ 2. When inserting a retention catheter, after the RT has placed the sterile drape, prepared the lubricant, and poured antiseptic solution over the cotton balls, the next step is to
   a. Insert the catheter
   b. Inflate the balloon
   c. Cleanse the meatus
   d. Put on sterile gloves

_____ 3. When removing a retention catheter, the most important consideration is
   a. Deflate the balloon
   b. Cleanse the meatus
   c. Maintain privacy
   d. Explain the procedure to the patient

_____ 4. When transporting a patient with a retention catheter with closed-system drainage in place, the RT must remember
   a. To keep the drainage bag below the level of the bladder
   b. To prevent tension on the catheter
   c. To keep the excess tubing coiled at the level of the patient's hips, not below

   d. a and b
   e. a, b, and c

_____ 5. The RT may disconnect the catheter from the closed-system drainage before transporting the patient.
   a. True
   b. False

_____ 6. When caring for a patient with a suprapubic catheter, the RT does not need to follow the same rules of asepsis as for a retention catheter.
   a. True
   b. False

_____ 7. If a urinary drainage bag must be lifted over a patient in order to prepare for transport, the RT must
   a. Empty the drainage bag
   b. Disconnect the drainage bag
   c. Do it quickly
   d. a and b

_____ 8. If a retention catheter is to be taped onto a male patient, it must be taped
   a. To the inside of the leg
   b. To the scrotum
   c. To the lateral aspect of the thigh
   d. To the lower abdomen

Laboratory reinforcement

1. Demonstrate in the school laboratory on the female or male mannequin (depending on the student's sex) a catheterization procedure. You are to insert a retention catheter.

2. Using a mannequin, demonstrate in the school laboratory the removal of a Foley catheter.

3. Using a mannequin, demonstrate in the school laboratory the proper means of transporting a patient who has a retention catheter with closed-system drainage and who is to be transported by gurney to the diagnostic imaging department.

Chapter Eleven
Assisting with Drug Administration

Goal of this chapter:

The RT student will learn to assist safely with the administration of drugs used in diagnostic imaging.

Behavioral objectives:

When the student has completed this chapter, he will be able to do the following:
1. List the precautions necessary when assisting with drug administration
2. List the physical factors that influence drug action
3. List the methods of drug administration
4. Select the correct equipment for administering any drug requested by the physician in diagnostic imaging
5. Define basic medical abbreviations and terminology related to drug action and administration
6. List the anatomic sites most commonly used in administration of parenteral medications by intravenous (IV), subcutaneous, intramuscular (IM), and intradermal routes
7. List the symptoms that indicate that an intravenous infusion may be infiltrating into the surrounding tissues
8. Describe the symptoms of an adverse drug reaction

Glossary

Absorbent a substance capable of taking in another substance through its surface

Analgesic a drug that relieves pain

Anorexia loss of appetite caused by anxiety, depression, or illness

Anti-inflammatory an agent that suppresses inflammation of living tissue

Antipyretic an agent that reduces fever

Antitussive an agent preventing or relieving coughing

Apnea temporary cessation of breathing for various medical reasons

Arrhythmia irregularity or loss of rhythm of the heart beat

Ataxia defective muscular coordination

Baroreceptor sites sensory nerve endings stimulated by changes in pressure found in the walls of the atria of the heart, vena cava, aortic arch, and carotid sinus

Blepharitis inflammation of edges of eyelids

Candida yeastlike fungi; part of normal flora of mouth, skin, intestinal tract, and vagina; may become infected as a result of the administration of antibiotics for other unrelated infections

Cardiovascular pertains to heart and blood vessels working together to circulate blood throughout the body

Conjunctivitis inflammation of the mucous membrane that lines underside of eyelids (conjunctiva)

Dermatophytosis fungal infection of skin of hands and feet, rarely penetrating deeper than hair and nail follicles

Diplopia double vision

Diuretics agents that increase the natural secretion of urine by increasing glomerular filtration and decreasing tubular absorption

Drug dependence an emotional or physical state resulting from interaction of body and drug; produces a compulsion to take the drug continuously to avoid the discomfort of its absence

Drug sensitivity unusually susceptible to antigen or foreign protein; can result from an allergy or can occur by continual, repeated injections of a substance

Dyscrasia an abnormal blood or bone disorder

Dyskinesia defect in voluntary movement

Embolism obstruction of a blood vessel by a foreign substance or a blood clot

Erythema small spot or colored spot producing redness over the skin; caused by nerve mechanisms within body, inflammation, or some external influence

Eunuchism condition resulting from complete lack of male hormone

Glaucoma disease of eye characterized by intraocular pressure; can result in atrophy of optic nerve and blindness

Gonadism congenital endocrine disorder of the sex gland before differentiation into definite testis or ovary

Habituate becoming accustomed to anything from frequent use

Hemolysis destruction of red blood cells

Hemophilia a hereditary blood disease in which blood fails to clot, and abnormal bleeding occurs

Hepatotoxic toxic to liver cells

Hirsuitism excessive growth and presence of hair in unusual places, especially in women

Hyperkinesia increased muscular movement and physical activity

Hypertrophy abnormal increase in size of an organ or body structure not caused by tumor growth

Hyponatremia decreased concentration of sodium in the blood

Hypovolemic reduced blood volume

Jaundice characterized by yellowness of skin and whites of eyes; a symptom indicating dysfunction of liver cells or bile passageways

Keratitis inflammation of the cornea

Methemoglobinemia a condition in which the iron in hemoglobin has been oxidized to ferric iron

Mydriatic causing pupillary dilatation

Natural flora plant life that normally lives in body areas and is adapted to that specific environment

Nephrotoxicity a toxic substance that damages kidney tissues

Neurotoxicity having the capability of harming nerve tissue

Nystagmus constant, involuntary, cyclical movement of the eyeball in any direction

Osteoporosis increased pores (able to admit fluids) and softening of bone seen most often in the elderly

Otitis media inflammation of the middle ear

Ototoxic harmful to the eighth cranial nerve or the organs of hearing

Paradoxical excitement a condition in which stimulation should not exist but does

Parkinson's disease chronic nervous disease characterized by a fine, slowly spreading tremor, muscular weakness, rigidity, and an abnormal gait

Phlebitis Inflammation of a vein

Photosensitivity sensitive to light

Prophylaxis observance of rules necessary to prevent disease

Prostatic concerning prostate gland that surrounds the neck of bladder and urethra in the male

Proteinuria protein, usually, in the urine

Pruritis severe itching caused by allergy or emotional factors

Resistant strain inherent ability to oppose disease against antibiotic treatment

Septicemia presence of pathogenic bacteria in blood

Thrombocytopenia abnormal decrease in number of blood platelets

Tinnitus ringing or tingling sound in the ear

Vagotomy incision of a section of the vagus nerve

Vasodilators a nerve or drug that dilates the blood vessels

Vertigo dizziness

Drugs are chemical agents selected for use by physicians to perform specific physiologic actions in the body. The study of all aspects of drug effects, properties, origins, and preparation is a particular scientific discipline called *pharmacology*. A detailed study of pharmacology is beyond the scope of this text; however, the RT must learn particular aspects of this science in order to be a safe assistant in drug administration.

The RT does not administer drugs because he is neither trained nor licensed to do so. A violation of this restriction is professional malpractice. However, the RT will be asked to assist with drug administration in diagnostic imaging, and he is expected to be a competent assistant. He must familiarize himself with safety measures to be taken when drugs are being given.

Drugs administered by any route have the potential of causing adverse reactions. Since the RT will often be the only person to observe the patient for some time after a drug has been administered, he must be an accurate observer and learn to assess symptoms of adverse reactions to drugs and take correct action should they occur. The RT must familiarize himself with the desired effects and the potential adverse reactions of any drug that is administered in his department.

Drug names

The same drug may be sold under many different proprietary or trade names. The *trade name* is assigned to a drug by a particular manufacturer. The same drug may be manufactured by another company and be given a different proprietary name. The trade name of a drug is copyrighted and cannot be used by another manufacturer.

The *chemical name* of a drug represents its exact chemical formula and remains the same always. A drug's *generic name* is the name given the drug prior to its official approval for use. Like the chemical name, it remains unchanged. Drugs are also given *official names,* and frequently the official and generic names are the same. The official name is the way the drug is listed in official publications like the *United States Pharmacopeia.*

The RT must be aware that any drug used in his department may be represented by several trade names. If he checks the generic name, which is always listed on the container label under the trade name, he will be able to identify the drug, regardless of which proprietary name is used.

In the tables that follow, the RT will find a description of the common drug categories and examples of drugs in each category. The intended purpose for which each drug is administered, the routes of administration, and the possible adverse effects of the drugs are also included. In a text such as this, it is not possible to list every drug in each category. The aim is to acquaint the RT with the drugs he is likely to encounter in his work. The drugs are listed by their generic names, and some of the common proprietary names are listed below the generic names. The drugs listed have been randomly chosen and are not indicative of the preference of the author.

Several of the drugs listed are found on the emergency drug trays or carts in the diagnostic imaging department. If this is the case, the RT must check these drugs daily to be certain that they have not reached the expiration date listed on the container. He must also be certain that the liquid drugs are clear and colorless. Any sediment or discoloration of any medication must be questioned, and the drug must be returned to the hospital pharmacy. If the medication has reached its expiration date or is used, it must be replaced immediately.

Contrast agents are the drugs that the RT will work with most often. They will be discussed in the following chapter.

Drugs used to treat infections

Anti-infective (antimicrobial) drugs do not all react in the same way, nor do they all destroy the same types of microorganisms. They are chosen selectively for use by the physician according to their ability to inhibit or destroy particular bacteria, fungi, or protozoal infections.

Although it is widely believed that anti-infective drugs can cure any infection without ill effect, this is not entirely true. There are continuing problems with administration of antimicrobial drugs that remain unsolved. They are as follows:

1. *Tissue damage.* The gastrointestinal (GI) mucosa becomes irritated when these drugs are taken by mouth, resulting in nausea, vomiting, and diarrhea. Local reactions at parenteral sites of injection may also occur. The most serious effects to body tissues are those that result in kidney damage and neurotoxicity. Neurotoxic symptoms can range from vertigo and deafness to convulsive seizures.

2. *Allergic reactions.* These may range from mild hypersensitivity to severe, life-threatening anaphylactic shock and may result from any anti-infective drug.

3. *Superinfections.* When anti-infective drugs are used, they inhibit the growth of the natural flora of the body. In the absence of these natural inhabitants of the body, stronger microbes, or those that are not susceptible to antimicrobial medications, grow uncontrollably and produce life-threatening infections.

4. *Misuse of anti-infective drugs.* Many people who have common upper respiratory infections, such as the common cold, which are caused by viruses unresponsive to these agents, request treatment with anti-infective drugs. This may result in a sensitivity to the drug prescribed, and when the drug is needed for treatment of a serious infection, an allergy to the drug requires that it be discontinued. Another result might be development of a resistance to the drug that renders it ineffective at a time when it is needed.

When anti-infective drugs are used, they should be used in a concentration and dosage high enough to destroy or inactivate the bacteria and for sufficient time for this action to result. If this is not done, resistant strains develop, and the treatment is not successful.

Since all anti-infective drugs are not effective against every type of microorganism, the physician chooses the drug for use based on the initial diagnosis. A culture and sensitivity study of affected body tissue is performed to ascertain the drug of choice; however, this laboratory test takes 2 to 3 days to complete. In the meantime, without treatment, the microbe population will increase; therefore, an anti-infective drug is prescribed that is presumed will be effective.

The development of drugs for the treatment of viral infections has been more difficult to develop. Recently, however, there have been several antiviral agents produced that are of some benefit in the treatment of herpes simplex virus.

Interferon harvested from human sources has proven effective against viral infections, but this source is obviously restricted. Currently there is hope that production of interferon in large quantities will make it available for more widespread use in the treatment of viral diseases. Prevention of viral diseases by immunization is the most reliable method for control at the present time.

Table 11-1 gives the RT student an idea of which drugs are used to treat specific infections.

TABLE 11-1.
Drugs used to treat infections

DRUG	PURPOSE	ROUTE	POSSIBLE ADVERSE EFFECTS
PENICILLINS			
Penicillin G	Treats skin and soft tissue abscesses; Streptococcus and *Staphylococcus aureus* infections; meningitis; pneumonias; *Hemophilus influenzae* infections	Parenteral	Anaphylactic drug reactions—may be fatal; rash; urticaria; mild GI disturbances; neurotoxicity; take careful drug history
Ampicillin	Treats paratyphoid; typhoid; invasive Salmonella pediatric infections	Oral, parenteral	Same as listed above
Carbenicillin	Treats urinary tract infections; Pseudomonas and Proteus infections	Oral, parenteral	Same as listed above
Cephalosporins			
Cefaclor	Treats otitis media; tracheal bronchitis; urinary tract infections	Oral	Acute anaphylactic reactions; rash; urticaria; nephrotoxicity in large doses; blood dyscrasias; neurotoxicity; phlebitis
Cefoxitin sodium	Treats lower respiratory tract infections; gynecologic infections; gonorrhea	Parenteral	Same toxic reations for all cephalosporins
Cephalexin monohydrate	Respiratory tract infections; genitourinary tract infections; soft tissue infections	Oral	Same as listed above
Cephalothin sodium	Treats respiratory infections; bone and joint infections; septicemia; nosocomial infections	Parenteral	Same as listed above
ALTERNATIVES TO PENICILLINS AND CEPHALOSPORINS			
Erythromycin	An alternative for patients hypersensitive to penicillin; also *Mycoplasma pneumoniae, Entamoeba histolytica,* and legionnaires' disease	Oral and occasionally IM	Abdominal cramps, nausea, vomiting; jaundice; a form of hepatitis
Clindamycin	Same use against gram-negative cocci as penicillins	Oral	Diarrhea; GI reactions; drug-induced bowel damage
CHLORAMPHENOCOL AND TETRACYCLINES			
Doxycycline hyclate; Minocycline hydrochloride Tetracycline hydrochloride	Prophylaxis against acute respiratory infections in patients with chronic lung disease; psittacosis; Q fever; Rocky Mountain spotted fever; acne; several types of typhus; venereal infections caused by gram-negative bacilli; and Chlamydial infections	Oral and parenteral	GI irritations; discoloration of children's teeth; photosensitivity; liver damage; super infections
Chloramphenicol	Treats typhoid fever and other Salmonellosis infections; rickettsial infections	Oral, parenteral, topical	Nausea; vomiting; diarrhea; severe blood dyscrasias—patient should have frequent blood counts; use with extreme caution in infants and children
Aminoglycosides Polymyxins Streptomycin sulfate injection	Pulmonary and other forms of tuberculosis; plague; tularemia	Parenteral	All potentially ototoxic and nephrotoxic; all may produce hypersensitivity; vertigo; ataxia; newborn deafness
Neomycin sulfate Kanamycin sulfate	For superficial and joint infections; to reduce GI flora preoperatively; to supress *E. coli* infection	Oral, topical	Same as above
Gentamicin sulfate	Treats infections caused by gram-negative bacteria; sepsis; infected burns; Pseudomonas and Proteus infections	Parenteral	Resistant strain has developed; use in combination with other anti-infective drug; same adverse effects as listed above

TABLE 11-1 (continued)

DRUG	PURPOSE	ROUTE	POSSIBLE ADVERSE EFFECTS
ANTIMYCOBACTERIAL DRUGS: DRUGS USED TO TREAT TUBERCULOSIS AND LEPROSY (MYCOBACTERIUM LEPRAE INFECTIONS)			
Isoniazid (INH)	Most active drug to treat tuberculosis	Parenteral, oral	Fever; skin rash; peripheral and central nervous system symptoms; these rare if given with pyridoxine
Rifampin	Used with INH to treat tuberculosis; prophylaxis for meningitis	Parenteral, oral	Rash; thrombocytopenia; proteinuria; "flu syndrome"; anemia
Dapsone Other sulfones	Treats leprosy	Oral	Hemolysis; GI intolerance; methemoglobinemia; fever; pruritis; erythema nodosum
SULFONAMIDES TRIMETHOPRIM			
Sulfasalazine	For treatment of ulcerative colitis; enteritis; inflammatory bowel disease	Oral	Fever, skin rashes, photosensitivity; vomiting; diarrhea; arthritis; conjunctivitis
Sulfisoxazole	Urinary tract infections	Oral	Same as above
Trimethoprim	Acute urinary tract infections	Oral	Same as above
Trimethroprims	Treats *Pneumocystis carinii* pneumonia; Shigella; systemic Salmonella infections	Oral, IV	Anemia; blood dyscrasias; other adverse effects listed above
ANTIFUNGAL INFECTIONS			
Amphotericin B	Used to treat fungal meningitis; candidiasis; coccidioidomycosis	IV, Intrathecal	Chills; fever; vomiting; headache; renal and hepatic dysfunction
Griseofulvin	For treatment of severe dermophytosis involving skin, hair, and nails	Oral	Fever; skin rash; blood dyscrasias; hepatic toxicity; mental confusion
Nystatin	For use in Candida infections	Topical, oral	Usually nontoxic; may cause gastric distress; sensitivity reaction vaginally

Analgesics/antipyretics, nonsteroidal anti-inflammatory drugs, and drugs used to treat allergies

The inflammatory response of the body is a natural reaction to attack from invading antigens or organisms. If this response is allowed to progress, the body part affected, usually a joint, becomes incapable of normal function as a result of pain and structural change. When this type of invasion occurs, the body's enzymes react by producing prostaglandins and other related substances that are responsible for the signs and symptoms of an inflammatory response, *i.e.*, pain, fever, and malaise.

When an allergic response is activated in the body, histamine is released that engorges peripheral blood vessels and causes leakage of plasma proteins and fluid into the surrounding tissues. When this occurs, if the reaction is acute, blood pressure falls, and bronchial smooth muscles contract, thereby restricting the flow of oxygen into the lungs. Histamine release may also affect the GI, respiratory, and lacrimal glands. Epigastric distress, nausea, vomiting, and diarrhea are often initial symptoms of an allergic (anaphylactic) reaction. There are medications available that help to relieve the symptoms of allergic response. Most of these work to combat the effects of histamine released when these reactions occur (see Table 11-2).

There are many drugs being marketed that are effective in reducing inflammation and its effects on the body. These drugs are not narcotics and may be used over long periods of time for chronic inflammatory conditions with relative safety. All of these drugs are not useful for the same medical problems, however, and there may be some harmful side effects from each that must be considered.

TABLE 11-2.
Analgesics/antipyretics, nonsteroidal anti-inflammatory drugs, and drugs used to treat allergies

DRUG	PURPOSE	ROUTE	POSSIBLE ADVERSE EFFECTS
ANALGESIC/ANTIPYRETICS			
Aspirin	Used to ease pain; reduce fever and inflammation; prolong bleeding time and reduce incidence of trans-ischemic attacks	Oral	GI bleeding; vomiting; affects hearing; vertigo hypersensitivity contraindicated in patients with hemophelia
Acetaminophen	Treats moderate pain without anti-inflammatory effects; used to reduce fever	Oral	Liver toxicity in large doses; dizziness; excitement; disorientation; renal tubular necrosis
NONSTEROIDAL ANTI-INFLAMMATORY DRUGS (NSAID)			
Ibuprofen	Analgesic for treatment of mild to moderate pain; anti-inflammatory for osteoarthritis; pain of dysmenorrhea	Oral	GI irritation; bleeding; rash; tinnitus; anxiety; headaches; aseptic meningitis; allergic reactions
Indomethacin	Anti-inflammatory used to treat gouty arthritis; osteoarthritis; acute gout	Oral	Severe headache; abdominal pain; diarrhea; GI hemorrhage; contraindicated for children or in pregnancy
Colchicine	Used to relieve inflammation of acute gouty arthritis; to prevent Mediterranean fever and sarcoid arthritis	Oral, IV	Diarrhea; nausea and vomiting; abdominal pain; large doses (more than 8 mg in 24 hours) may be fatal
DRUGS USED TO TREAT ALLERGIES			
Bronspheniramine Maleate	Treats seasonal rhinitis; perennial allergic and vasomotor rhinitis and urticaria	Oral, parenteral	Drowsiness; dizziness; do not fly airplanes or drive; do not combine with use of alcohol
Diphenhydramine hydrochloride (Benadryl)*	Blocks action of released histamine; produces sedation of the central nervous system; to treat nasal, drug, food, and skin allergies; also to treat motion sickness and radiation sickness due to effects of radiation exposure, and for acute anaphylaxis	Oral, parenteral	Drowsiness; dizziness; GI disturbances; patient must be warned that reaction time may be affected; driving, flying airplanes, and working with machinery may be hazardous
Promethazine hydrochloride (Phenergan)	Relief of motion sickness; apprehensiveness; potentiates action of central nervous system depressants and makes reduction in their dosage possible	Oral, parenteral, rectal	Disturbed coordination; drowsiness; blurred vision; dry mouth

*Found on emergency drug trays

Drugs that act on the autonomic nervous system

The automatic nervous system may also be called the visceral or involuntary nervous system. One has little or no self-initiated control over the organs and systems that are controlled by these nerves.

The autonomic nervous system is divided into the *sympathetic* and *parasympathetic* nervous system. Drugs are used selectively to depress or to stimulate the organs or glands regulated by this part of the nervous system. These include glands that form secretions (the liver, the salivary glands, the sweat glands, the lacrimal glands, and the nasopharyngeal glands), the smooth muscle organs (the stomach, the intestines, the uterus, urinary bladder blood vessels, the cardiac muscle, the ciliary muscle, male sex organs, and bronchial muscle) (see Table 11.3).

Drugs that act on the central nervous system

The central nervous system controls the skeletal muscles and the reasoning and memory functions of the brain. This group of drugs is extensively used in medical practice and is also the most widely used without prescription by a physician. They are used generally to relieve anxiety, decrease pain, and alter

TABLE 11-3.
Drugs that act on the autonomic nervous system

DRUG	PURPOSE	ROUTE	POSSIBLE ADVERSE EFFECTS
Pilocarpine hydrochloride Neostigmine bromide	Constricts the pupil of the eye; used in open-angle glaucoma	Topical	Dehydration; nausea and vomiting
Atropine*	Used in gastric disease as an antispasmodic, antisecretory drug; counteracts bradycardia by increasing the heart rate; a mydriatic for opthalmologic examinations	Oral, parenteral, topical	Dry mouth; blurred vision; tachycardia; constipation; CNS symptoms; contraindicated for patients with narrow-angle glaucoma, prostatic hypertrophy
Dicyclomine (Bentyl)	Antispasmodic; relaxes gastric smooth muscle in gastritis and peptic ulcer	Oral, IM	Dry mouth; blurred vision; urinary retention; nausea and vomiting
Glycopyrrolate (Robinul)	Used as adjunct in treatment of peptic ulcer; reduces bronchotracheal, salivary, and pharyngeal secretions in preparations for anesthesia	Oral, parenteral	May increase heart rate; dry mouth; urinary retention; blurred vision; ocular tension; nausea; vomiting; anaphylactic reaction
Scopolamine	Prevents motion sickness; occasionally preoperatively used to increase the effect of a narcotic analgesic	Transdermal	Tachycardia; dry mouth; blurred vision; central nervous system toxicity; contraindicated for patients with wide-angle glaucoma
Dopamine hydrochloride*	Increases cardiac output, blood pressure, (BP) and urinary output in septic, hypovolemics; treats cardiogenic shock and heart failure	IV	Cardiac arrhythmia, extreme hypertension; will cause tissue necrosis if extravasation occurs
Isoproterenol hydrochloride*	Potent bronchodilator used to treat asthma, shock, and cardiac arrest as heart stimulant	Sublingual, IV	May be harmful in cardiogenic shock; tachycardia; palpitations; angina-type pain; flushing; tremors; headache; nausea
Norepinephrine bitartrate (Levophed)*	Increases BP and coronary blood flow in cases of profound hypotension	IV	Not a substitute for fluid and electrolyte replacement; bradycardia; headache; extreme hypertension
Ephedrine sulfate	Increases BP by increasing cardiac output and systemic vasoconstriction; bronchodilator used to treat allergic disorders and bronchial asthma	Parenteral	Extreme hypertension resulting in intracranial hemorrhage; tachycardia; cardiac arrhythmias; circulatory collapse; anxiety; pallor
Aminophylline	Relaxes bronchial smooth muscle; manages acute and chronic asthma	Oral, parenteral	Epigastric distress; nausea and vomiting; GI bleeding; delerium; convulsions; cardiovascular collapse
Epinephrine* (Adrenalin)	Bronchodilator and vasoconstrictor used to treat acute asthmatic attacks and anaphylactic shock	Parenteral	Hypertensive headache; intracranial hemorrhage; cardiac arrythmias; pallor; palpitations; anxiety; dizziness
Propranolol hydrochloride*	Treats cardiac arrythmias; angina pectoris and essential hypertension; for prevention of migrane headaches	Oral, parenteral	Bradycardia; decreased myocardial contractility; contraindicated in bronchial asthma; use with caution in COPD
Tilnolol maleate	Treats hypertension; chronic open-angle glaucoma	Oral, topical	Bradycardia; bronchial spasms; fatigue; dizziness; headache; blepharitis; conjunctivitis; keratitis
Succinylchlorine chloride injection	Produces skeletal muscle paralysis; used as adjunct to anesthesia to facilitate endotracheal intubation	IV	Profound respiratory distress; apnea; bradycardia; cardiac arrythmias; increased intraocular pressure
Tubocurarine chloride	Same as succinylchlorine	IV	Same as above; hypersensitivity reaction

*Found on emergency drug trays

TABLE 11-4.
Drugs that act on the central nervous system

DRUG	PURPOSE	ROUTE	POSSIBLE ADVERSE EFFECTS
SEDATIVE–HYPNOTICS (NONBARBITURATE TYPE)			Potential for all drugs in this class to produce dependence and dangerous withdrawal symptoms
Chloral hydrate	Produces sedation and relieves anxiety	Oral, rectal	Nausea and vomiting; gastric irritation
Flurazepam hydrochloride (Dalmane)	Treats insomnia	Oral	Contraindicated in pregnancy or with alcohol; prolonged administration not recommended; headache; disorientation; coma
Temazepam (Restoril)	Treats insomnia	Oral	Diarrhea; dizziness; euphoria; tremors; ataxia; anorexia; hallucinations
ANTIANXIETY AGENTS			All drugs in this category can produce dependence; use with alcohol should be avoided; patients using these drugs must not operate motor vehicles after taking them
Lorazepam (Ativan)	Relief of anxiety and insomnia caused by anxiety	Oral, parenteral	Excessive drowsiness; restlessness; coma; skin rash; nausea
Diazepam (Valium)	Antispasmodic; anticonvulsant; relief of acute agitation; short-term relief of anxiety; sedation	Oral, parenteral	Contraindicated in narrow-angle glaucoma; respiratory distress; hypotension; paradoxical excitement and insomnia
Alprazolam (Xanax)	Short-term relief of anxiety disorders	Oral	Contraindicated in patients with narrow-angle glaucoma; light-headedness; drowsiness; seizures if withdrawal is too rapid
ANTIEPILEPTIC DRUGS Phenytoin* (Dilantin)	Controls partial or generalized seizures	Oral, parenteral	Nystagmus; diplopia; ataxia; sedation; hirsuitism; gingval hyperplasia; peripheral neuropathy; blood dyscrasias; hypersensitivity reactions
LOCAL AND GENERAL ANESTHETICS Nitrous oxide Halothane Isoflurane	General anesthetics; all used in combination with another IV or general inhaled anesthetic to achieve a total anesthetic state	Inhalation	Cardiac depressants; respiratory depression; may be hepatotoxic and nephrotoxic
Thiopental sodium	Ultra–short-acting for use in introduction of general anesthetic	IV	Same as above
Lidocaine*	Area anesthetic block for a particular area; blocks nerve fibers making them insensitive to pain; used in treatment of ventricular arrythmias	Topical; parenteral	Sleepiness; light-headedness; visual and auditory disturbances; convulsions; central nervous system depression; cardiovascular collapse; death
DRUGS USED IN MANAGEMENT OF PARKINSONISM Levodopa Carbidopa (Sinemet)	Improves Parkinsonian symptoms: posture, balance, speech, and tremors in combination or alone	Oral	Dyskinesia; involuntary movements; mental changes; nausea; vomiting; loss of appetite
Benztropine Mesylate (Cogentin)	Supplement for symptomatic relief of Parkinsonian symptoms; also used with phenothiazine-type antipsychotic agents to control extrapyramidial symptoms	Oral	Dry mouth; nausea and vomiting; nervousness; blurred vision
DRUGS USED TO TREAT MENTAL ILLNESS			
Thioridazine hydrochloride	Controls agitation and psychotic episodes	Oral	Drowsiness; hypotension; extrapyramidial symptoms

TABLE 11-4 (continued)

DRUG	PURPOSE	ROUTE	POSSIBLE ADVERSE EFFECTS
Chlorpromazine hydrochloride (Thorazine)	Same as above	Oral, parenteral	Blood and liver disorders
Amitriptyline hydrochloride Imipramine hydrochloride	Relieves episodes of major depression	Oral	Dry mouth; blurred vision; orthostatic hypotension; tremors; convulsions
Lithium carbonate	Controls acute manic episodes	Oral	Muscle weakness; nausea and vomiting; tremors; twitching; coma; cardiovascular collapse
OPIATE ANALGESICS Codeine Propoxyphene (Darvon) Oxycodone (Percodan)	All used for pain control; codeine used as an antitussive	Oral	All opiates may result in tolerance and are addictive; may cause nausea; restlessness; hyperactivity; respiratory depression; postural hypotension; constipation; urticaria; hypersensitivity; shock; depressed renal function; death
Morphine hydrochloride Meperidine hydrochloride (Demoral)		Oral, parenteral	
Naloxone hydrochloride (Narcan)	Narcotic antagonist; to reverse respiratory distress, coma, and hypotensive effects of narcotics	Parenteral	In narcotic-addicted patients, may produce rapid withdrawal symptoms
STIMULANTS Amphetamine	Increases mental alertness; elevates spirits; reduces fatigue; depresses appetite	Oral	A controlled substance as a result of abuse; increased nervousness; excitability; overdose can cause chills; rapid heart rate; collapse; may be habituating
Caffeine	Increases mental alertness; elevates spirits; reduces fatigue; used to alleviate postspinal headache	Oral, IM when combined with sodium	Highly abused; tachycardia; cardiac arrythmias; irritability; insomnia; may be habituating

*Found on emergency drug trays

the mental state. Drugs included in this group are central nervous system stimulants and depressants; drugs that affect behavior; drugs used to control hyperkinesia, epilepsy, skeletal muscle spasm, and Parkinson's disease; and drugs used to treat nausea (see Table 11-4).

Drugs used to treat cardiovascular disease

Cardiovascular drugs act to change the rate, force, and rhythm of the heart. They include drugs that act on the blood and blood-forming organs, drugs that act on the blood vessels, drugs used to treat hypertension, drugs that affect blood coagulation, and the diuretic drugs (see Table 11-5).

Drugs that act on the gastrointestinal system

Drugs used to treat diseases of the GI system include drugs that inhibit and reduce secretion of gastric acid, stimulate and decrease gastric muscle motility, protect

gastric mucosa, replace pancreatic enzymes, reduce gallstones, treat chronic inflammatory bowel disease, diarrhea, and constipation (see Table 11-6).

Drugs used to treat endocrine disorders

The endocrine system comprise a network of glands that work with the nervous system and other body systems to regulate body function. The endocrine glands are the adrenals, the pituitary, the thyroid, the hypothyroid, the pancreas, the ovaries, and testes. They produce hormones (complex chemical substances), which are then released into the circulatory system and transported to particular body systems and cells in the body where they perform their specified function.

An example is the thyroid gland, which secretes the hormone thyroxin, which is essential to normal body growth in infancy and childhood and throughout life controls metabolic processes in the body. Insulin, digestive enzymes, and glucagon are secreted from the pancreas; epinephrine and norepinephrine, from the adrenal medulla; steroids, from the adrenal

TABLE 11-5.
Drugs used to treat cardiovascular disease

DRUG	PURPOSE	ROUTE	POSSIBLE ADVERSE EFFECTS
DRUGS THAT AFFECT THE RATE, FORCE, AND RHYTHM OF THE HEART			
Digitalis*	Used in treatment of congestive heart failure and of some cardiac arrythmias	Oral, parenteral	Cardiac toxicity after prolonged use; anorexia; nausea and vomiting; abdominal pain; diarrhea; gynecomastia; cardiac arrest
Quinidine Procainamide*	Controls cardiac arrythmias	Oral	Cardiac toxicity; fainting; cardiac arrest; headache; nausea and vomiting; tinnitus
DIURETICS Furosemide* (Lasix) Acetazolamide (Diamox) Hychlorthiazide	All are used to treat conditions that affect fluid and electrolyte abnormalities; each drug acts at a different site in the renal system to increase urine production and excretion of sodium and chloride ions; manages diseases such as hypertension, glaucoma, and congestive heart failure	Oral, parenteral	Hypersensitivity reaction; depletion of electrolytes; skin rashes; blood dyscrasias
ANTIHYPERTENSIVE AGENTS Clonidine	All act at one or more baroreceptor sites to interfere with normal blood pressure (BP) regulation mechanisms	Oral	Range from nausea and vomiting to hypotension, depression, hypersensitivity, blood dyscrasias, dry mouth, dizziness, to cardiac symptoms
Reserpine		Oral, parenteral	
Prazosin		Oral, parenteral	
Atenolol		Oral	
Diazoxide		Oral, parenteral	
DRUGS THAT AFFECT BLOOD COAGULATION Heparin sodium	To prolong blood-clotting time; prevents formation of new thrombi but does not dissolve existing ones; used when rapid action is desired	Parenteral	Thrombi can develop if withdrawn rapidly; alopecia and osteoporosis occur rarely with prolonged use; overdose may cause bleeding
Courmarin	Same as Heparin except prescribed for long-term anticoagulation	Oral	Excessive bleeding
Streptokinase	Breaks down emboli in cases of myocardial infarction, deep vein and artery thrombosis, and acute massive pulmonary embolism	Parenteral	Hemorrhage
Vitamin B$_{12}$	Treats pernicious anemia and deficiency caused by partial or total gastrectomy	Parenteral	None known
Folic acid	Manages megaloblastic anemias and dietary folic acid deficiency	Oral, parenteral	None known
Ferrous sulfate (Feosol)	Treats iron-deficiency anemia	Oral	Gastric irritation; nausea; diarrhea; headache
Iron-dextran injection			
VASODILATORS Nitroglycerin	Rapid-acting vasodilator; reduces vascular resistance and lowers BP; counteracts pain resulting from circulatory disturbance of angina pectoris	Sublingual, topical, transdermal	Dizziness; weakness; headache; tachycardia; orthostatic hypotension
Isosorbide dinitrate	Same uses as nitroglycerin	Sublingual, oral (long-acting)	

*Found on emergency drug trays

TABLE 11-6.
Drugs that act on the gastrointestinal system

DRUG	PURPOSE	ROUTE	POTENTIAL ADVERSE EFFECTS
Aluminum hydroxide Magnesium hydroxide Simethicone	Relieves gastric acidity	Oral	Constipation; intestinal obstruction; systemic alkalosis in patients with renal disease; large doses may produce diarrhea
Sodium bicarbonate*	Relieves gastric hyperacidity; also used in emergencies when patient is acutely acidotic	Oral, parenteral	Do not use for long periods of time; promotes systemic alkalosis and fluid retention
Sucralfate (Carafate)	Treats ulcers by forming a protective coating at ulcer site preventing further damage	Oral	None known
Cimetidine (Tagamet)	Treats duodenal ulcers by inhibiting gastric acid secretion	Oral, parenteral	Sexual dysfunction in males; confusional states; blood dyscrasias
Metoclopramide (Reglan)	Increases gastric motility in patients with gastric motor failure resulting from vagotomy, gastroesophageal reflux disease, and others	Oral, parenteral	Nervousness
LAXATIVES Psyllium hydrophilic mucilloid (Metamucil)	Induces evacuation; bulk cathartic; not absorbed, but increases bulk in intestinal tract by absorbing GI fluid	Oral	All cathartics: dependence; electrolyte imbalance; should not be used in undiagnosed abdominal pain
Castor oil	Induces evacuation; irritant cathartic; irritates mucosa of intestinal tract to produce catharsis; frequently prescribed as cathartic of choice before radiologic procedures requiring that the bowel be free of fecal material	Oral	
Cascara sagrada	Irritant cathartic	Oral	
Magnesium hydroxide mixture (Milk of Magnesia)	Saline cathartic; prevents absorption of water out of intestinal tract; draws fluid in, thereby increasing bulk	Oral	
Mineral oil	Lubricant cathartic; not absorbed; mechanical aid that lubricates intestinal tract and prevents absorption of water	Oral	
Dioctyl sodium sulfosuccinate (Colace)	Detergent laxative; acts as wetting agent to soften fecal material	Oral	
Bisacodyl	Contact laxative; acts directly on large intestine to increase peristalsis	Rectal suppository	
ANTIDIARRHEAL DRUGS Kaolin mixture with pectin (Kaopectate)	Antidiarrheal	Oral	
Diphenoxylate hydrochloride with atropine sulfate (Lomotil)	Synthetic antidiarrheal; relieves cramping pain of diarrhea; decreases peristalsis	Oral	Drowsiness; dry mouth; nausea
Loperamide hydrochloride	Treats diarrhea	Oral	Abdominal pain; nausea and vomiting; drowsiness; dizziness; constipation

*Found on emergency drug trays

TABLE 11-7.
Drugs used to treat endocrine disorders

DRUG	PURPOSE	ROUTE	POTENTIAL ADVERSE EFFECTS
PITUITARY HORMONES AND DRUGS			
Oxytocin	Induces uterine contractions in order to begin or strengthen labor; used in preeclampsia near term; uterine inertia; incomplete abortion; also used to control postpartum hemorrhage	Parenteral	Acute hypotensive episodes; uterine rupture; fetal death
Vasopressin	Treats pituitary diabetes insipidus; in some cases of esophageal variceal bleeding and colonic diverticular bleeding	Parenteral	Headache; abdominal cramps; allergic reactions; hyponatremia
FEMALE SEX HORMONES			
Conjugated estrogens	Treats estrogen deficiency caused by menopause; female gonadism; dysfunctional uterine bleeding	Oral, parenteral, transdermal	Nausea and vomiting; vaginal discharge; depression; malaise; withdrawal bleeding; endometrial carcinoma with prolonged use without adjunct therapy
Polyestradial phosphate	Treats inoperable prostatic carcinoma	Parenteral	Pulmonary emboli; thrombophlebitis; allergic reactions; nausea and vomiting
MALE SEX HORMONES			
Methyltestosterone	Treats eunuchism; male climacteric symptoms caused by androgen deficiency; inadequate sexual development in females; inoperable breast cancer that may be hormone-dependent; prevention of breast engorgement postpartum	Oral, buccal	In women, hirsuitism, acne, male characteristics; in males, chronic priapism; increased libido; prostate growth; nausea, vomiting; hepatotoxicity
THYROID HORMONES			
Levothyroxine sodium (Synthroid, Levothoid)	Used for long-term replacement therapy in cases of hypothyroidism	Oral, parenteral	Hypermetabolism with weight loss, cramps, diarrhea, vomiting, tremors, sweating, heart palpitations, cardiovascular disease
Sodium iodide I-131	Destroys glandular tissue in cases of hyperthyroidism	Oral, parenteral	Thyroid cancer; leukemia; chromosome damage; hypothyroidism
DRUGS USED TO TREAT DIABETES			
Insulin	Pancreatic hormone; increases ability to utilize glucose, thereby lowering blood sugar levels; aids in conversion of fat to glycogen and promotes protein synthesis; used to control diabetes mellitus; many types, which are prescribed according to onset of action, duration, and patient tolerance	Subcutaneous	Rash, tissue atrophy at injection site, coma; patient must be observed closely until regimen is regulated; any changes in daily living schedules may give rise to severe reaction
Glucagon	Pancreatic extract, antagonistic to insulin; to treat hypoglycemia	Parenteral	Nausea; vomiting; hypotension; possible hypersensitivity
Chlorpropamide (Diabinese) Tolbutamide (Orinase)	Antihypoglycemic agents used to treat mild diabetes mellitus	Oral	Allergic skin reaction; heartburn; nausea; alcohol intolerance
ADRENOCORTICOSTEROID DRUGS			
Hydrocortisone	Treats diseases caused by chronic and acute adrenal insufficiency; manages inflammatory, immunologic and nonendocrine problems	Oral, topical, parenteral (route depends on purpose and type of preparation)	Symptoms of acute metabolic disease are masked, metabolic toxicity; infections; ocular toxicity; hyperglycemia; osteoporosis

cortex; and gonadal and pituitary hormones, from the pituitary gland.

After isolation and purification of chemical synthesis, these hormones are used in medical practice to replace deficient supplies in the body or, in large doses, to increase the available amount to an above-normal supply. They are also used to alter function in order to diagnose pathology of the adrenals and to treat nonendocrine diseases by increasing or decreasing normal endocrine activity (see Table 11-7).

Nutrients, fluids, and electrolytes

This group is composed of replacement fluids and nutrients for those normally present in the body that have been lost as a result of disease or injury. They may also be used to supplement normal volumes in order to achieve a specific physiologic effect.

Drug absorption

In order for a drug to achieve its desired effect on the body, it must reach the site of action. Most drugs must be absorbed into the body's systemic circulation in order to reach the intended receptor site. The exceptions to this are drugs intended for topical effect. The way a drug enters the body affects the speed and intensity of its absorption and action.

Routes of drug administration

The routes of drug administration are as follows:

ORAL ROUTE

The oral route is the safest and most desirable route of drug administration when it can be used. The oral route is used if the drug is one that will not be

TABLE 11-8.
Drugs used as nutrients, fluids, and electrolytes

DRUG	PURPOSE	ROUTE	POTENTIAL ADVERSE EFFECTS
Amino acid injection High-calorie solutions for injection	Used as fluid, electrolyte replacement	Parenteral	Infection; tissue sloughing
Calcium*	Treats tetany; with vitamin D to treat hypocalcemia	Oral, parenteral	GI irritation; peripheral vasodilatation resulting in hypotension; cardiac arrythmias
Phosphorus	Treats diet-deficiency diseases	Oral	
Vitamins	Treats diet-deficiency diseases	Oral, parenteral (some B-complex vitamins are administered IM)	Excessive doses of vitamin A may cause skin changes; later, fatigue; muscle, bone, and joint pain; liver and spleen enlargement; gingivitis; intracranial pressure; congenital abnormalities; acute toxicity in infants given vitamin A
Sodium chloride	Replaces sodium and chloride	Parenteral, oral replacement possible	Anorexia; cellular dehydration; distention; edema; hypertension; nausea; oliguria; pulmonary edema; weakness
Dextrose (concentration in solution varies with need)	In solution with sodium chloride	Parenteral, usually IV	Rare in small doses; may produce hypoglycemia or hyperglycemia; convulsions, loss of consciousness
Sodium bicarbonate	Treats metabolic acidosis as in cardiac arrest; ketoacidosis; and hyperkalemia	IV	Rare when used cautiously, may produce alkalosis, hyperexcitability, irritability, tetany
Potassium	Treats potassium deficiency	Oral, parenteral	Bradycardia; cardiac arrest; dysphagia; respiratory distress; weakness; muscle paralysis leading to death
Magnesium	Treats convulsive states and cerebral edema; corrects nutritional deficiency and uterine tetany	Parenteral	Absence of knee-jerk reflex; cardiac arrest; circulatory collapse; flushing; hypotension; respiratory depression; profuse perspiration

destroyed by gastric secretions and when slower absorption and longer duration of drug activity are desired.

PARENTERAL ROUTE

There are several methods of parenteral (any means that bypasses the digestive tract) drug administration. Topical drug administration may theoretically be included here but, in this text, will be addressed separately following discussion of common parenteral methods. Parenteral drug routes are used when rapid action is desired. The RT must be able to assist with medication administered by the following parenteral routes:

1. Subcutaneous—injected into the subcutaneous, or loose connective layers under the skin (Fig. 11-1); absorption and effect are rapid by this route

2. Intramuscular (IM)—through the skin and subcutaneous tissues into the muscle (Fig. 11-2)

3. Intradermal—between the layers of the skin (Fig. 11-3)

4. Intravenous (IV)—into the vein

Other parenteral routes used in special diagnostic imaging procedures will be discussed in Chapter 12.

The RT must be aware of the injection sites most commonly used for each method described above. He must know the type and size of needle generally preferred when parenteral drugs are to be given and the other equipment needed for each method.

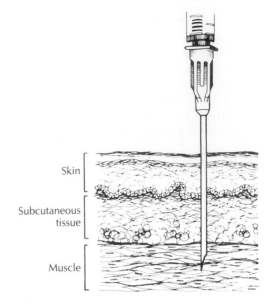

Figure 11.2

TOPICAL ROUTE

Topical drug administration includes drugs administered for local treatment of skin, eyes, nose, throat, the respiratory mucosa, the vagina, and, in some cases, the rectum. Rectal administration of drugs is occasionally used for systemic effect if the patient is unable to retain a drug administered orally or if gastric secretions would destroy the drug.

The skin, when unbroken, is slow to absorb drugs into the systemic circulation. The rate is accelerated if there is an open lesion or if the drug is applied to the mucous membranes. Some drugs are applied to the skin for intended systemic effect. When this is the case, the route is called *transdermal.* When this method is used, it is believed that drugs are absorbed slowly, and a constant blood level of the drug is achieved.

Buccal administration of a drug refers to the placing of a drug in the mouth between the teeth and the mucous membranes of the cheek and allowing it to

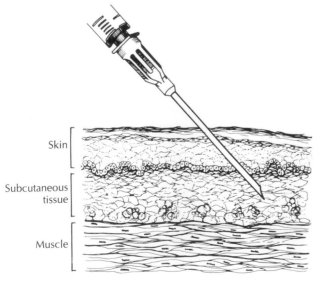

Figure 11.1

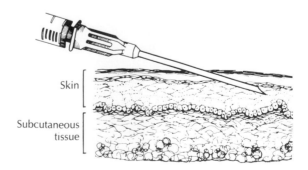

Figure 11.3

dissolve. This method is used when rapid absorption directly into the systemic circulation is desired.

Sublingual administration of a drug refers to drugs placed under the tongue for absorption. Both the sublingual and buccal routes are used when rapid drug absorption and action are desired for drugs destroyed by the liver or by gastric secretions.

Inhalation is used for drugs that vaporize readily. The absorption rate is high in the pulmonary mucosa; however, the types of drugs administered in this manner are relatively restricted and are not frequently used or seen in diagnostic imaging.

Procedures for drug administration

Subcutaneous administration

Subcutaneous medications are given at a 45-degree angle by injection into the tissues beneath the skin. If the physician requests that a medication be prepared to be given subcutaneously, the RT will need the following equipment:

1. A syringe of the correct size (a tuberculin syringe for an amount of less than 1 ml; a 2 ml to 3 ml for a 2-ml amount)

2. A ⅝- or ½-inch-long hypodermic needle with a 23- to 25-gauge lumen

3. Three alcohol wipes

4. The correct medication

Subcutaneous injections are given in the outer aspect of the upper arms, the abdomen, the scapulae, and the anterior thighs (Fig. 11-4). Only small amounts of drugs, 1 ml to 2 ml, should be administered in these areas. Subcutaneous drugs should be highly soluble and nonirritating to the tissues into which they are injected. Since this is an invasive procedure, sterile or surgical aseptic technique is used.

Oral administration

Oral administration of drugs is the safest and most efficient method and the one most often used. Nevertheless, there are several valid reasons for not giving drugs orally: The drug may have an unpleasant taste; it may cause nausea and vomiting; it may be destroyed by digestive juices; there is a danger of aspiration; the patient is uncooperative; or more rapid absorption is desired.

Oral medications are available in liquid, tablet, or capsule form.

When the physician desires an oral medication to

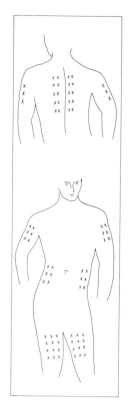

Figure 11.4. Appropriate sites for subcutaneous injections. (Walsh J, Persons CB, Wieck L: Manual of Home Health Care Nursing. Philadelphia, JB Lippincott, 1987)

be given, the RT must wash his hands and obtain a tray, the proper medication, a graduated medicine glass, and a glass of water (if the patient is permitted to swallow water). It is desirable to prepare an identifying ticket that states the patient's name and the drug ordered by the physician, as well as the strength and amount of the drug ordered. This ticket is placed on the tray with the medication.

When the RT has obtained the drug for administration, he takes the tray to the physician and asks him to verify the label on the drug bottle. The RT then pours the desired amount of the drug into the graduated medicine glass and has the physician check the dosage (Fig. 11-5). The RT may then be requested to give the drug to the patient. If so, he once again identifies the patient and then gives him the medication. Stay with the patient in order to be certain that the drug has been swallowed. Offer the patient a glass of water if it is permitted, then return the tray to the proper area. Discard the medicine cup or glass and again wash your hands.

When the correct medication and equipment are arranged on the tray, the RT should notify the physician. Together they approach the patient, identify him, and explain the procedure to him. The RT may open the vial and present it to the physician with the label facing him so that he can read it and draw up the medication. While the physician is doing this,

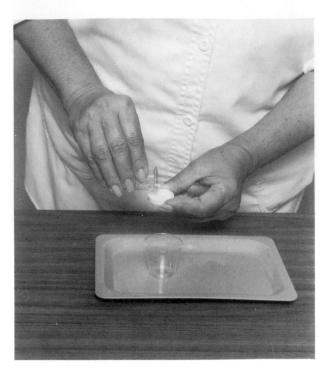

Figure 11.5

the RT will expose the area that the physician selects for the injection. The medication is administered by the physician. The RT can then make the patient comfortable, correctly dispose of the equipment, and wash his hands. He continues to observe the patient for any adverse effects from the medication for at least 30 minutes.

Intramuscular administration

Intramuscular (IM) injections are used when prompt absorption of a drug is desired. Larger amounts of medication may be administered IM than subcutaneously (1 ml to 3 ml), although 3 ml should not be injected into a patient who is small or whose muscles are poorly developed.

The length of the needle required for IM injection is largely determined by the patient's weight. For the average adult patient, a needle 1½ inches long is usually adequate, depending on the size of the patient and the muscle selected for the injection. The gauge varies from 18 to 22 depending on the viscosity of the drug. A 22-gauge needle should be used whenever possible, because it causes the least pain. The materials required for an IM injection are as follows:

1. A 3- to 5-ml syringe

2. An 18- to 22-gauge needle 1½ inches in length

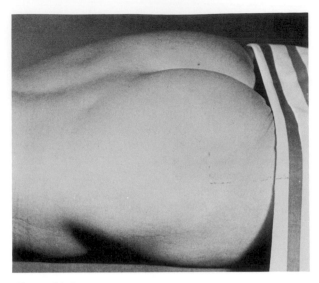

Figure 11.6

3. Three alcohol wipes

4. Correct medication

The procedure following the preparation of equipment is the same as for a subcutaneous injection. The usual sites for intramuscular injection are the upper–outer quadrant of the gluteus maximus muscle or the gluteus medius muscle (Fig. 11-6). Other areas where IM injections may be given are the deltoid muscle (Fig. 11-7), the ventral gluteal area, and the vastus lateralis muscle (Fig. 11-8).

If the medication is to be given in the gluteal muscle or in the thigh, while the physician is drawing up the medication, the RT will position the patient for the injection. For administration in the gluteal area, the patient is instructed to turn to the prone position or to the Sims' position. He is draped so that only the area needed for injection is exposed. After the physician has given the drug, return the patient to a comfortable position, dispose of the equipment correctly, wash your hands, and continue to observe the patient for at least 30 minutes for symptoms of an adverse drug reaction.

Intradermal administration

Intradermal injections may also be called intracutaneous injections. This type of injection is usually used for purposes of testing for sensitivity to a drug or antigen. When these test doses are given, the patient must be watched carefully for an anaphylactic reaction. They are usually given into the dermis of the inner aspect of the forearms. A very short needle, about ½ inch in length, is used. The lumen of the

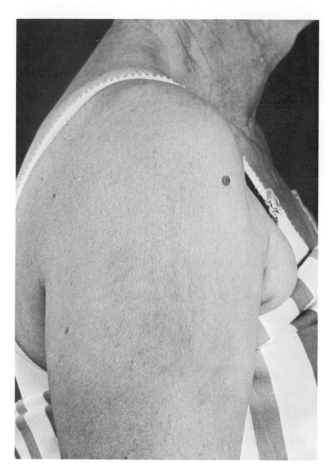

Figure 11.7

needle should be approximately 26-gauge. Only very small amounts of medication are given intradermally, and absorption is relatively slow. These minute amounts of medication are most accurately measured in a 1-ml tuberculin syringe. The procedure is the same as for an IM or subcutaneous injection. Usually the drug administered at this site will cause a burning pain for a brief time. This should be explained to the patient before the injection is given.

Intravenous administration

The intravenous (IV) method of drug administration is selected when the effect of a drug is desired immediately or if a drug cannot be injected into body tissues without damaging them. This may be considered one of the most hazardous routes of drug administration, because once a drug is injected directly into the circulatory system, reaction to it is instantaneous. Most drugs given in diagnostic imaging are given by this route. The RT must observe the patient continuously when he is receiving a drug by this method. Pulse rate and blood pressure should be taken prior to and frequently during IV drug administration. Any change in the vital signs or patient behavior should be reported to the physician in charge of the patient immediately.

The procedure for IV drug administration varies somewhat, depending on the type and amount of medication or solution to be administered. The use of surgical asepsis is mandatory for all intravenous drug administration to prevent introduction of microorganisms into the bloodstream.

Some IV drugs are given in small amounts through a pre-existing IV line. This intravenous line can be a heparin lock or an IV "piggyback." A *heparin lock* is a venous catheter that is left in place in the vein for long periods of time for the purpose of administering IV medication. There is a reservoir at the top of the catheter into which a small amount of heparin is added following each drug administration to prevent blood clotting in the needle. The medication is administered into this reservoir. When a drug is given directly into a heparin lock or into a pre-existing IV line, it is called giving a *bolus* of medication intravenously (Fig. 11-9).

An IV "piggyback" is another method of administering IV drugs through an established line. A piggyback is a small intravenous infusion (usually 100 ml to 250 ml), which is attached to an adjoining or already existing line. This solution is attached to the pre-existing line in such a manner that it flows into the vein at the intended rate. When it is completed, the original solution is begun again (Fig. 11-10).

If the drug is to be administered slowly by bolus, the RT will need the following items:

1. A syringe large enough to hold the amount of medication

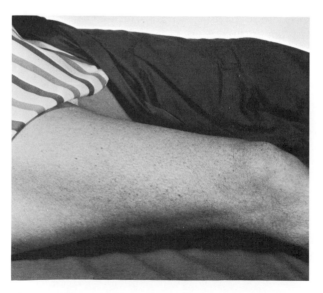

Figure 11.8

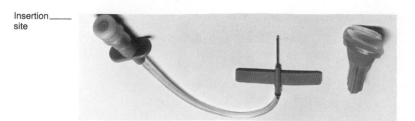

Insertion
site

Figure 11.9.   Equipment for a heparin lock. (Walsh J, Persons CB, Wieck L: Manual of Home Health Care Nursing. Philadelphia, JB Lippincott, 1987)

2. A 25-gauge needle, usually 1 inch in length (2.54 cm if the bolus it is to be administered through is a heparin lock or into an existing IV line

3. Four or five antiseptic alcohol wipes

4. The drug to be administered

The RT prepares the equipment and proceeds to the patient's room. The physician will draw up the drug after he identifies it and the patient with the RT. The physician then cleanses the site and administers the drug slowly. The RT and the physician observe the patient carefully for adverse reactions to the drug during this type of drug administration because the effects of the medication are immediate and irreversible. The patient is to be observed following medication administration for at least 30 minutes.

INTRAVENOUS INFUSIONS

If the drug is to be infused intravenously over a long period of time and is dissolved in 250 to 1000 ml of fluid, a plastic venous catheter or a butterfly needle is used. This type of needle has plastic "wings," which are taped flat against the skin following insertion to keep it in place and comfortable while an IV infusion is in progress. These are available in various sizes, but an 18- to 20-gauge needle 1 inch in length is most commonly used in diagnostic imaging (Fig. 11-11).

A venous catheter, also called an *angiocatheter*, is a plastic tubing with a needle through the tubing for insertion into the vein. Once the needle is in the vein,

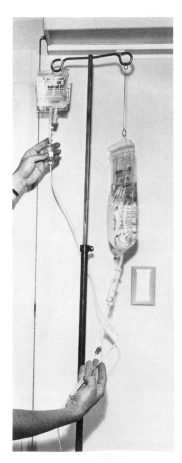

Figure 11.10.   Giving intravenous medication, using the "piggyback" method. The medication in the small container will enter the venous system before the solution in the larger container. (Walsh J, Persons CB, Wieck L: Manual of Home Health Care Nursing. Philadelphia, JB Lippincott, 1987)

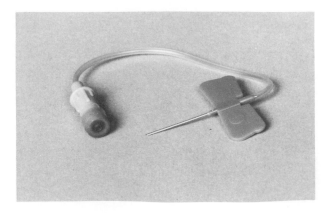

Figure 11.11.   A butterfly needle.

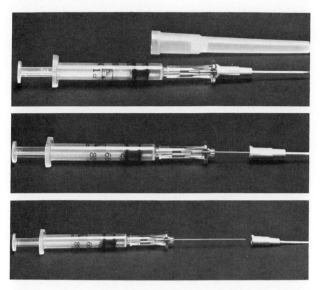

Figure 11.12

the catheter is moved into place within the vein and the needle removed. The catheter is then connected to the IV tubing. This type of venous catheter is flexible and will tolerate some movement without becoming dislodged from the vein (Fig. 11-12).

The injection site for IV infusion will vary depending on the drug to be administered and the duration of the infusion. If the amount to be administered is a small one, or one that requires less than 1 hour for administration, the antecubital vein may be used, because it is easily accessible in the majority of patients. This site is not recommended for extended IV therapy, because it inhibits the patient's ability to flex his arm and can become very uncomfortable. For prolonged IV infusions, veins in the forearm and the back of the hand are preferred (Fig. 11-13).

The type of solution to be administered also influences the selection of an infusion site. Hypertonic solutions, those to be administered rapidly, and viscid solutions (thick and sticky) should be administered into a large vein in the forearm such as the antecubital vein.

Items needed to begin an intravenous infusion are as follows:

1. A tourniquet

2. Several alcohol wipes and several iodophor wipes

3. Adhesive tape, precut

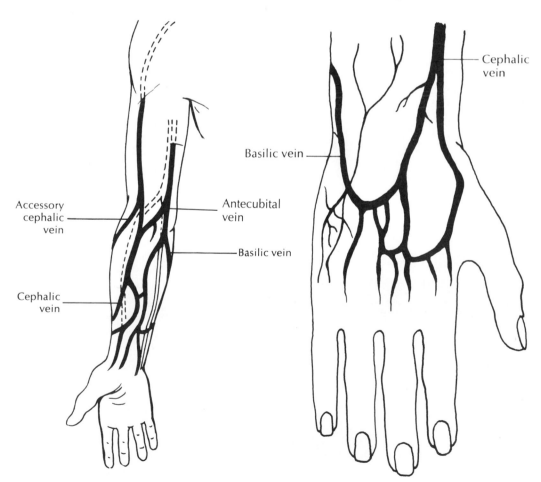

Figure 11.13

4. The correct fluid or drug

5. A sterile, disposable intravenous infusion set (tubing)

6. An IV standard.

7. The type of intravenous catheter or needle requested by the physician

8. Sterile gloves

The procedure for assisting with beginning an IV infusion is as follows:

1. The RT notifies the physician when the necessary items are assembled and explains the procedure to the patient.

2. If the solution to be administered is in a glass vacoliter, the RT may remove the metal cap and the rubber diaphragm from the bottle (Fig. 11-14).

3. The IV tubing may be opened, and the protective covering may be removed from the insertion of the drip chamber. Do not contaminate this tip, because it is placed into the sterile solution. Insert the drip-chamber tip into the rubber stopper (Fig. 11-15).

4. Clamp the tubing with the clamp supplied and attached to the tubing. Have a receptacle or a sink at hand.

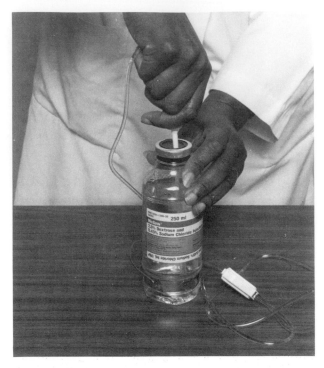

Figure 11.15

5. Invert the bottle of solution and hang it on the tubing. Do not contaminate this tip (Fig. 11-16). Open the clamp and allow fluid to run through the tubing until all air is removed (Fig. 11-17).

6. Reclamp the tubing. Replace the protective tip on the tubing, using sterile technique.

If the solution is in a plastic bag, remove the container from its protective covering (Fig. 11-18). Remove the protective cap from the tip of the drip chamber on the tubing and its port of insertion on the bag (Fig. 11-19). Place the tip into the port, then invert and hang the bag on the IV standard. Open the valve, and clear the air from the tubing. Replace the sterile protective cap. The procedure is the same from this point on, regardless of the container used.

The physician's gloves should be ready for him to put on. After he is gloved, apply the tourniquet above the area planned as an injection site. Next, hand the physician an iodophor wipe so that he may begin cleansing the area. The skin being prepared should be washed in a circular motion from the injection site outward. This is repeated with three iodophor wipes and followed with three alcohol wipes to free the skin from as many microorganisms as possible. Following the skin prep, the area should be permitted to dry.

When the skin is dry, the RT may apply the tourniquet about 6 inches (12 cm) above the area prepped for injection. The tourniquet should be applied by

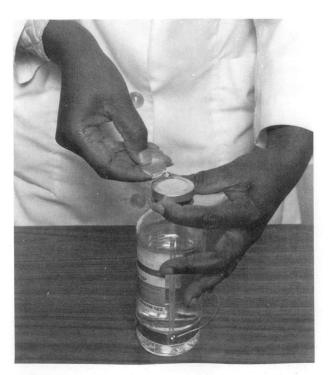

Figure 11.14

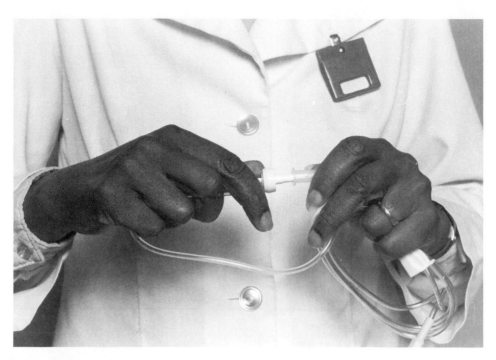

Figure 11.16

looping it so that it may be released with one motion and so that it obstructs only the venous, not the arterial, blood flow. It should be a flat piece of rubber that stays flat upon application (Fig. 11-20).

Next, offer the physician the IV needle or catheter attached to the IV tubing, making certain that the sterility of the needle is maintained by leaving the needle in its protective sheath until ready for use. After the infusion has been started, the physician will tape the needle or catheter in place and inform the RT how quickly he wants the fluid to infuse (drops per minute). This should be noted and the IV monitored so that the timing is correct (Fig. 11-21).

If the IV infusion site is the antecubital vein, place the patient's arm on an arm board so that the elbow joint is immobilized. The arm may be attached to the arm board with plain or elasticized gauze. Check the arm frequently to be certain that the arm board is not applied so tightly that it interferes with circulation. The signs and symptoms of impaired circulation for a patient with a casted extremity in Chapter 3 may be used. Also check the infusion site for any signs of infiltration of the fluid into the surrounding tissues.

The IV standard should be placed 18 to 24 inches above the level of the vein, because the height at which the container of solution is suspended affects the rate of flow. If the bottle of solution is positioned lower than the vein, blood will flow into the tubing. The rate of flow of an IV infusion may also be affected by the position of the catheter or needle in the vein. If the bevel of either is positioned against the wall of

the vein, it will slow or stop the infusion. Changing the position of the patient's arm will often correct the problem.

If there is a question about rate of infusion, a safe rule to follow is to allow the solution to infuse at 15 to 20 drops/min. If a large amount of solution infuses too quickly, there is danger of fluid intoxication or pulmonary edema. Unless the physician has ordered a rapid infusion, the IV solution that is flowing very rapidly should be slowed down. This can be done by simply tightening the control mechanism on the tubing slightly.

Occasionally, a patient may come for diagnostic imaging with an IV infusion pump in place. There are many types of them on the market, and each institution selects the pump that best suits the needs of its patients. The IV infusion pump, whatever the type, monitors rate of flow of IV fluid to prevent the solution from infusing too rapidly. When the flow stops, becomes too rapid, or the container empties, an alarm will sound. The RT must remember that when he hears this alarm, he must notify the nurse in the area or the physician, if there is not a nurse available.

Any complaint of pain or discomfort at the site of insertion of an IV needle should be heeded, and the site should be checked immediately. Swelling around the site or cold, blanched skin is an indication that the needle or catheter has become dislodged from the vein, and the fluid or medication is infiltrating into the surrounding tissues. The RT should turn the IV off immediately and notify the physician in charge

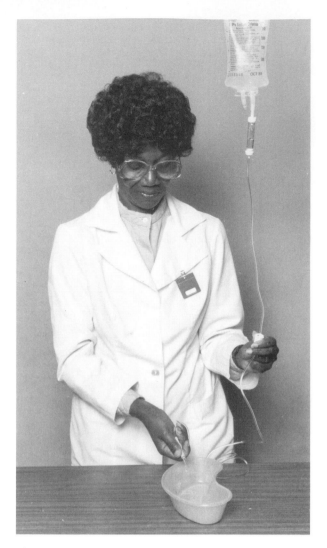

Figure 11.17

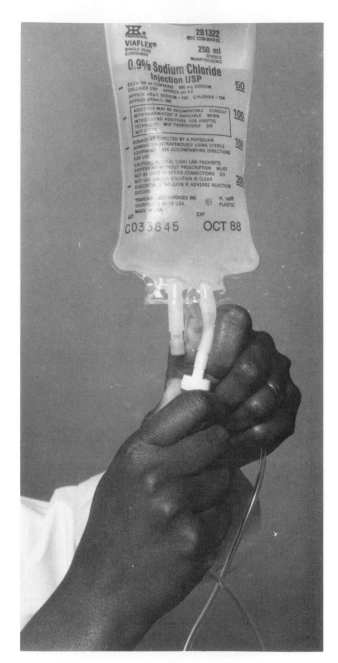

Figure 11.19

of the patient. Severe tissue damage may result from infiltration of IV drugs and fluids. Drugs administered intravenously act very rapidly. Any complaint of itching or feeling of congestion or fullness in the chest or throat is cause to discontinue administration of an IV drug. Do not wait for further evidence of complications. Stop the infusion immediately, and then notify the patient's physician.

DISCONTINUING IVS

An IV infusion is not discontinued without a physician's order to do so. The patient who must receive IV drug therapy endures varying amounts of discom-

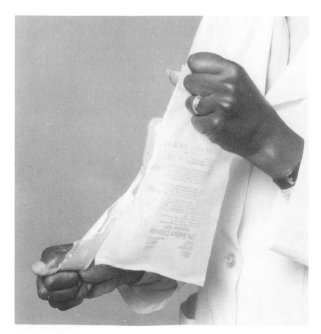

Figure 11.18

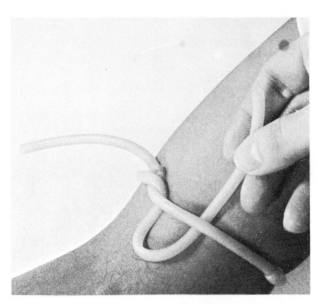

Figure 11.20. A correctly applied tourniquet can be removed rapidly by pulling one end. (Spencer RT, Nichols LW, Lipkin GB et al: Clinical Pharmacology and Nursing Management, 2nd ed. Philadelphia, JB Lippincott, 1986)

fort to begin the procedure, because venipuncture can be painful. The RT must be certain that the procedure is to be discontinued so the patient does not have to endure such discomfort a second time as a result of carelessness or misunderstanding.

In order to discontinue an IV, the RT will need the following equipment:

1. A pack of dry, sterile, 2-inch by 2-inch gauze sponges

2. Clean, disposable gloves

3. Scissors to cut the tape

4. Tape

5. A tourniquet

The following procedure should then be observed:

1. The RT goes to the patient and carefully identifies him.

2. Clamp off the intravenous solution and prepare two strips of tape, and place them where they can be reached easily later.

3. Loosen the tape that holds the venous catheter or needle in place so that the hub is clearly visible and free of tape.

4. Open the sterile gauze sponges, being careful not to contaminate them.

5. Put on the clean gloves.

6. Gently withdraw the needle or catheter from the vein until it is completely removed (Fig. 11-22).

7. Immediately after the catheter is removed, apply pressure to the site of withdrawal with a dry, sterile sponge until the bleeding stops.

8. Inspect the needle or catheter that has been removed from the vein to be certain that it has emerged intact. If there is a possibility that a portion of it has broken off and remains in the

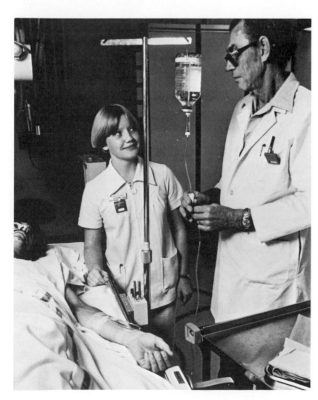

Figure 11.21

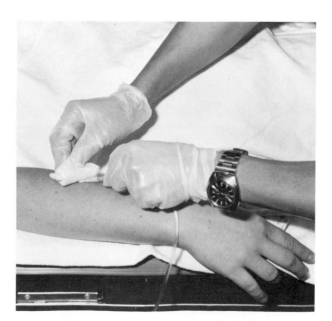

Figure 11.22

vein, immediately apply the tourniquet above the site of needle or catheter insertion, and notify the physician; do not leave the patient.

9. When the bleeding stops, use another sterile gauze pad, fold a sterile dry sponge, and tape it in place over the insertion site with some pressure applied. A Band-Aid may be used for this purpose.

10. Explain to the patient that this dressing may be removed in 1 or 2 hours.

11. Place the used syringe and needle into the "contaminated sharps" disposal container. Do not recap the needle. Remove your gloves.

12. Dispose of the vacoliter, and wash your hands.

Needles, syringes, and medicine glasses

Needles range in length from ½ inch to 6 inches. The size of the lumen is called the *gauge* of the needle, and it ranges from sizes 13 to 30. The most commonly used sizes range from 18- to 23-gauge and ⅝- to 1½-inch length. Needles and syringes are generally meant for single use and are disposed of after this. The gauge and length of the needle is printed on the outside of the packaging, which keeps it sterile until time for use.

Syringes are also disposable. The parts of the syringe are pictured in Figure 11-23. They are available in sizes from 1 ml to 50 ml. Syringes are calibrated in milliliters and in minims (minim, singular); 1 ml equals 16 minims. They are packaged in paper wrappers to maintain sterility, and needles are often already attached. The size of the syringe and the size of needle are printed on the package (Fig. 11-24).

After a needle is used, it should be placed into a container prepared for this purpose. These containers are labeled for "contaminated sharps" and are made

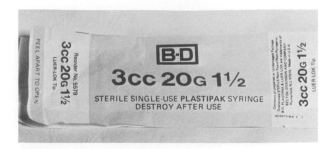

Figure 11.24

of a hard, red plastic. The RT must consider all used needles as potentially lethal. Do not recap a used needle: It must be held carefully by the syringe to which it is attached, with the needle pointed down and carried immediately to one of these containers and deposited, needle first, into it. Never place a used syringe and needle back on a tray to be disposed of at a later time (Fig. 11-25). The RT must be careful not to stick himself when handling used needles. This is considered a very hazardous medical accident that must be reported as a "critical incident" and attended to immediately. AIDS, hepatitis B, and hepatitis non-A non-B can be contracted in this manner.

Most medicine glasses are made of disposable plastic. All are of 1-ounce size and are calibrated for

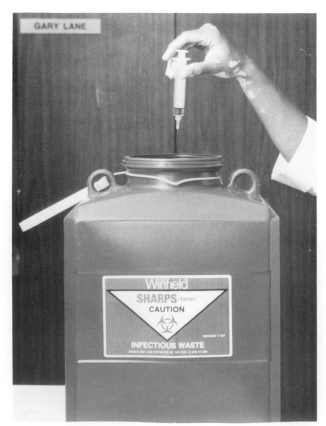

Figure 11.25

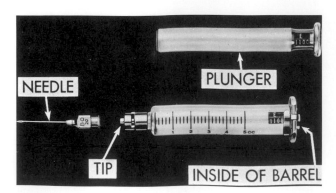

Figure 11.23

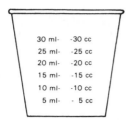
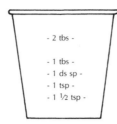
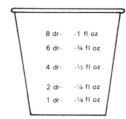

Figure 11.26

household, apothecary, and metric measures. The RT must learn to convert from one system to another (Fig. 11-26).

Packaging of injectable medication

Injectable medications are packaged in ampules, vials, and vacoliters.

Vials

A vial is a glass container with a rubber stopper circled by a metal band; the band holds the rubber stopper in place. Vials are generally available in 5-, 10-, 20-, 30-, and 50-ml sizes. On the label is found the name of the medication, the dosage per milliliter, and the route by which it may be administered (*e.g.,* morphine sulfate—1 ml = 15 mg). Multidose vials are not frequently used because of the hazards of contamination.

The needle is inserted through the rubber stopper into the solution. The solution runs into the syringe more quickly if air is injected into the vial before the solution is drawn up (Fig. 11-27).

Ampules

An ampule is always a single-dose container and is made entirely of glass. The indented area at the neck is opened by filing the neck with a small metal file (Fig. 11-28). The top then easily snaps off the container. The RT must never attempt to snap the top off an ampule without protecting his hands with a sterile gauze pad, because the glass may break unevenly and cut the hand (Fig. 11-29). The ampule is labeled, like the vial, with the name of the medication, the dosage per milliliter, and the route of administration. If all of the medication is not used, the remainder must be discarded, because it does not remain sterile once the ampule has been opened.

Vacoliters

The vacoliter is a glass bottle that has been filled under vacuum pressure; it is available in sizes of 250 ml, 500 ml, and 1000 ml. Like the vial, it has a rubber stopper surrounded by metal. A spot marked "X" inside the circle on the rubber stopper indicates the place where the drip chamber is to be inserted into the bottle, a procedure that must be done by firmly pushing into the stopper. After the drip chamber has been inserted, the bottle is inverted for use. The name and quantity of solution are stated on the label. The vacoliter is calibrated in cubic centimeters or milliliters so that the quantity of solution being infused may easily be monitored (Fig. 11-30).

Precautions in drug administration

All drugs are potentially dangerous. The RT must never become casual or careless when assisting with drug administration and must never give a drug on his own authority. In order to assist the physician with drug administration responsibility, the RT must

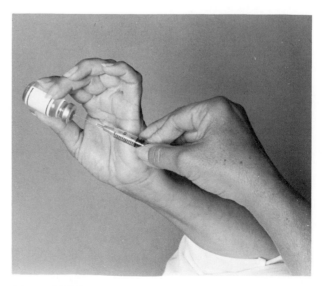

Figure 11.27

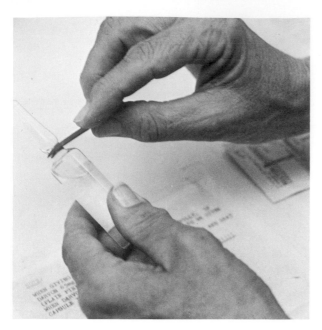

Figure 11.28

understand the fundamentals of this very complex science. It is recommended that the RT read the literature packaged with drugs used commonly in diagnostic imaging. This includes the potentially adverse reactions to drugs, the contraindications for administration of a particular drug, and the correct method of storing each one.

When assisting with drug administration, the RT with the physician must adhere to the *Five Rights* of drug administration as follows:

1. The right patient
2. The right drug

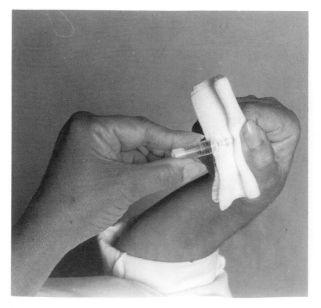

Figure 11.29

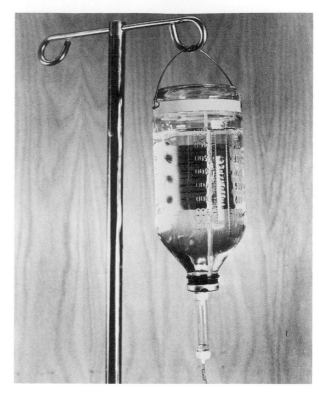

Figure 11.30

3. The right amount
4. The right route
5. The right time

Any drug administered in the diagnostic imaging department must be ordered in writing by the physician caring for the patient and administered by a registered nurse, a licensed vocational nurse, or by a physician. The order may be written in a designated area on the patient's chart or on a prescription form and signed by the physician giving the order. In some instances, a telephone order or a verbal order for a drug or treatment may be given to a registered nurse who in turn writes it on the chart and designates it as a verbal or telephone order that the physician will sign within 24 hours after giving the order.

Other precautions that must be taken by the RT when he assists with drug administration are as follows:

1. The patient must be observed for adverse reactions to the medication during drug administration and for 30 minutes thereafter.

2. A history of adverse reactions or allergic reactions to drugs must be taken for each patient before drugs are administered (as described in Chapter 5). Drug reactions occur frequently, most of them during the first 30 minutes following adminis-

tration if the drug was given orally, IM, subcutaneously or intradermally; more quickly if given IV. Report complaints of itching, shortness of breath, dizziness, or extreme drowsiness to the patient's physician immediately and prepare for an emergency. Do not leave a patient who may be having a drug reaction unattended.

3. The patient must not be allowed to drive himself home following a drug reaction or after receiving a sedative or narcotic analgesic medication. Patients must be observed for at least 30 minutes before leaving the department alone after receiving any drug.

4. When assisting with drug administration, read the drug label carefully and make certain that the physician administering the medication reads the label before administering the drug.

5. Check the strength, dosage, and name of the drug.

6. If a drug contains a sediment or appears to be cloudy, it must not be used until the pharmacist has approved it. If in doubt, discard the drug.

7. The expiration date of all medications is written on the label. If the medication is beyond the prescription date, it must be discarded.

8. If the RT is requested by a physician to record a drug given on a patient's chart, he must list the name of the drug, the strength, the amount given, the route, and the site of administration. The physician signs his name after the entry on the chart.

9. The patient's name must be checked with the medication order to be certain that the right patient is receiving the right medication. Hospital patients wear an identifying name band, which should be read for verification.

10. Never use medications from unmarked or poorly marked bottles. Destroy these drugs.

11. Measure exact amounts of every drug used.

12. Store drugs in accordance with manufacturer's specifications. No drugs should be stored in an area where temperature and humidity vary greatly or are extreme. Low room temperature is always advised.

13. If the medication is a liquid, it should be poured away from the label of the bottle.

14. Two medications must not be mixed together unless this is authorized by the physician.

15. If an error is made during drug administration, notify the physician in charge of the patient immediately.

16. Before selecting a medication on behalf of a physician, check the label of the container three times: before it is measured, before you leave the area of drug preparation, while the physician is reading the label.

17. Take only one drug to one patient at one time.

18. Never leave the patient until he has taken the drug offered him.

19. If an IV or intraspinal drug is being administered, the patient should be observed continuously and never left alone.

20. When approaching a patient who is to receive a drug, ask him to state his name. Do not accept the fact that a patient answers to what is thought to be the correct name. When the patient is anxious, he may not hear clearly.

Factors that influence drug dosage

Medication history

The patient's medication history also influences drug dosage. Usually, persons who take drugs frequently and in large quantities are less sensitive to them than those who rarely or never use them.

Allergies

Allergy or susceptibility to drugs must be noted, and precautions must be taken.

Temperament and occupation

A person's temperament and occupation may also influence his reaction. The following questions are to be asked: What is the condition of the patient? Is he young and vigorous? Is he old and weak? Is the patient a child? If so, how old is the child? Why is the medication being given? Does the patient have to be fully sedated, or does he simply need to be relaxed so that the procedure can properly be performed? Obviously, more medication is needed to achieve full sedation than is needed for relaxation.

Time of day

The time of day influences drug action. A drug given in the morning, when a patient is well rested, may not be as effective as it might be later in the day.

Route of administration

The channel or route of drug administration is also an important factor, since far less medication is required by IV than by mouth. IV drugs are immediately absorbed into the bloodstream and circulated to all parts of the body, whereas oral drugs are absorbed more slowly, and some of the drugs may be inactive during the period of absorption.

Abbreviations and equivalents

The following are prescription abbreviations commonly used in hospitals throughout the United States with which the RT should become familiar:

a.c.—before meals

A.D.—right ear

ad lib.—as desired

AK—above knee

ant.—anterior

A&P—anterior and posterior

BaE—barium enema

b.i.d.—two times a day

c̄—with

cc—cubic centimeter

D.C.—discontinue

EEG—electroencephalogram

ER—emergency room

Fe—chemical symbol for iron

FBS—fasting blood sugar

g—gram

GB—gallbladder

gr—grain

gtt—drop

HCl—hydrochloric acid

H&P—history and physical

h.s.—at bedtime

I and O—intake and output

kg—kilogram

lb—pound

liq—liquid

M—minim

mcg or **μg**—microgram

mg—milligram

ml—milliliter

NaCl—sodium chloride

NSAID—nonsteroidal anti-inflammatory drug

O.D.—overdose

O.S.—left eye

OTC—over the counter drug (nonprescription)

O.U.—each eye

oz—ounce

p̄—after

p.c.—after meals

pH—hydrogen concentration or activity of a solution

p.o.—by mouth; orally

p.r.n.—whenever necessary

q. 4 h.—every 4 hours; **q. 2 hr** — every 2 hours, etc.

q.d.—every day

q.h.—every hour

q.s.—sufficient quantity

q.i.d.—four times per day

R.B.C.—red blood cell

s̄—without

ss.—one half

stat.—immediately

supp.—suppository

TB—tuberculosis

t.i.d.—three times a day

tsp—teaspoon

U.—unit

U.S.P.—United States Pharmacopeia

ʒ—fluidram

℥—fluid/ounce

W.B.C.—white blood cell

The following measures are used interchangeably in many hospitals. The RT should be able to convert from one to the other immediately.

1 tsp = 1 ʒ = 4 ml to 5 ml

2.2 pounds = 1 kg (kilogram)

1 inch = 2.54 cm (centimeters)

30 ml = 1 ʒ

15 ml = ½ ʒ

gr ¹/₂₀₀ = 0.3 mg

gr ¹/₁₅₀ = 0.4 mg

gr ¹/₁₀₀ = 0.6 mg

gr ¹/₆ = 10 mg

gr ¹/₄ = 15 mg

gr ¹/₃ = 20 mg

gr ½ = 32 mg

gr 1 = 60 mg

gr 15 = 1 g = 1000 mg

1 minim = ¹/₁₆ ml or ¹/₁₅ ml

15 or 16 minims = 1 ml

500 ml = 1 pint

1000 ml = 1 quart

30 grams = 1 ounce

Summary

The RT is not permitted by law to administer drugs, but he will be expected to assist with drug administration in the course of his work. Any person who assists with the administration of drugs must know the potential hazards of drug administration and the precautions that must be taken when they are administered. He should also understand the intended effect or the purpose of the drug administered.

Each drug that is marketed for medical use has several names. It has a chemical name, which is derived from its chemical formula; a generic name, which is given prior to official approval; and a trade name, which is the name given to it by a particular manufacturer. The chemical name and the generic name do not change, but the same drug may have more than one trade name. The RT should acquaint himself with the generic name and the various trade names of the drugs used frequently in his department.

Drugs may be categorized in various ways. In this chapter they are categorized according to their intended purpose and the manner in which they affect the body systems. The RT should review these and become familiar with the drugs that will be found on the emergency drug trays in his department as well as throughout the hospital.

Most drugs must be absorbed into the systemic circulation in order to reach the desired site of action. The exceptions to this are topical drugs whose desired effect is at the site of application such as the eye, the nasal passages, or, in most situations, the skin. The way a drug enters the body determines the rate at which it is absorbed and begins to achieve its desired effect. The routes of drug administration are oral and parenteral.

Oral administration is safe and efficient. This is the route used when medication will not be destroyed by gastric secretions or the patient is not suffering from nausea and vomiting, and a prolonged period of effectiveness is sought.

The most common parenteral routes of drug administration are subcutaneous, intramuscular, intradermal, and intravenous. These routes of drug administration are used when rapid action and a shorter duration of action is desired.

Medications for parenteral use are packaged in vials, ampules, and vacoliters. The trade name of the drug, the generic name of the drug, the route of administration, and the quantity per milliliter are listed on the drug label.

All drugs administered by parenteral routes must be administered by means of sterile technique. The size of needle and syringe or vacoliter selected will depend on the type of medication and the route by which it has been ordered. The RT must take meticulous precautions when disposing of used hypodermic needles so that he does not prick his skin or another person as he disposes of the used equipment. Immediately following an injection, the used syringe and needle must be placed, needle first, into the correct receptacle. Needles are not recapped. Any injury that results from a needle stick from a contaminated needle must be reported as a critical hospital incident, and the injured person must have immediate care.

All drugs are potentially harmful and may be life-threatening. The RT must always take every precaution when assisting with drug administration. The right patient must receive the right drug in the right dose at the right time by the right route. A drug history must be taken on every patient who receives a drug in the diagnostic imaging department. The patient who receives a drug must be observed for at least 30 minutes following administration. Any symptom of an unfavorable drug reaction must be reported to the physician in charge of the patient immediately. Patients who are receiving drugs must never be left unattended. If they have received a sedative or had a drug reaction, they must not be allowed to drive themselves home. Patients receiving IV infusions or an IV bolus of a drug must have their vital signs taken prior to the IV being started and several times during the administration and must be continuously observed.

The patient's age, weight, sex, medication history, history of allergy, emotional status, occupation, and overall physical condition, as well as the reason for the drug administration and the route and time, are factors that must be taken into account in determining the strength and quantity of drug to be prescribed. The RT must be aware of these factors and be alert to any deviation from normal reactions to drugs by patients when in the diagnostic imaging department.

Chapter 11, pre-post test

_____ 1. What is a safe rate of infusion for intravenous fluid?
   a. 5 to 10 drops/min
   b. 25 to 30 drops/min
   c. 15 to 20 drops/min
   d. 30 to 40 drops/min

_____ 2. A patient comes to the diagnostic imaging department with an IV infusion in place and infusing. After the patient has been in the department for about 30 minutes, he begins to complain that his hand feels cold and painful. You examine it and see that it is also swelling. The RT should
   a. Explain to the patient that the IV seems to be infiltrating into surrounding tissue
   b. Stop the infusion
   c. Remove the catheter from the vein
   d. Stop the infusion and notify the physician

_____ 3. When a patient is receiving a medication in the diagnostic imaging department, it is the RT's responsibility to
   a. Administer the drug
   b. Observe the patient during and after the drug has been administered
   c. Decide on the dose to be administered
   d. Plan the route of administration

_____ 4. The drug name given it by a particular manufacturer is the
   a. Trade name
   b. Generic name
   c. Chemical name
   d. Proper name

_____ 5. An analgesic is a drug used for
   a. Vasodilatation
   b. Decongestion
   c. Relief of pain
   d. Enuresis

_____ 6. Factors that may influence the effect of a drug are
   a. Age and weight
   b. Sex and time of day
   c. Medication history and the patient's temperament
   d. a and b
   e. a, b, and c

_____ 7. The channel of drug administration does not influence the amount of drug administered.
   a. True
   b. False

_____ 8. Parenteral drug routes may include
   a. Intramuscular
   b. Intravenous
   c. Oral
   d. a and c
   e. a and b

_____ 9. An abnormally rapid heart beat is called
   a. Tachypnea
   b. Tachycardia
   c. Tetany
   d. Teratogenic

_____ 10. A drug that increases the flow of urine is called a
   a. Derivative
   b. Diuretic
   c. Digestant
   d. Demulcent

_____ 11. Match the word, phrase, or symbol with the most appropriate word or medical abbreviation below.

1. Short needle; ⅝ inches long with 23 to 25 gauge	a. IM
2. Needle 1½ inches long with 18 to 22 gauge	b. IV
3. Needle 1 inch long with 18 to 20 gauge	c. Subcutaneous
4. Needle 3½ inches long with 20 to 22 gauge	d. Intrathecal
5. Needle ½ inch long with 26 gauge	e. Intradermal

12.
1. p.r.n.	a. immediately
2. gtt.	b. before meals
3. stat.	c. twice a day
4. b.i.d.	d. whenever necessary
5. a.c.	e. drop

13.
1. 2.2 pounds	a. 1 gram
2. 60 mg	b. before meals
3. 15 grains	c. 1 grain
4. 30 milliliters	d. 1 kilogram
5. 1 ounce	e. 1 cubic centimeter

_____ 14. IV drug administration is an example of
   a. Local drug administration
   b. Subcutaneous drug administration

c. Parenteral drug administration
d. Sublingual drug administration

—— **15.** All drugs given by parenteral routes are given by:

a. Medical aseptic technique
b. Surgical aseptic technique

—— **16.** List the five "rights" of drug administration

Laboratory reinforcement

1. In the school laboratory, draw up 4 ml of sterile normal saline for IM injection. You have several sizes of needles and syringes from which to choose. Choose the correct needle and syringe size.

2. In the school laboratory, prepare to assist the radiologist with administration of 250 ml of a contrast medium for IV instillation.

3. In the school laboratory, prepare to assist the radiologist with administration of ½ ml of sterile water for subcutaneous injection. You have a series of needles and syringes from which to select. Choose the correct needle size and syringe size.

4. In the school laboratory, position a patient for administration of an IM injection.

Chapter Twelve

Care of Patients During Special Procedures

Goal of this chapter:

The RT student will understand the emotional and physical problems of patients undergoing special diagnostic imaging examinations and be able to care for them safely and with sensitivity.

Behavioral objectives:

When the RT student has completed this chapter, he will be able to do the following:
1. Recognize a normal electrocardiograph pattern and the medical implications of one that is abnormal
2. Explain the properties of iodinated contrast agents and the medical complications that may result from their administration
3. Describe the medical complications, emotional implications, and patient-teaching responsibilities for the patient undergoing cardiac catheterization or angiography
4. Identify the medical complications, patient care, and teaching responsibilities during myelography
5. Explain the medical complications, emotional implications, patient care, and teaching responsibilities for the patient during computerized tomography
6. Describe the patient care, teaching responsibilities, and emotional implications for the patient receiving magnetic resonance imaging.
7. Describe the patient care and teaching responsibilities for the patient during ultrasonography
8. Identify the medical side effects, the emotional implications, patient care, and teaching responsibilities for the patient receiving external radiation therapy.

Glossary

Adverse reactions the development of unwanted side effects or toxicity caused by administration of drugs; onset may be sudden or take days to develop

Ectopic in an abnormal position; out of sequence

Hypertension a condition in which patient has a higher blood pressure than that judged to be normal

Ionic strength pertains to atomic weight of a substance; *i.e.*, number of positive- or negative-charged particles

Multiple myeloma progressive, malignant tumors originating in cells of bone marrow

Occlusion the acquired or congenital closing of a passage, often a blood vessel

Paresthesia sensation of numbness or tingling, usually in an extremity

Percutaneous through the skin

Pheochromocytoma a vascular tumor that produces hypertension and other medical problems

Pott's disease tuberculosis of the spine; form of inflammatory arthritis affecting vertebrae of children and young adults

Rhinitis inflammation and congestion of the mucous membrane of the nose
Sickle-cell disease a hereditary chronic form of anemia, character-ized by abnormal, crescent-shaped red blood corpuscles, prominent among the black population
Stylet a thin probe, solid or hollow, used to maintain an opening for a catheter or needle during a medical procedure
Submaxillary below the upper jaw
Urography a roentgenogram of any part of the urinary tract

The patient undergoing special diagnostic imaging procedures requires special consideration, as do patients receiving magnetic resonance imaging, external radiation therapy, and ultrasonography. Many of them have been informed that they may have a life-threatening illness, and the special diagnostic procedure that they are about to undergo will either confirm or rule out this threat.

Special diagnostic imaging procedures and treatments are not without risk and are anxiety-provoking to most patients. The patient is received into a surgery-type atmosphere in which the health-care team is either masked and gowned or hidden behind protective glass and addressing the patient by microphone. This, combined with a prospect of a shortened life span, results in feelings of helplessness and fear.

Patients receiving radiation therapy may be in various stages of the grieving process. They know that they have a potentially terminal illness and are being treated with radiation in an attempt to prolong their lives or obtain some relief from pain during their final days.

The RT working in these diagnostic imaging areas must have exceptional technical skill, and he must also have superior communication and patient-teaching skills. In these areas of patient care, the physician, the registered nurse, and the RT work together as an interdependent team. Each depends on the other for safe and successful diagnostic and treatment outcomes. All patient care skills presented in the previous chapters of this text will be applied in these areas.

The RT who assists with special procedures must understand the properties of iodinated contrast agents and be acquainted with basic electrocardiogram (ECG) monitoring, because many patients receiving these diagnostic imaging procedures will be monitored by cardiac monitors continuously. Most will also receive iodinated contrast agents to aid in the visualization of organs and tissues.

Expertise in advanced radiologic techniques is required to work in most of the departments discussed in this chapter. The intent of this text is to give the beginning RT student an overview of patient care in these areas so that he may benefit by observational experiences there. Detailed technical discussion of the procedures described is beyond the scope of this text and will only be mentioned when relevant to patient care and instruction.

Cardiac monitoring

Some diagnostic imaging procedures and treatments such as cardiac catheterization require continuous cardiac monitoring during the entire procedure. Although the RT is not the member of the health-care team in these areas who is responsible for this monitor, he should be able to recognize an aberrant reading as such. The discussion of cardiac monitoring presented here is not extensive and will not prepare the RT to assume the responsibility of cardiac monitoring. The interpretation of ECGs is a specialty area and requires a lengthy course of study. The several diagrams listed here are ominous, and if the RT sees one, he must report it to the registered nurse or physician caring for the patient immediately.

An ECG is the most frequently used test for evaluating the functional status of the heart. ECG tracings assist with identification of disturbances in the rhythm (dysrythmias), conduction, and electrolyte balance of the heart. It also assists with diagnosis and treatment of heart disease.

As the heart is monitored by an ECG machine, a tracing is made on electrically sensitive paper or on a monitor (like a television screen) of the electrical activity of the heart for the purpose of detecting abnormal transmission of cardiac impulses from the heart through surrounding tissue to the skin. When the impulses reach the skin, electrodes, which have been strategically placed, sense the electrical impulses and transmit them to the ECG machine, which in turn records the impulses in graphic form.

The RT must remember that the ECG is only measuring the electrical activity of the heart; therefore, all ECG readings that are not normal are not necessarily indicative of heart disease. Conversely, a normal ECG pattern is not always an indication of a healthy heart, since mechanical events in the myocardium (the heart muscle) cannot be detected by this machine.

There are several types of ECG tests and monitors. All require that electrodes be positioned on various parts of the body in varying numbers and positions. The only type that will be discussed in this text will be those used for continuous cardiac monitoring, which is generally the type that the RT will be exposed to in his work.

Continuous cardiac monitoring is done to detect

patterns of cardiac impulses and to display them on a monitor screen for continuous observation and analysis. If the patient's heart rate or rhythm deviates from the normal rate or rhythm, an alarm sounds to alert the team caring for the patient. In this manner, any life-threatening problem is detected instantly. This monitor will also provide printouts of the patient's cardiac rhythms at selected sites.

Preparation for cardiac monitoring

When the patient is to have continuous cardiac monitoring during a special diagnostic procedure or treatment, he is informed of what is to take place. If the RT assists with the placement of electrodes, he must be directed by a person who has been trained to do this.

Wherever the electrodes are to be positioned, the patient's skin must be prepared by removing the dirt and oils present with alcohol. Hair in those areas is sometimes removed by physician's order to reduce skin resistance. Electrodes used for continuous monitoring usually come prelubricated in a prepared package. If the electrodes are not prelubricated, an electroconductive paste must be applied to each electrode before placement. Patterns of placement of

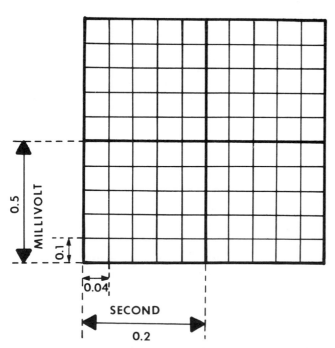

Figure 12.1.   Time and voltage lines on ECG paper. Vertically: 1 mm = 0.1 mV; 5 mm = 0.5 mV; 10 mm = 1.0 mV. Horizontally: 25 little boxes = 1 second; 1500 little boxes = 60 seconds. (Patrick ML, Woods SL, Craven RF et al: Medical-Surgical Nursing. Philadelphia, JB Lippincott, 1986)

electrodes vary, but three electrodes are placed on the anterior chest wall (Fig. 12-1). Once the electrodes are applied, an alarm is set on the ECG machine for 30% above and 30% below the patient's baseline heart rate, and then the monitor and machine are activated. Any deviation from the setting will activate the alarm.

ECG rhythms

The cardiac monitor screen will display the heart rate, rhythm, and patterns of impulses. The components of cardiac rhythm are expressed in waves called *P waves,* the *QRS complex,* the *T wave,* the *ST segment,* and the *PR* and *QT intervals.* A *U wave* is sometimes present following the T wave. When a U wave is present it is usually indicative of an abnormality (Fig. 12-2).

When the cardiac monitor displays a pattern in which P, QRS, and T waves are present in a normal rate and rhythm sequence, it is referred to as a *normal sinus rhythm.* All P waves should be upright, rounded, and similar in size and shape. A P wave should exist for, and be equidistant from, every QRS complex. All QRS complexes in a normal sinus rhythm are of equal size and shape, point in the same direction, and are equidistant from the P wave (Fig. 12-3).

Some rhythms that the RT may see and should recognize as ominous and point out to the physician or registered nurse with whom he is working are shown in Figures 12-4 to 12-9.

Iodinated contrast agents

Iodinated contrast agents are used in diagnostic imaging for assessment of location, size, and stability of the structure of the gastrointestinal (GI) tract, the kidneys, the gallbladder, the pancreas, heart, adrenal glands, arteries, veins, and joints. They are considered to be drugs because they are chemical substances introduced into the body to help in the diagnosis or assessment of disease conditions, to assist in treatment planning, and to facilitate treatment. They are used to increase visibility of body cavities, organs, and vasculature on radiographic film and on fluoroscopy. When an iodinated contrast agent (also called contrast medium) is injected or instilled into the circulatory system or into a body cavity, it increases the radiographic density (opacity) of the area, because the atomic density of iodine is high and can provide the visual contrast needed to allow visualization. Iodinated contrast agents are administered

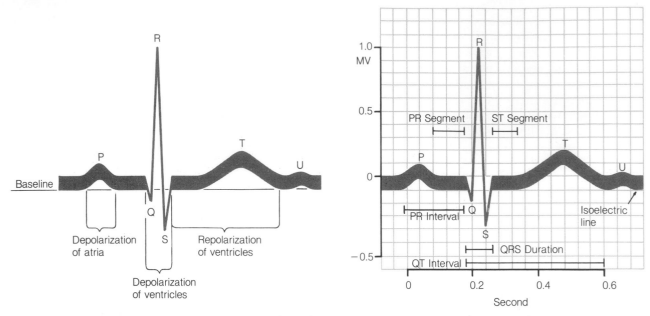

Figure 12.2. *Diagram of the electrocardiogram (lead II) and representative depolarization and repolarization of the atria and ventricle. The P wave represents atrial depolarization; the QRS complex, ventricular depolarization; and the T wave, ventricular repolarization. Atrial repolarization occurs during ventricular depolarization and is hidden under the QRS complex. (Patrick ML, Woods SL, Craven RF et al: Medical-Surgical Nursing. Philadelphia, JB Lippincott, 1986)*

Figure 12.3. Normal sinus rhythm. *(Patrick ML, Woods SL, Craven RT et al: Medical-Surgical Nursing. Philadelphia, JB Lippincott, 1986)*

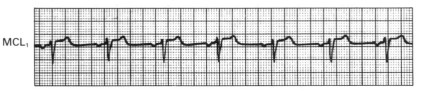

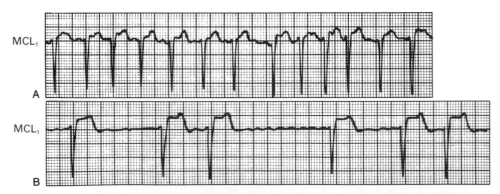

Figure 12.4. *(A) Atrial fibrillation with uncontrolled ventricular response (more than 100 beats/min). (B) Atrial fibrillation with controlled ventricular response (fewer than 100 beats/min). (Patrick ML, Woods SL, Craven RF et al: Medical-Surgical Nursing. Philadelphia, JB Lippincott, 1986)*

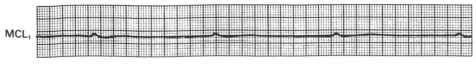

Figure 12.5. *Ventricular asystole. (Patrick ML, Woods SL, Craven RF et al: Medical-Surgical Nursing. Philadelphia, JB Lippincott, 1986)*

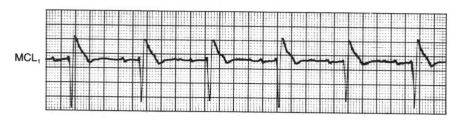

Figure 12.6. First degree heart block. (Patrick ML, Woods SL, Craven RF et al: Medical-Surgical Nursing. Philadelphia, JB Lippincott, 1986)

by oral, vaginal, intravenous, and intra-arterial routes, or they may be instilled directly into body cavities (percutaneously).

When the physician selects an iodinated contrast agent, he considers the area of the body to be visualized and the agent that will allow maximum visualization of that area. He must also consider the general physical condition and health status of the patient. Similarly, the patient's age, weight, and size are vital to the selection process, as is the route by which the medium will be excreted. Most iodinated contrast agents are excreted through the kidneys; therefore, if the patient has poor kidney function, this factor must be considered. Other important variables in selection are the ability of the agent to mix with normal body fluids, the viscosity, osmolarity, ionic strength, and potential toxicity. Most contrast agents currently used are in aqueous solution (are water-soluble); however, there are a few diagnostic imaging examinations that require the use of contrast agents with an oil base.

Patient care considerations

Regardless of their area of use, iodinated contrast agents have the potential for producing adverse reactions, which range from mild to severe. Although the choice of media is the physician's to make, the RT will be assisting with administration and must be aware of potential adverse reactions. He must do all that is within his professional capacity to prevent problems and keep the patient as comfortable as possible while iodinated contrast agents are in use.

Adverse reactions to iodinated contrast agents may affect all body systems. Most reactions occur within 2 to 5 minutes following administration, and almost all within 10 minutes. Delayed reactions are infrequent, and the RT will usually not be aware of them, because the patient will have returned to his hospital room or his home when they occur. He must be aware that delayed reactions can occur and therefore should instruct the patient in the signs and symptoms of such reactions and what action to take should they occur.

Symptoms of mild reactions to iodinated contrast agents

Flushing or a feeling of warmth, metallic taste, nausea, vomiting, light-headedness, sensitivity to touch around the mouth (perioral dysesthesia), pain at injection site or in the extremities, headache, and parotid or submaxillary swelling

Symptoms of severe reactions

Central Nervous System
Paresthesias, convulsions, paralysis, shock, coma

Cardiovascular
Bradycardia, hypotension

Integumentary System
Urticaria, tissue necrosis

Hematologic
Blood dyscrasias and inhibition of coagulation

Renal
Renal failure

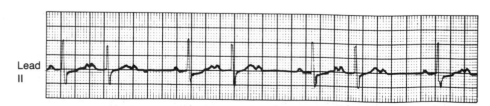

Figure 12.7. Second degree heart block, Mobitz type I. (Patrick ML, Woods SL, Craven RF et al: Medical-Surgical Nursing. Philadelphia, JB Lippincott, 1986)

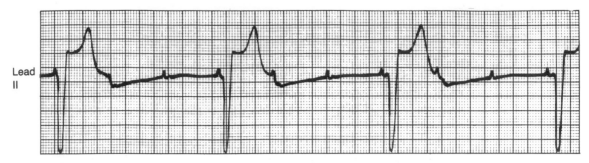

Figure 12.8.   Complete heart block, third degree. (Patrick ML, Woods SL, Craven RF et al: Medical-Surgical Nursing. Philadelphia, JB Lippincott, 1986)

Respiratory

Rhinitis, dyspnea, bronchospasm, asthma, laryngeal and pulmonary edema, subclinical pulmonary emboli

Other problems are: irritated, itching eyes; conjunctivitis; and all signs and symptoms of anaphylactic shock listed in Chapter 5.

Patients who have a history of allergic reactions to iodinated contrast agents have twice the risk of adverse reactions as those who do not. It is urgent that the RT ask the patient the questions pertaining to allergy listed in Chapter 5 before these agents are administered by any route. If the patient's answers are positive, the physician must be informed and the agent not administered until the matter is resolved.

Other patient care precautions and considerations

The RT should instruct the patient receiving an iodinated contrast agent to inform his physician of the following conditions, or he must do so himself:

1. If the patient is pregnant

2. If the patient has a medical diagnosis of diabetes mellitus, multiple myeloma, pheochromocytoma, sickle-cell disease, or a thyroid disorder

3. If the patient is currently taking any drugs, whether they are by prescription or not

All the conditions listed above may affect the pharmocologic action of iodinated contrast agents and must be considered by the physician.

It is recognized that nonionic, low osmolar (determined by the number of particles in the solution) iodinated contrast agents decrease the potential for adverse reactions. Use of this type of contrast agent decreases the incidence of cardiovascular symptoms, nausea and vomiting, pain during injection, and adverse effects on the circulating blood volume. Whenever possible, low osmolar, nonionic agents are chosen for use for the safety and comfort of the patient.

Many iodinated contrast agents are quite viscid (thick, sticky). This property contributes to discomfort during injection. Some are so viscid that they must be administered by power injector (Fig. 12-10). The RT must remember that all iodinated contrast agents are most comfortable for the patient when administered at body temperature. This is particularly true of the viscid agents. When a power injector is used, there is a heating mechanism in place. When this machine is not used, a simple solution to raising the temperature of contrast agents to body temperature is placing the solution to be injected into a basin of tepid water for 10 to 15 minutes prior to administration. This reduces the viscosity of the agent and thereby decreases the amount of physiologic vasoconstriction and pain produced by administration at room temperature. The RT must ascertain that the temperature of the contrast agent is not higher than body temperature when administered.

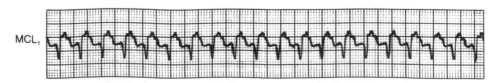

Figure 12.9.   Paroxysmal atrial tachycardia. (Patrick ML, Woods SL, Craven RF et al: Medical-Surgical Nursing. Philadelphia, JB Lippincott, 1986)

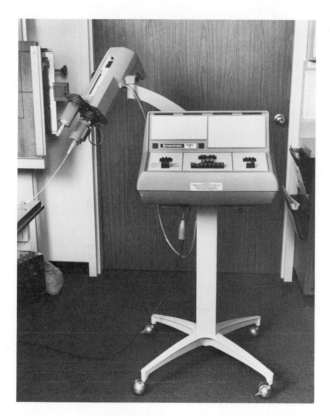

Figure 12.10. An injector pump.

When the RT assists with administration of iodinated contrast agents, he should carefully inspect each vacoliter or vial of solution for the presence of particulate matter. If there are any particles seen, the contrast agent should not be used. Return it to the pharmacy of origin for evaluation.

Contrast agents should be drawn up into the syringe for administration immediately before injection. They should not be drawn up and left for a period of time prior to use because they may become contaminated.

If the patient is to have a procedure repeated that involves an iodinated contrast agent, a sufficient period of time for excretion of the first injected contrast agent from the body should be allowed. If the medium from the previous examination has not been cleared from the body, the chances of an adverse reaction may increase.

Patients who are to receive iodinated contrast media should have adequate fluid intake to hydrate the body prior to administration, because sufficient hydration helps to prevent adverse reactions.

Hyperosmolar iodinated contrast agents administered orally to persons who are dehydrated or to infants may result in life-threatening electrolyte imbalance. In addition, the RT must take great care to prevent gagging and choking when the patient is drinking these agents because, if aspirated, they may cause pulmonary edema.

When a patient is to receive an iodinated contrast agent, his vital signs should be taken prior to administration to establish a baseline as described in Chapter 4. Vital signs should then be taken frequently during the time that the patient is receiving the contrast agent.

Patient care and instruction after receiving iodinated contrast agents

Following procedures during which iodinated contrast agents are administered, the RT should instruct the patient to increase fluid intake to 3000 ml for at least 24 hours to assist with the dilution and excretion of the agent from the body. Patients who are returning to their homes should be allowed to rest following the examination and be assisted with dressing as needed. The patient should be instructed in the potential symptoms of a delayed adverse reaction, *i.e.*, the central nervous symptoms described, urticaria, shortness of breath, or dyspnea. They should be instructed to return to the hospital immediately if these or any of the adverse reactions described earlier in this chapter should occur.

Use of specific iodinated contrast agents

Table 12-1 lists some of the iodinated contrast agents and the diagnostic imaging examinations for which they are used. The agents listed were randomly chosen and do not indicate author preferences or recommendation.

Cardiac catheterization and angiography

The RT will be a part of the health-care team when patients have invasive diagnostic procedures that involve cardiac catheterization and angiography. A registered nurse is also part of the team for these special procedures and will be assigned to administer medications and generally monitor the patient's condition as the procedure evolves. However, the RT, as part of this highly technical team, must take part in patient assessment and patient care as well. He must be alert to any symptoms of respiratory or cardiac arrest, be able to monitor vital signs accurately, assist with medication administration, be able to apply the principles of medical and surgical asepsis, and communicate with the patient in a therapeutic man-

TABLE 12-1.
Iodinated contrast agents used in diagnostic imaging examinations

BODY SYSTEM	CONTRAST AGENT	METHOD OF ADMINISTRATION
Gastrointestinal	Iopanoic acid	Oral
	Ipodate calcium	
	Diatrizoate sodium	Oral, Rectal
Genitourinary	Meglumine diatrizoate	Percutaneous
	Meglumine Iothalamate	
	Meglumine Iodipamide	
Cardiovascular	Diatrizoate meglumine and Diatrizoate sodium 370	Intravenous
	Metrizamide	
Spinal Cord	Metrizamide	Intrathecal
	Iohexal	
Lymphatic	Ethiodized oil	Percutaneous

ner. Each member of the team must have special education in the problems and potential complications that may result from these procedures.

Medical indications for cardiac catheterization are numerous. A special legal consent form must be signed by the patient prior to these procedures. During the procedure, one or more catheters are passed by way of the femoral or brachial artery into the cardiac chambers, the valves, or great vessels of the heart. Iodinated contrast agent is injected through the catheter, and fluoroscopy is used for visualization. Cineangiographic films are taken to monitor progression of the contrast agent and to detect pathology. This procedure is done to confirm the diagnosis of heart disease, to determine the exact location and extent of the disease process, to determine the necessity of cardiac surgery, to evaluate the effects of medical cardiac treatment, to place an internal cardiac pacemaker, or to eliminate arterial occlusion by performing percutaneous transluminal coronary angioplasty.

Angiography is done to visualize the vascularity of all areas of the body in order to diagnose pathology of the blood vessels such as aneurisms and occlusions caused by stricture, masses, or other deformities. Iodinated contrast agent is injected, and serial radiographs are taken as it infiltrates the vessels being studied. A long catheter is often inserted to reach the area. The catheter insertion is monitored and guided to its destination by fluoroscopy. Peripheral vessels are injected directly with iodinated contrast media. The vasculature most often visualized during angiography are the renal system, the carotid and cerebral vessels, and the peripheral vascular system of the legs.

Patient care during the procedure

Patients having cardiac catheterization have usually been fasting for approximately 8 hours prior to the examination. A mild sedative or tranquilizing drug is sometimes prescribed before the procedure, but may not be if it might prevent accurate diagnosis. When the patient arrives in the cardiac catheterization laboratory or special procedures room, the RT should spend a few minutes acquainting him with the machinery, explaining the procedure, and allowing the patient to ask any questions that he may have. The patient's anxiety may be relieved by allowing him to bring a favorite musical tape to play while being cared for. If the patient is a child, allow him to bring a favorite toy or story tape. Encourage him to play the tapes, especially if the procedure extends beyond 1 hour.

Patients undergoing cardiac catheterization and angiography are usually extremely anxious as the procedure begins. If the time of the procedure extends and does not seem to be going smoothly, the patient will become increasingly anxious. The RT, in the midst of his technical work, must not forget the patient. He must take a few moments frequently to discuss the patient's feelings with him and to inform him in a simple manner of what is going on. This will do a great deal to alleviate patient anxiety. Patient complaints must be listened to carefully and not be dismissed as insignificant. Any complaints registered by the patient must be relayed to the physician in charge of the procedure at once. The patient should be instructed to inform the physician of any unusual sensations that he may have during the procedure. The patient undergoing these diagnostic procedures and treatments is subjected to physical discomfort that must also be recognized by the RT. During cardiac catheterization, the patient must often lie in one position on a very firm surface with arms folded up over the head for a long period of time. If a catheter is to be inserted, the area of insertion is shaved and prepped as for a surgical procedure as described in Chapter 9. The cardiac monitor is observed continuously for any changes in cardiac activity that would indicate potential problems. The iodinated contrast agent injected into the coronary arteries may cause the patient to feel nauseated. A warm, flushing sensation is felt as the medium is injected and will last about 30 seconds. The patient may complain that his heart feels as if it is "fluttering" or that he feels light-headed. These feelings are caused by ectopic (premature or out-of-sequence) heartbeats as the catheter is moved or manipulated by the physician.

During coronary arteriography, the patient may complain of chest pain or a feeling of tightness in his chest. If this does occur, or if the patient's blood pressure changes in any way, the patient must be instructed to cough as rapidly and with as much effort as possible to aid in clearing the contrast agent from the coronary arteries and to mechanically stimulate the heart in case of ectopic beats. Coughing may also help to dispel the feeling of nausea and light-headedness that results from the injection of the iodinated contrast agent.

Patient care and education after cardiac catheterization or angiography

Patient care following angiography and cardiac catherization is relatively uniform and must be followed meticulously in order to prevent circulatory deficit, thrombus formation, or hemorrhage. In most institutions, the patient is transported to the hospital postanesthesia recovery area or to an intensive coronary care area to be monitored following cardiac catheterization and angiography. However, the RT must understand the monitoring and care required following these examinations so that he can instruct the patient and so that he can begin to monitor the patient immediately.

The patient will be extremely fatigued, and any movement required of him must be done with adequate assistance and with little patient assistance demanded. The patient's pulse must be monitored on the side of the invasive procedure every 15 minutes for 1 hour and then every 30 minutes for the next 3 hours. The blood pressure is monitored on the side opposite the invasive procedure at the same time intervals. The pulses distal to the site of catheter insertion must also be monitored at frequent and regular intervals for 24 hours following the procedure. Following femoral catheterization, the patient should be instructed to move his toes and dorsiflex his feet frequently. The extremities must be assessed for coldness, cyanosis, pallor, numbness, and tingling; the patient should be instructed to inform the nurse if he has any of these symptoms. If there should be a circulatory deficit, surgical intervention may be necessary to correct the problem.

If a femoral artery was used for catheter insertion, the patient is informed that he must remain at bedrest for 12 to 24 hours following the procedure to prevent hemorrhage. A weight, a sandbag, or an ice bag is often placed over the site of catheter insertion. The patient's head should not be raised more than 30 degrees during the immediate postcatheterization period.

If the brachial site was used for catheter insertion, the arm on the side of insertion is kept straight with an arm board for several hours, but the patient may be up as soon as his vital signs are stable. Regardless of the site of insertion, the patient must be monitored for 24 hours for external bleeding or for bleeding into the tissues surrounding the insertion site.

The patient who has received iodinated contrast media must be instructed to increase his fluid intake to prevent dehydration and hypotension. Patients are often given intravenous fluid replacement therapy following these procedures, but the patient should be made aware of his need for increased fluid intake.

The time that the procedure began and ended, any drugs or contrast agents administered, and the patient's tolerance of the procedure are recorded on the patient's chart. Also recorded are the instructions given to the patient following the procedure.

Myelography

Myelography (myelograms) is a diagnostic imaging examination of the spinal cord in which an iodinated contrast agent, as well as air on some occasions, is injected into the subarachnoid or epidural spaces of the spinal cord. This examination is done to detect pathologic conditions of the spinal cord such as ruptured intravertebral disks, tumors, malformations, arthritis, and other extraspinal diseases.

Patient care and education prior to myelography

A special legal consent form must be signed by the patient for this procedure. The patient must be instructed to increase clear fluid intake and omit solid foods for 3 to 4 hours before the myelogram in order to be well hydrated and to prevent nausea and vomiting. The patient must also be instructed to stop taking all drugs for 24 hours prior to the examination and to take no drugs that are monoamine oxidase inhibitors for 2 weeks before the myelogram.

Myelograms should not be performed on patients with multiple sclerosis, inflammation of the meninges, Pott's disease, infections or bloody subarachnoid fluid, increased intracranial pressure, recent myelogram, or allergy to iodinated contrast media. Myelograms may also be contraindicated in patients who are seizure-prone. Seizure-prone patients may receive medication to reduce the possibility of seizures prior to the examination. Physicians may order medication to reduce the patient's anxiety in preparation for this procedure.

The area into which the iodinated contrast agent is to be injected intrathecally is shaved if necessary and prepped as for other sterile invasive procedures. The RT should inform the patient that the table will be tilted during the examination but that a foot rest and shoulder harness will prevent him from falling. The patient's privacy must be protected by having him wear pajamas or by taping a draw sheet in place to prevent it from sliding off during the table movement.

Baseline vital signs should be taken before the myelogram begins and then monitored during the examination. The patient should be informed that the examination will take from 1 to 2 hours to complete.

Intrathecal drug administration

Intrathecal (intraspinal) injections are given with a needle that is 3½ inches long with a 16- to 25-gauge lumen. A stylet within the needle remains in place until the physician has completed the spinal puncture. When the needle is in the desired position in the spinal column, the stylet is removed, and the syringe containing the medication or contrast agent is attached to the needle.

Intrathecal drugs are administered by the physician who is performing the special procedure or by an anesthesiologist. An open sterile tray containing the necessary equipment and drugs will be available. The RT assists by obtaining any extra articles needed by the physician and placing them on the sterile field and by positioning the patient.

For lumbar myelography the patient is usually positioned in a prone position with a pillow under the abdomen to raise the lumbar area slightly (Fig. 12-11). Other positions that may occasionally be used for administration of intrathecal drugs are the bent sitting position (Fig. 12-12) and the side-lying position with knees pulled up and spine curved forward as much as possible (Fig. 12-13). All these positions make the spinal column more accessible.

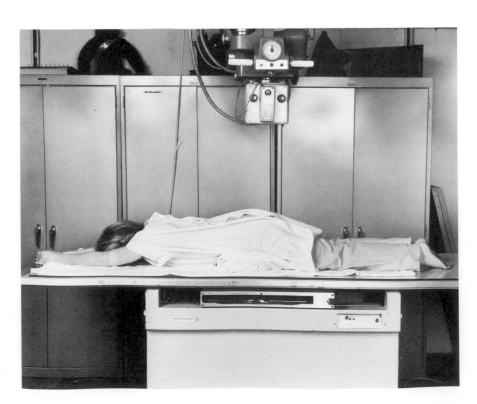

Figure 12.11. Patient positioned for myelography.

Many patients who receive myelograms are in severe pain as a result of injury or disease. The RT must assist the patient with any movement he must make during the procedure and return him to a normal physiologic position as quickly as possible. The patient must also be kept warm. Placing booties on his feet often helps.

Any unusual symptoms or complaints that the patient has while the myelogram is in progress should be reported to the physician performing the procedure. Specimens of spinal fluid are often collected during this procedure and should be correctly labeled, bagged, and taken or sent to the laboratory immediately.

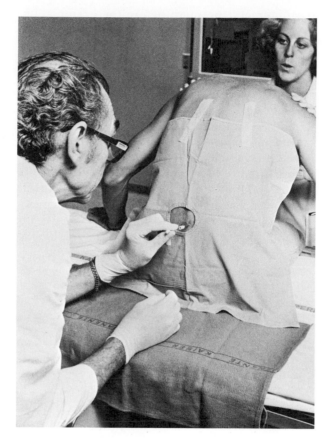

Figure 12.12. Intrathecal administration with the patient in a bent sitting position.

Patient care and education following myelography

Following the myelogram, the patient who received a water-soluble contrast agent should be cautioned to remain at bed rest for from 8 to 24 hours with the head of the bed slightly elevated at a 35- to 45-degree angle. This will prevent the contrast agent from being dispersed upward and possibly prevent headache following the examination.

The patient should be informed that he may have increased lumbar pain following a lumbar myelogram. He should also be encouraged to increase his fluid intake. The RT should inform the patient to notify his physician immediately if he is unable to urinate or if he develops a fever, drowsiness, stiff neck, seizures, or paralysis. Other complications of myelography are arachnoiditis (inflammation of the delicate spinal cord covering) and meningitis. Any unusual reactions that the patient had to the contrast agent or in general are recorded on the patient's chart. The time the procedure began and ended, specimens sent to the laboratory, and the patient's tolerance of the procedure are also recorded. Instructions given to the patient for postmyelogram care are to be included on the chart.

Computerized tomography

Computerized tomography (CT) is also called computerized transaxial tomography (CTT). In this section it will be referred to as CT. This is a diagnostic imaging procedure that can be used to scan the brain and head or the entire body. CT scans produce pictures of multiple cross-sectional views of body organs that, when displayed on radiographic film, are three dimensional in appearance. This is a highly effective

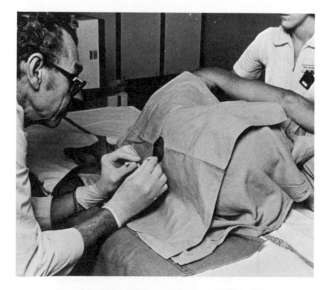

Figure 12.13. Intrathecal administration of drug with the patient lying on his side. The RT helps the patient to maintain this position. The patient's knees are flexed, and his head is brought down close to his knees so that his back arches.

method of diagnosing pathologic intracranial and organic pathology.

Iodinated contrast agents are used to increase tissue density for body and brain scans. Barium solutions are used to increase organ density of the GI tract.

Patient care and instruction before computerized tomography

In preparation for CT of the brain, the patient should be instructed not to eat or drink for 2 to 3 hours prior to the examination. Any medications that the patient is taking routinely may be taken. If the patient has diabetes mellitus, his CT should be arranged so that his regular meal pattern and insulin administration are maintained. The patient will be receiving an iodinated contrast agent, so all precautions and questioning that precede administration of that drug are included in pre-CT patient care.

The RT must spend a few moments explaining the procedure to the patient in order to alleviate his anxiety. The patient should be told that he will be expected to lie very quietly as he is being scanned to ensure clear images. The patient should be allowed to inspect the machine and allowed to express any feelings of claustrophobia that he may have. The RT must inform the patient that he may communicate with him through a microphone placed above the machine portal. The RT must show the patient where he will be sitting behind the glass window where he can observe, hear, and communicate with the patient at all times. The RT must establish a feeling of trust in the patient, because it is very frightening for patients to feel that they are in a room alone, receiving a drug to which they may have a reaction with nobody in close observation whom they can trust. The extremely anxious patient may prefer to receive an antianxiety or sedative drug prior to the examination. Those who are in pain or those who are unable to lie quietly, particularly children, may need an analgesic or sedative drug.

The patient should be informed of the feelings of nausea, warmth, flushing, and the metallic taste he may have following administration of the iodinated contrast agent. An emesis basin should be placed near the patient where he can pick it up easily if need be. The patient should know that this examination usually takes about 1 hour. A special legal consent form is signed by the patient receiving these studies.

Computerized tomography of the body

Patients who are to have CT of the bowel and abdominal organs are to have nothing to eat or drink from midnight the night before the examination. They may receive a barium contrast agent mixed in orange juice to drink the night before the examination and more (1000 ml) immediately prior to the scan. An iodinated contrast agent is also injected intravenously immediately before the CT scan begins.

The RT must spend the same amount of time explaining the procedure to the patient before beginning this examination as for the head CT scan. For the bowel and abdominal CT scan, the patient must also be instructed to listen carefully for instructions to breathe, hold his breath, and release his breath. He must be told that these instructions will be numerous.

Whichever area of the body is being scanned, the RT should pause from time to time and ask the patient how he is feeling and inform him of the time remaining for examination. If the patient is made to feel that he is the major focus of the procedure and is kept informed, he will be more cooperative and relaxed while the examination is in progress.

Patient care after computerized tomography

Patients who have come from their homes and plan to return home should be accompanied by a person who can drive them or assist them to get there safely. Patients who have received sedative or antianxiety medication may not drive themselves.

When the procedure is complete, the intravenous contrast agent is discontinued by order of the physician as described in Chapter 11. The patient is then allowed to sit up with assistance. He should sit quietly on the table for several minutes before he is assisted back to the dressing room, wheelchair, or gurney. If the patient is hospitalized, he may be returned to his room with assistance. If he is going home, assist him to the dressing room and give him the help he needs to get dressed. Observe the patient for at least 30 minutes for adverse reaction to drugs received and for general instability before discharging him from the department.

If the patient has received an iodinated contrast agent, he must be instructed to increase his fluid intake to at least 3000 ml for the next 24 hours to aid in excretion from the body and to prevent dehydration. If barium has been administered, the instructions in Chapter 7 concerning post-barium administration should be followed.

Any adverse reactions that occurred during CT and any medications that the patient received must be recorded on the patient's chart. The time that the procedure began and ended, the patient's tolerance of the procedure, and the instructions that the patient received for postprocedure care must also be recorded.

Urography

Preparation for intravenous urography requires that the patient not eat or drink after the early evening meal the previous day. If the patient is weak, debilitated, or extremely young, this procedure may be altered. The patient is also instructed to take a mild laxative drug of the physician's choice the night before the examination so that the bowel is partially cleansed for adequate visualization. A cleansing enema may also be ordered the morning of the examination.

The RT explains to the patient that the contrast medium will be administered either by bolus or as an infusion and that a series of films will then be taken. He should also be told that he may be asked to empty his bladder at some time during the examination so that the bladder-emptying time can be measured. In many departments, CT may also be included with intravenous urography. If this is the case, the procedure should also be explained to the patient.

The posturography care follows the same directions as for all special procedures in which iodinated contrast agents are administered. Recording the procedure is also the same.

Magnetic resonance imaging

Magnetic resonance imaging (MRI) is a generally noninvasive method of diagnosing neoplastic, vascular, and central nervous system pathology. A con-trast agent, Gadolinium diethylenetriaminepenta-acetic acid (Gd[DTPA]) is awaiting approval to be used for patients receiving MRI for diagnosis of central nervous system pathology. This is not an iodinated contrast agent.

MRI is performed by placing the entire body of the patient or, if the problem is with an extremity, only the extremity in a magnetic field that puts out measurable radio signals, which are then displayed on a computer monitor or magnetic tape to be replayed on a video screen (Fig. 12-14).

If a limb or limbs are being diagnosed for measure of blood flow to extremities, the patient sits or lies quietly while the limb being examined is placed in a cradle in a flow cylinder. The limb or limbs are moved in and out of the cylinder as the extremity studies are completed. If both legs and arms are to be examined, the legs are usually examined first.

If entire body imagery is to be done, the patient is placed on a pallet that moves slowly through a large magnetic cylinder (Fig. 12-15). If the head is to be scanned, a clear plastic cylinder with antennae are placed around the head.

Patient care and instruction for magnetic resonance imaging

Patient education is the key to successful imaging when MR is the technique used. Claustrophobic fears are common and come to light when the patient is faced with spending 1 hour or more in a rather close

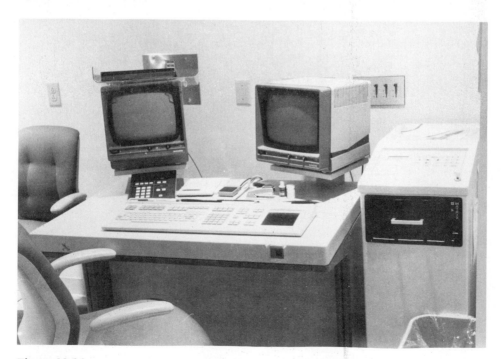

Figure 12.14

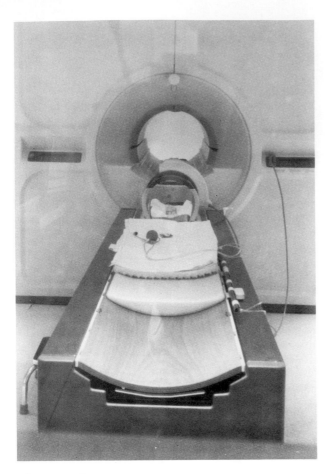

Figure 12.15

cylinder in a large room alone. Accurate information and instruction help to alleviate these fears.

The adult patient must be informed that the examination will take from 60 to 90 minutes, during which time he must lie in a supine position and remain completely still. The patient should be informed that, although he may feel that he is completely alone, there will be at least two persons just on the other side of a glass window who are constantly observing him, and that they can and will be communicating with him frequently during the examination. The patient should also be shown that there is a microphone through which he can communicate to the staff. The patient should be allowed to examine the machine and ask any questions he may have before beginning the examination. This is especially necessary for children. The patient should also be informed that he will hear a pounding noise during the entire examination.

If the patient is a child, the parent may be allowed to sit beside the cylinder and talk to the child during the examination. Infants may be fed shortly before the examination and may then sleep during the entire time. Some adults benefit by keeping their eyes closed during the time in the cylinder. The RT can assist

patients during the examination by speaking to them frequently and letting them know how much time is left for the examination to be completed.

The RT must remember that many patients who are having MRI are anxious and fearful because of possible ominous diagnostic outcomes, as are the parents of children who are having this examination. Patients may focus on their claustrophobic feelings in an attempt to deny the possibility of a threatening-outcome diagnosis. The RT must be patient, sensitive, and nonjudgmental when communicating with these patients and their family members. Making the patient's feelings seem foolish or offering reassuring cliché responses will only increase the patient's anxiety. Time must be spent discussing the process and the patient's or the parents' feelings and concerns before beginning the examination. If this is not done, the patient may be unable to remain as quiet as is necessary for a successful examination.

Patients must be instructed to remove all metal jewelry, dental bridges, clothing with metal closures, belts, metal-containing prosthesis, hair clips, and shoes before entering the MRI room. Purses and wallets containing credit cards must be left outside in a secure place. The RT will be responsible for placing these items safely away for patients and informing them of where their belongings are being kept.

The patient should also be informed that this procedure does not expose him to radiation and that there will be no painful stimuli. There may be some tingling sensations felt if the patient has metal dental work in place.

MRI is contraindicated for patients who have internal pacemakers, implanted heart valves, metal orthopedic implants, or surgical clips. It is also contraindicated at this time for pregnant patients, because the effects of MRI on pregnancy are unknown at present. Patients on life-support pumps or who are critically ill cannot have this examination because they cannot be monitored while in the magnetic scanner.

There are so special patient instructions or teaching responsibilities following the procedure. The RT should make certain that the patient is cared for and does not forget to take his belongings with him when he leaves the area.

External radiation therapy

At least one half of the patients with a diagnosis of cancer will receive external radiation therapy during the course of the disease. This form of treatment is used to cure the disease, to control malignant tumors that cannot be removed, to prevent spread of the tumor to the brain and spinal cord, and to decrease pain when the cancer metastasizes to the bones, brain, or soft tissues. RTs who work in the area of radiation therapy should receive specialized education; however, the RT student may rotate to this area in the course of his education and must have some understanding of patient care in radiation therapy.

When external radiation therapy is prescribed by the patient's physician, the patient is sent to the radiation treatment area for preparation known as treatment simulation. During this simulation, the patient is evaluated, and treatment is mimicked with machines that determine the exact treatment field, the volume of tissue to be radiated, and the radiation dosage necessary to accomplish the treatment purpose. When these decisions have been made, the patient's external skin is marked with indelible pen so that the same area of tissue receives the radiation therapy with each treatment. A plan of treatment is outlined for the patient, which usually extends daily for several weeks. The patient is instructed to refrain from removing or altering the markings. If they are accidentally removed, patients are asked not to redraw them, but to notify the radiation team so that they can reconstruct them according to plan.

At the time that the treatment plan is made, the patient should be shown the treatment room and be allowed to ask any questions concerning the treatment that he wishes. The treatment rooms are large, impersonal rooms in which the patient must remain alone during the radiation treatment. He should be informed that he can communicate by microphone with the radiation team and they with him. He should also be informed that the treatment table is somewhat uncomfortable and hard. If the patient is in pain, it should be suggested that he receive pain medication 30 minutes before each treatment so that he will be more comfortable. The RT must also explain to the patient that the radiation treatments themselves are painless and that there is no danger of the patient carrying radiation with him out of the treatment area.

Patient care

The RT caring for patients receiving radiation therapy must be aware that these patients are in various stages of the grieving process. They have received a diagnosis of a disease from which they may or may not recover. Some will have hope of recovery and perhaps be in a phase of denial of the seriousness of their problem. Patients who are in this phase must never be confronted with their denial, since this may be their only means of coping with the problem. Others will be in the later stages of the grieving process. Many have had radical surgical procedures that

have altered their body image. This is particularly the case for a man or woman who has had reproductive organs or external genitalia altered by the surgery during the reproductive years.

Some patients receiving external radiation therapy are in the terminal stages of cancer and have metastasis of the disease to their bones. When this occurs, the structure of the bone weakens and becomes very fragile. There is a high incidence of pathologic fractures with this condition. The RT caring for the person in the terminal stages of cancer must remember this and must allow the patient to move at his own pace with as much assistance as necessary. The RT must be extremely cautious when lifting or moving cancer patients. Be certain to have adequate assistance to prevent abrupt, jarring, or pushing movements because this may cause fractures and a great deal of unnecessary pain for the patient. Allow the patient to direct all moves at his own pace.

Patients with cancer often have weakened immune systems. This must be taken into consideration because these patients are highly susceptible to infections. RTs must practice judicious medical asepsis, and, when the occasion calls for it, meticulous surgical asepsis during patient care.

The RT must also remember that the patient undergoing a course of radiation therapy has localized toxic reactions to the treatment. This toxicity usually affects only the tissues surrounding the area being radiated as the cells in the treatment area are destroyed by radiation. However, generalized systemic reactions may also occur. Some of the local reactions that may occur, depending on the irradiation site, are alopecia (loss of hair); erythema (redness and inflammation of the skin or mucous membranes); loss of appetite; alterations in oral mucous membranes (xerostomia and stomatitis); decreased salivation; difficult swallowing; chest pain and cough; esophageal irritation; nausea and vomiting; diarrhea; and blood dyscrasias.

Generalized systemic side effects include fatigue, nausea, vomiting, and headache. The patient may be reassured that all these effects will subside when the treatments are completed. There are some changes in the area of the radiation treatment that are produced called fibrous tissue formation (scar tissue). This is due to the destruction of the blood supply in the area of radiation, and that tissue will not regenerate.

Use of therapeutic communication techniques by RTs caring for patients having external radiation therapy is of utmost importance. The RT should make himself available to answer questions that he can answer and assist patients to find answers when he does not know. Allow patients to express their concerns and explore their feelings with the use of simple reflective statements.

Patients with a diagnosis of cancer have a heightened awareness of their bodies. Problems that would have been ignored in previous times are suddenly of great concern. Patients have a great need for a feeling of security and reassurance concerning the present and the future. The RT must make himself available for communication at any time. If the RT simply ushers the patient into and out of the radiation treatment room and neglects to communicate with the patient, he is omitting an extremely important aspect of his professional responsibility.

Ultrasound

Ultrasound is a method of visualizing the soft-tissue structures of the body for diagnosis of disease processes without use of radiation. It is a relatively noninvasive, painless procedure that requires the skill of a specially trained individual, usually an RT. Ultrasound employs high-frequency sound waves to examine body organs in search of malpositioning or malformation.

As the ultrasound examination is being done, the images are displayed on a cathode ray tube. Permanent copies of the examination results are produced either as photographs or on sensitized paper with results somewhat like those from an ECG reading.

This form of diagnostic imaging is extremely useful in obstetrics to determine fetal development; in neurology to diagnose brain disorders; in urology for diagnosis of urinary bladder, scrotal, prostatic, and renal lesions. It is also used to diagnose vascular aneurisms as well as pancreatic, gallbladder, thyroid, parathyroid, lymph node, eye, and breast pathology. This is not an all-inclusive list, and new uses for ultrasonography are being found constantly. The RT who is not trained as an ultrasonographer must have some awareness of the process of ultrasound in order to correctly schedule diagnostic imaging procedures to his patient's best advantage.

Patient care

Patient care considerations for ultrasound include instruction in preparation for the procedure, an explanation of the procedure itself, and correct scheduling to prevent unsatisfactory examinations. There is little postexamination instruction needed.

If a patient is to have barium studies as well as an ultrasound examination, the ultrasound examination should be scheduled to precede the barium studies because residual barium in the GI tract will interfere with effective ultrasound examinations. If a patient has a tendency to have large amounts of gas in his bowel, the gas will interfere with visualization. A patient with this problem should be instructed to eat low-residue foods for 24 to 36 hours prior to the examination and be scheduled at a time when the bowel will be relatively gas-free, as is the case in the early morning before breakfast.

Active children or patients who are unable to remain quiet because of pain, emotional illness, or anxiety must be scheduled at a time when they can be accompanied by a person who can keep them calm and relaxed. Use of sedative drugs may also be recommended by the physician.

Patients should be informed that this is a painless, noninvasive procedure that takes from 15 minutes to 1 hour to complete. A lubricating gel or water is used as the conductive agent. The gel will be applied by the ultrasonographer if it is used. If water is used, the patient will be immersed in water, or a water bath is hung over the area to be scanned.

A transducer is held by the sonographer and is moved over the surface to be examined as the screen is watched and images are produced. The patient must be shown the transducer and reassured that it will cause no pain.

Some examinations require a preparatory cleansing enema and fasting for several hours prior to the scheduled time. Others require a full urinary bladder. If either of these is required, the RT sonographer must explain the preparation to the patient.

Wound dressings, scars, and obesity are all factors to be considered when ultrasound is the imaging technique prescribed. Dressings must be removed, and lubricating gel cannot be applied over an open wound. Scars and obesity prevent good visualization.

Patient care following ultrasonography is the same as thoughtful patient care following any diagnostic imaging procedure. The lubricating gel must be carefully removed so that the patient's clothing is not soiled by it. If the patient was immersed in water, he must be provided with towels and a private area in which to dry and dress. Patients who are in a weakened condition must not be left alone, and any assistance the patient needs must be provided. Patients who have had sedative medication must not be allowed to drive home or return to their hospital room unattended.

Summary

RTs working in the special procedures area of diagnostic imaging are members of a highly skilled technical team. As a member of this team, the RT must work with the other team members to ensure positive patient outcomes to examinations and treatments done as special procedures. A successful outcome includes clear imaging and physical and emotional safety for the patient.

The RT is not responsible for reading ECGs; however, the RT who works with patients having special procedures must be able to recognize a normal ECG and recognize an ominous reading. The electrocardiograph measures the electrical activity of the heart in order to detect patterns of cardiac impulses and display them on a monitor or on graphic paper for observation and analysis. The components of cardiac rhythm are the P wave, the QRS complex, the T wave, the ST segment, and the PR and QT intervals. When the P, QRS, and T waves are all present in a normal rate and rhythm sequence, it is referred to as *normal sinus rhythm.*

Iodinated contrast agents are used for many special procedures. They are considered to be drugs because they are chemical substances introduced into the body to diagnose and assess disease conditions and to facilitate treatment. The physician chooses the contrast agent for use depending on which will allow maximum visualization of the area being examined safely for the patient. The patient's age, weight, size, and state of health are some of the major considerations when a contrast agent is selected for use. The RT must always be aware of the potential for adverse reactions when an iodinated contrast agent is administered. He must assess patients for any adverse reactions whenever they have received this type of drug.

RT considerations when an iodinated contrast medium is administered are as follows:

1. Iodinated contrast agents are less painful for the patient if they are administered at body temperature. A simple way to attain this temperature is to place the solution in a basin of tepid water for 10 to 15 minutes prior to its administration.

2. Contrast agents should be examined for particles present in the solution. If there are any present, the agent should not be used.

3. Iodinated contrast agents should be drawn up and administered immediately, not left for a period of time and then injected.

4. Repeating procedures in which iodinated contrast agents are used should be done with caution. A period of time long enough for the first contrast agent to be excreted from the body should be allowed before a second agent is administered. If this is not done, the chances for an adverse reaction to the contrast agent increases.

5. Adequate fluid before and after iodinated contrast medium administration is important. Patients who are well hydrated have fewer adverse reactions to these drugs than do those who are dehydrated. The RT should instruct the patient to increase fluid intake to 3000 ml for 24 hours after receiving an iodinated contrast agent and instruct him in the symptoms of adverse reaction to these agents.

Special procedures and diagnostic imaging techniques in which the RT will participate involve specialized education. The RT participating in these procedures must be aware of the increased patient anxiety that must be dealt with when the patient is undergoing these procedures. He must be a highly skilled technologist; however, he must also have excellent therapeutic communication skills, so that he can alleviate the patient's anxiety and fear before, during, and after the special procedure.

One-half of the patients who are diagnosed as having cancer receive external radiation therapy for treatment or control of symptoms. The RT caring for these patients must understand that they are in varying stages of the grieving process and will need extra time for communication. The RT must also realize that the cancer patient has an increased awareness of his body functions and will focus on physical symptoms that he would have ignored in previous times. The RT should make himself available to discuss these problems with the patient at any time the patient desires. If the RT omits time for communication when caring for the patient receiving external radiation therapy, he is neglecting a vital professional obligation.

Chapter 12, pre-post test

1. List the components of a normal ECG pattern.

2. List the medical complications that may occur following administration of an iodinated contrast agent.

3. List three physical conditions that may affect the pharmacologic action of an iodinated contrast agent that must be reported to the patient's physician if present.

4. List three precautions that the RT must take if he is assisting with administration of an iodinated contrast agent.

5. Discuss patient care that the RT is responsible for prior to and following cardiac catheterization.

6. List two major subjects the RT should cover when instructing the patient after an angiogram.

7. List three patient instructions necessary prior to a myelogram.

8. List three positions in which the patient can be placed for intrathecal drug administration.

9. List three physical symptoms that the RT should instruct the patient to report immediately to his physician following myelography should they occur.

10. List four symptoms the RT should inform the patient receiving iodinated contrast agents to expect when an intravenous or intra-arterial iodinated contrast agent is injected.

11. Describe patient care following CT.

12. List three aspects of patient care and education that the RT must include when a patient is receiving MRI.

13. List four generalized systemic reactions that may occur when a patient is receiving external radiation therapy.

14. List the special patient care considerations for the RT when the patient is receiving external radiation therapy.

Laboratory reinforcement

In the school laboratory, select a fellow student and role play a patient-teaching situation. Instruct a patient before and after CT that involves a scan of the upper and lower GI tract.

Answers for Pre-Post Tests

Chapter 1

1. d

2. b

3. c

4. d

5. a

6. a. 3
   b. 1
   c. 4
   d. 5
   e. 2

7. a

8. b

9. c

10. d

11. a

12. b

13. c

14. b

15. *The five stages of the grieving process:*

   shock and denial   bargaining
   anger   depression
       acceptance

16. b

17. *Problem-solving process:*
    1. Perform assessment or data collection
    2. Analyze data
    3. Set a goal
    4. Establish plan for achievement of goal
    5. Evaluate plan. Was goal attained? What went well? What could be better next time?

18. *The patient's legal rights:*
    1. Right to confidential, considerate care
    2. Right to informed consent
    3. Right to refuse treatment
    4. Right to transfer to facility of choice
    5. Right to examine all medical records and know names of health workers
    6. Right to follow-up care
    7. Right to examine all financial statements

19. *Professional obligations of the RT:*

    Maintaining the patient's physical privacy
    Maintaining the patient's confidentiality
    Protecting the patient from unnecessary radiation
    Exercising sound judgment in his professional practice
    Refraining from criticism of his fellow professionals
    Avoiding wasteful use of materials used for patient care
    Guarding the medications used for patient case

Chapter 2

1. d

2. d

3. false

4. a

5. b

6. a

7. c

8. d

9. d

10. c

11. a. 1
    b. 5
    c. 4
    d. 2
    e. 3

12. *The seven categories of isolation:*

Drainage/Secretion   Contact
    Precaution   Blood/Body Fluid
Enteric   Strict Isolation
AFB
Respiratory

Chapter 3

1. e

2. a

3. d

4. e

5. b

6. a. 2
    b. 3
    c. 5
    d. 4
    e. 1

7. b

8. d

9. c

10. *Signs of circulatory impairment in a patient with a plaster cast:*

Pain
Coldness
Tingling
Burning in fingers or toes of extremity on which cast is applied
Swelling
Color changes in skin (pale or bluish)
Inability to move toes or fingers or a feeling of numbness

11. d

12. *Rules for correct posture:*

Stand with feet parallel and at right angles to the lower legs
Keep knees slightly bent
Keep buttocks in and abdomen up and in
Hold chest up and slightly forward
Hold head erect and chin in

13. b

14. Arm, leg

15. Pull, push

16. *Rules for moving patients:*

Give only needed assistance
Transfer across shortest distance
Move patient toward his strongest side
Lock wheels on all equipment used to transport patients
Protect patient's feet with shoes during move
Inform patient of plan and destination
Give short, simple directions

17. *Methods of transferring patients:*

Walking
Wheelchair
Gurney

18. c

19. *Areas of the body most susceptible to skin breakdown:*

Scapulae   Knees
Trochanters   Heels of the feet

20. Signs of circulatory impairment are the same as for a patient wearing a cast (see question 10).

Chapter 4

1. a

2. b

3. c

4. d

5. b

6. d

7. b

8. b

9. c

10. 1. c
     2. d
     3. b
     4. a

11. *Devices for oxygen delivery:*

Nasal cannula   Mask
Nasal catheter   Tent

12. *Hazards of oxygen administration:*

Oxygen supports combustion
Oxygen may be toxic to patient

Chapter 5

1. c

2. b

3. c

4. e

5. b

6. c

7. d

8. a

9. 1. e
2. a
3. b
4. d
5. c

10. *Questions RT must ask a patient receiving an iodinated contrast agent:*

Are you allergic to any foods or drugs?
If yes, which ones?
Have you ever had asthma or hay fever?
Have you ever had hives or other allergic skin reactions?
Have you ever had an x-ray examination using an iodinated contrast agent?
If yes, was the reaction during or after the exam and what was the nature of the reaction?

11. *Symptoms of diabetic ketoacidosis:*

Weakness
Drowsiness
Dull headache
Lethargy
Sweet odor to breath
Hypotension
Fatigue
Warm, dry skin
Dry tongue
Dry mucous membranes
Thirst
Deep, rapid respirations
Flushed face
Tachycardia
Weak pulse
Ultimately, coma (onset slow because of lack of insulin)

Symptoms of hypoglycemia:

Shakiness
Nervousness and irritability
Dizziness and hunger
Headache
Profuse, cold, clammy perspiration
Tremors and numbness of lips and tongue
Blurred vision
Slurred speech
Impaired motor functions
Convulsions
Diminishing level of consciousness
Coma comes rapidly (onset rapid as a result of too much insulin and no food)

Symptoms of hyperosmolar coma:

Extreme dehydration with increased thirst
Skin dry
Eyes sunken
Increased body temperature
Polyuria
Muscle twitching
Slurred speech
Mental confusion
Coma (usually results from changes in diet or from being placed on nothing by mouth)

Chapter 6

1. d
2. b
3. d
4. e
5. e
6. c
7. a
8. b
9. e

10. *Factors the RT must consider in caring for the patient with acute abdominal stress:*

The patient is in severe pain
The patient is nauseated and may be vomiting
The patient may develop hypovolemic shock as a result of internal hemorrhage

11. d
12. d

Chapter 7

1. *Positive contrast agents:*

Increase organ density
Improve radiographic visualization

Negative contrast agents:

Decrease organ density in order to produce contrast

2. a
3. a
4. b
5. b
6. d
7. e
8. a

9. *Equipment needed for a cleansing enema:*

Clean, disposable gloves
Drape sheet for patient
Disposable pad for under hips
Disposable towels
Enema set
Water and castile soap (if ordered)
Water-soluble lubricant
Bedpan
Patient's robe and slippers

10. d

Chapter 8

1. d
2. d
3. d
4. b
5. a
6. e
7. b
8. *Reasons for NG or NI intubation:*

   1. Maintain gastric or intestinal decompression
   2. Diagnose diseases of the GI tract
   3. Feed or medicate patients unable to swallow food or drugs

   Responsibilities of the RT caring for a patient with such a tube in place:

   1. Verify and understand physician orders concerning whether suction is to be continuous or intermittent
   2. Know length of time permissable to discontinue suction
   3. Know amount of suction pressure required
   4. Understand how to disconnect and reconnect suction apparatus

9. d
10. b

Chapter 9

1. c
2. e
3. b
4. b
5. e
6. c
7. c
8. b
9. b
10. c
11. a
12. b
13. e
14. a
15. b
16. b

Chapter 10

1. c
2. c
3. a
4. e
5. b
6. b
7. a
8. a

Chapter 11

1. c
2. d
3. b
4. a
5. c
6. e
7. b
8. e
9. b
10. b
11. 1. c
    2. a
    3. b
    4. d
    5. e
12. 1. d
    2. e
    3. a
    4. c
    5. b
13. 1. d
    2. c
    3. a
    4. e
    5. b
14. c
15. b
16. *The five "rights" of drug administration:*

The right patient	The right route
The right drug	The right time
The right dose	

Chapter 12

1. *Components of a normal ECG pattern:*

The P wave	The ST segment
The QRS complex	The PR and the QT
The T wave	intervals

2. *Complications that may occur following administration of an iodinated contrast media:*

   Flushing and feeling of warmth
   Metallic taste in mouth
   Nausea and vomiting
   Light-headedness
   Perioral dysesthesia
   Pain at injection site
   Pain in extremities
   Headache
   Parotid or submaxillary swelling
   Paresthesias
   Convulsions
   Paralysis
   Shock and coma
   Bradycardia
   Hypotension
   Urticaria
   Tissue necrosis
   Blood dyscrasias
   Renal failure
   Rhinitis
   Dyspnea
   Bronchospasm
   Asthma
   Laryngeal and pulmonary edema
   Subclinical pulmonary emboli

3. *Physical conditions that may affect the pharmacologic action of iodinated contrast agents:*

Pregnancy	Pheochromocytoma
Diabetes mellitus	Sickle-cell anemia
Multiple myeloma	Thyroid disorder

4. *Precautions that the RT must take if he is assisting with administration of an iodinated contrast agent:*

   Administer at body temperature for patient comfort
   Examine the solution for particles, discoloration or cloudiness
   Draw up the agent into the syringe or open immediately before use
   If second examination using contrast agent is to be performed, allow enough time for first agent to be excreted from body before second agent is administered
   Ensure adequate patient hydration pre- and post-examination using iodinated contrast agents
   Do not administer hyperosmolar contrast agents to infants or dehydrated persons as this may produce life-threatening electrolyte imbalance.

5. *Patient care responsibilities for the RT prior to and following cardiac catheterization:*

   1. Familiarize the patient with the machinery and procedure and encourage questions
   2. Alleviate anxiety by communication with patient as examination proceeds
   3. Report patient complaints of unusual sensations
   4. Monitor vital signs
   5. Assess patient continuously for adverse reaction to procedure and report to physician at once if noted
   6. Assess extremities for circulatory impairment postexam
   7. Assist patient with comfort and movement postexam
   8. Teach patient necessity of increased fluid intake following administration of iodinated contrast media

6. *Patient instruction following an angiogram should include:*

   Signs and symptoms of circulatory impairment and adequate hydration
   Signs and symptoms of anaphylactic reaction

7. *Patient instruction prior to a myelogram should include:*

   a. Increase clear fluid intake and omit solid foods 3 to 4 hours prior to exam
   b. Discontinue all drugs taken 24 hours prior to exam
   c. Discontinue all drugs that are monoamine oxidase inhibitors for 2 weeks prior to exam
   d. Make certain that a legal consent form has been signed, and that the patient has received informed consent

8. *Positions for intrathecal drug administration:*

   1. Prone
   2. Bent-sitting
   3. Side with knees pulled up and head and neck bent forward

9. *Symptoms that the patient should report to his physician immediately following myelography, should they occur:*

Inability to urinate	Stiff neck
Fever	Seizures
Drowsiness	Paralysis

10. *Four symptoms that the RT should inform the patient receiving IV iodinated contrast agents to expect:*

    Warmth
    Flushing, usually of neck or face
    Metallic taste
    Nausea
    Vomiting

11. *Patient care following CT:*

    Observe for 30 minutes for adverse reactions
    Assist patient to dress
    Return to wheelchair or gurney
    Increase fluid intake to 3000 ml for next 24 hours
    Do not allow a patient who has received a sedative or antianxiety drug to drive himself home
    If patient has received barium, instructions following barium intake must be given
    Any adverse reactions, drugs administered, or unusual events must be recorded on the patient's chart

12. *Patient care for MRI:*

Inform patient that this is a 60- to 90-minute
  examination
Assure patient that he is being continuously
  observed and may communicate by microphone
Encourage questions of patients or parents of
  patients
Inform of pounding noise heard during exam
Remove all metal, *e.g.,* jewelry, credit cards

13. *Systemic reactions to external radiation therapy:*

Fatigue
Nausea and vomiting
Headache
Loss of hair
Erythema
Loss of appetite
Alterations in mucous membranes
Decreased salivation

Dysphagia
Chest pain and cough
Esophageal irritation
Diarrhea
Blood dyscrasias

14. *Special considerations for the patient receiving external radiation therapy:*

High incidence of pathologic fractures makes
  gentle care during movement of patients
  mandatory
Patients are anxious or may be going through the
  grieving process and need time for therapeutic
  communication
Patients have increased awareness of all body
  functions and may complain of minor problems
  usually not considered
RT must respond thoughtfully to these complaints

Bibliography

Abernathy E: CE immunology: How the immune system works. Am J Nurs 456–473, 1987.

Abams AC: Clinical Drug Therapy, 2nd ed. Philadelphia, JB Lippincott, 1987.

Acquired Immunodeficiency Syndrome: Recommendations and Guidelines. Centers of Disease Control. Atlanta, Public Health Service Department of Health and Human Services, November 1982–November 1986.

Asperheim MK: Pharmacologic Basis of Patient Care, 5th ed. Philadelphia, WB Saunders, 1985.

Atkinson LJ, Kohn ML: Barry and Kohn's Introduction to Operating Room Technique, 6th ed. New York, McGraw-Hill, 1986.

Baptiste R, Koziol D, Henderson DK: Nosocomial transmission of hepatitis in an adult population. Infection Control, 8, No. 9: 364–369, 1987.

Beare PG, Rahr VA, Ronshausen CA: Nursing Implications of Diagnostic Tests. Philadelphia, JB Lippincott, 1985.

Bernzweig EP: The Nurse's Liability for Malpractice, 4th ed. Eli P. Bernzweig, 1987.

Billings, JA: Outpatient Management of Advanced Cancer. Philadelphia, JB Lippincott, 1985.

Birdsall C, Ruggio J: Mouth-to-mouth resuscitation—is there a safe, effective alternative? Am J Nurs, 87, No. 8: 1019, 1987.

Brammer LM: The Helping Relationship, 2nd ed. Prentice-Hall, 1979.

Brunner LS, Suddarth DS: Textbook of Medical-Surgical Nursing, 5th ed. Philadelphia, JB Lippincott, 1984.

Brunner LS, Suddarth DS: Textbook of Medical-Surgical Nursing, 6th ed. Philadelphia, JB Lippincott, 1988.

Carroll PF: The ins and outs of chest drainage systems. Nursing 86, 16, No. 12: 26–34, 1986.

Centers for Disease Control Guidelines: Nosocomial Infections: Infection Control. 4, No. 4: 47–78 and 283–290, 1983.

Chafee EE, Lytle IM: Basic Physiology and Anatomy, 4th ed. Philadelphia, JB Lippincott, 1980.

Christman C, Bennett J: Diabetes new names, new test, new diet. Nursing 87 17, No. 1: 34–41, 1987.

Cohen MR: Stay with the patient after giving the first dose of an I.V. Drug. Nursing 86, 23,

Cooney M, Perrone MT: Dysrhythmias: Interruption of the Heart's Normal Rhythm. Nursing Review: A Clinical Update System. Springhouse, PA, Springhouse Corporation, 1986.

Cooper D: Analyzing ABGs. California Nursing Review May/June 1987, pp. 32–38.

Cosgriff JH, Anderson DL: The Practice of Emergency Care, 2nd ed. Philadelphia, JB Lippincott, 1984.

Coughlin SH, Kahn R: Diabetes in America: Where do you fit in? Diabetes Forecast. 39(4):27–34, June 1986.

Craig CP: Preparation of the skin for surgery. Today's OR Nurse 8, No. 5: 17–20, 1986.

Delaat ANC: Microbiology for the Allied Health Professions, 3rd ed. Philadelphia, Lea and Febiger, 1984.

Dhundale K, Hubbard PM: "Home care for the A.I.D.S. patient: Safety first." Nursing 86, 16, No. 9: 34–39, 1986.

Dillman JB: The new immunology CE helping the body heal itself. Am J Nurs 87, No. 4: 455–474, 1987.

Edwards J, Krouse S: Helping the emergency colostomy patient through reality shock. Nursing 87: 63–64, July 1987.

Fader MI: Preheated contrast media: The advantage of intravenous injection. Radiol Tech 58, No. 2: 117–119, 1986.

Carrell J: Illustrated Guide to Orthopedic Nursing, 3rd ed. Philadelphia, JB Lippincott, 1986.

Fischbach F: Laboratory Diagnostic Tests, 3rd ed. Philadelphia, JB Lippincott, 1988.

Ford RD, (ed.): EKG Cards, A Clinical Reference. Keith Lassner, Publisher. Springhouse, PA, Springhouse Corporation, 1987.

Fowler S: Small hopes. Nursing 86:53–55, May 1986.

Fritz PA, Russell CG, Wilcox EM, Shirk FI: Interpersonal Communication in Nursing. New York, Appleton-Century-Crofts, 1984.

Gofman J: What nurses need to know about ionizing radiation. California Nurse 1987, pp 6–7.

Griffin JP: Be prepared for the bleeding patient. Nursing 86:34–40, June 1986.

Hahn AB, Oestreich S, Klarman J, Barkin RL: Pharmacology in Nursing, 16th ed. St. Louis, CV Mosby, 1986.

Hickey JV: The Clinical Practice of Neurological and Neurosurgical Nursing, 2nd ed. Philadelphia, JB Lippincott, 1986.

Hudak CM, Gallo BM, Lohr TS: Critical Care Nursing, 4th ed. Philadelphia, JB Lippincott, 1986.

Hunter TB: Fajardo LL: Outline of radiographic contrast agents. Applied Radiology 16, No. 11: pp. 137–158, 1987.

Jackson MM, Cummings MJ, Greenawalt NC: Why not treat all body substances as infectious? Am J Nurs 87, No. 9: 1137, 1987.

Jones S, Bagg AM: L-E-A-D drugs for cardiac arrest. Nursing 88: 34–41, January 1988.

Kaplan JC, Crawford DC, Durno AG, Schooley RT: Inactivation of human immunodeficiency virus by betadine. Infection Control 8, No. 10: 412–414, 1987.

Katzung BG: Basic and Clinical Pharmacology, 3rd ed. Norwalk, CT and Los Altos, CA, Appleton and Lange, 1987.

Kennedy M: AIDS: Coping with the fear. Nursing 87:45–55, April 1987.

Kim M-H M, Mindorff C, Patrick ML, Gold R, Ford-Jones EL: Isolation usage in a pediatric hospital. Infect Control 8, No. 5: 195–199, 1987.

Kotilainen HR, Gantz NM: An evaluation of three biological indicator systems in flash sterilization. Infect Control 8, No. 8: 311–316, 1987.

Kyba FN, Ogburn-Russell L, Rutledge JN: Magnetic Resonance. Nursing 87:44–47, January 1987.

Larson EL, Eke PI, Wilder MP, Laughon BE: Quantity of soap as a variable in hand-washing. Infect Control 8, No. 9: 371–375, 1987.

Lewis LW, Timby BK: Fundamental Skills and Concepts in Patient Care, 4th ed. Philadelphia, JB Lippincott, 1988.

Lewis SM, Collier IC: Medical-Surgical Nursing, 2nd ed. New York, McGraw-Hill, 1987.

McClennan BL: Low-osmolality contrast media: Premises and promises. Radiology 162, No. 1: 1–8, 1987.

McConnell EA: Meeting the challenge of intestinal obstruction. Nursing 87: 34, July 1987.

Millam DA: Tips for improving your venipuncture techniques. Nursing 87:46–49, June 1987.

Miller K: Advantages of a low-osmolality ionic contrast medium in intra-arterial applications. Radiol Technol 59, 43–47, 1987.

Montanari J, Spearing C: Tracheal cuff pressure. Nursing 86:46–49, July 1986.

Norsen LH, Fox GB: Understanding cardiac output—and the drugs that affect it. Nursing 85:34–41, April 1985.

Parker MD: Introduction to Radiology. Philadelphia, JB Lippincott, 1985.

Patrick ML, Woods SL, Craven RF, Rokosky J, Schnaidt B, Pauline M: Medical-Surgical Nursing. Philadelphia, JB Lippincott, 1986.

Peterson PJ: Respiratory distress after facial trauma. Nursing 88:33, January 1988.

Petty TL: Drug strategies for airflow obstruction. Am J Nurs 87, No. 2: 180–184, 1987.

Phipps WJ, Long BC, Woods NF: Medical-Surgical Nursing. St. Louis, CV Mosby, 1983.

Pisarcik G: Danger: You are facing the violent patient. Nursing 81:63–65, September 1981.

Porth CM: Pathophysiology Concepts of Altered Health States, 2 ed. Philadelphia, JB Lippincott, 1986.

Potter PA, Perry AG: Fundamentals of Nursing. St. Louis, CV Mosby, 1985.

Purtilo R: Health Professional/Patient Interaction. Philadelphia, WB Saunders, 1984.

Quinn A: Thora-drain III. Nursing 86:46–51, September 1986.

Raffensperger EB, Zusy ML, Marchesseault LC. Clinic Nursing Handbook. 1986.

Rahr B: Giving intrathecal drugs. Am J Nurs 86, No. 7: 829–831, 1986.

Randall BJ: Reacting to anaphylaxis. Nursing 86:34–39, March 1986.

Rankin S, Dufty K: Patient Education: Issues, Principles and Guidelines. Philadelphia, JB Lippincott, 1983.

Recommendations for Prevention of HIV Transmission in Health-Care Settings. 36, No. 25:35–175. Centers for Disease Control. Recommendations for prevention of HIV transmission in health-care settings. MMWR 1987, 36 (Suppl. No. 25:35–175.

Ribner BS, Landry MN, Gholson GL, Linden LA: Impact of a rigid puncture-resistant container system upon needlestick injuries. Infect Control 8, No. 2:63–66, 1987.

Robertson C: When an insulin-dependent diabetic must be NPO. Nursing 86:25–30, June 1986.

Rodman MJ, Smith DW: Clinical Pharmacology in Nursing, 2nd ed. Philadelphia, JB Lippincott, 1984.

Rosdahl CB: Textbook of Basic Nursing, 4th ed. Philadelphia, JB Lippincott, 1985.

Russell R, Dallas-Heitema C, Cohen MD: Magnetic resonance imaging techniques in children. Radiol Technol 57, No. 5:428–430, 1986.

Scharf L: Safe needle disposal: A timely reminder. RN 42, 1986.

Scherer JC: Nurses' Drug Manual. Philadelphia, JB Lippincott, 1985.

Shlaes DM, Lehman MH, Currie-McCumber CA, Floyd R: Prevalence of colonization with antibiotic-resistant gram-negative bacilli in a nursing home care unit: The importance of cross-colonization as documented by plasmid analysis. Infection Control 7, No. 11:538–545, 1986.

Sinnott JT, Cancio MR: Cytomegalovirus. Infection Control 8, No. 2:79–82, 1987.

Smith JA, Neil KR, Davidson CG, Davidson RW: Effect of water temperature on bacterial killing in laundry. Infection Control 8, No. 5:204–209, 1987.

Snydman DR, Donnelly-Reidy M, Perry LK, Martin WJ: Intravenous tubing containing burettes can be safely changed at 72-hour intervals. Infection Control 8, No. 3:113–116, 1987.

Sochurek H: Medicine's new vision. National Geographic, January 1987, pp. 2–40.

Spencer RT, Nichols LW, Lipkin GB, Waterhouse HP, West FM, Bankert EG: Clinical Pharmacology and Nursing Management, 2nd ed. Philadelphia, JB Lippincott, 1986.

Stuart GW, Sundeen SJ: Principles and Practice of Psychiatric Nursing, 3rd ed. St. Louis, CV Mosby, 1987.

Sumner SM: Septic shock. Nursing 87:33–37, February 1987

Surr CW: Teaching patients to use the new blood-glucose monitoring products, Part 1, Nursing 83: 42–45, January 1983.

Taylor DL: Hypoglycemia. Nursing 83:44–49, March 1987.

Thompson TL: Communication for Health Professionals. New York, Harper & Row, 1986.

Tong MJ, Howard AM, Schatz GC, Kane MA, Roskamp DA, Co RL, Boone C: A hepatitis B vaccination program in a community teaching hospital. Infection Control 8, No. 3:102–107, 1987.

Valenti RM: Lumber myelography: Contrast agents used in the past, present, and future. Radiol Technol 58, No. 6:493–496, 1987.

Van Parys E: Assessing the failing state of the heart. Nursing 87:42–49,

Vickers RM, Vu VL, Hanna SS, Muraca P, Diven W, Carmen N, Taylor FB: Determinants of legionella pneumophila contamination of water distribution systems; 15-hospital prospective study. Infection Control 8, No. 9:357–363, 1987.

Volk WA, Benjamin DC, Kadner RJ, Parsons JT: Essentials of Medical Microbiology, 3rd ed. Philadelphia, JB Lippincott, 1986.

Volk WA, Wheeler MF: Basic Microbiology, 4th ed. Philadelphia, JB Lippincott, 1980.

Walsh J, Persons CB, Wieck L: Manual of Home Health Care Nursing. Philadelphia, JB Lippincott, 1987.

Whaley LF, Wong DL: Essentials of Pediatric Nursing, 2nd ed. St. Louis, CV Mosby, 1985.

Wolff LV, Weitzel MH, Zornow RA: Fundamentals of Nursing, 7th ed. Philadelphia, JB Lippincott, 1983.

Zielinski XJ: Radiology—A Story of Contrasts. Unpublished.

Index